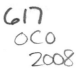

Handbook for Surgical Cross-Cover

Miss Isobel Fitzgerald O'Connor
Ear, Nose, and Throat Surgery Specialist Registrar, South East Thames Region, UK

Dr Michael Urdang
Emergency Medicine Resident,
Los Angeles County Hospital,
University of Southern California, USA

OXFORD
UNIVERSITY PRESS

OXFORD
UNIVERSITY PRESS

Great Clarendon Street, Oxford OX2 6DP

Oxford University Press is a department of the University of Oxford.
It furthers the University's objective of excellence in research, scholarship,
and education by publishing worldwide in

Oxford New York

Auckland Cape Town Dar es Salaam Hong Kong Karachi
Kuala Lumpur Madrid Melbourne Mexico City Nairobi
New Delhi Shanghai Taipei Toronto

With offices in

Argentina Austria Brazil Chile Czech Republic France Greece
Guatemala Hungary Italy Japan Poland Portugal Singapore
South Korea Switzerland Thailand Turkey Ukraine Vietnam

Published in the United States
by Oxford University Press Inc., New York

First published 2008

British Library Cataloguing in Publication Data

Data available

Library of Congress Cataloging in Publication Data

Data available

Typeset by Newgen Imaging Systems (P) Ltd., Chennai, India
Printed in Italy
on acid-free paper by
Legoprint S.p.A

ISBN 978–0–19–929648–4

10 9 8 7 6 5 4 3 2 1

Foreword

There can be nothing more terrifying for a young surgical trainee than being summoned to an unfamiliar ward to see a patient with a condition with which he or she is not familiar. The ability to dip into a handbook such as this book of surgical cross-cover may prove to be a lifeline.

Confidence comes from having a trusted reference document within easy reach, assuming doctors still have access to white coats with deep pockets.

Every new generation of doctors is accused of knowing less and less anatomy, physiology, and pharmacology, so it is refreshing to see that Michael Urdang and Isobel Fitzgerald O'Connor believe that this basic knowledge is important enough to remind its readers of the basic principles of surgical practice.

2008 will see the 48-hour European Working Time Directive implemented in full. The safe handover of surgical patients will prove even more exacting as full-shift systems are worked by all trainees. Communication skills will have to be improved and handover notes made legible. As a practising surgeon I am very aware of the problems that arise when these simple skills are overlooked.

The Oxford Handbooks are world renowned, and I am delighted that this practical guide-book, prepared by trainees for trainees, is joining the series.

Bernard Ribeiro CBE
President of the Royal College of Surgeons of England

Preface

It is 3am. You are an acute medical ST1, 2 months into your first job, and are bleeped to the general surgical ward: 'Doctor, doctor please come—Mr Smith's abdomen has burst open'. What do you do when you arrive? Having had 4 months surgical experience 18 months ago, you may be feeling worse than the patient!

By reducing the hours worked by junior doctors, introduction of the European Working Time Directive means that there are now not enough of us to provide full cover for each surgical specialty in the hospital for a round-the-clock service. Hospital management has therefore had to resort to innovative schemes such as the 'hospital at night' initiative to provide this cover for patients. Frequently this means a junior doctor with no postgraduate surgical training is the only doctor available to cover the overnight inpatient care for surgical patients.

If you haven't worked in a scheme like this then you are probably, to put it mildly, concerned at the implications of such a plan. If you have worked in such a hospital, you will understand the need for this book. This book, we hope, will live in the pocket of the junior doctor described above. It is a practical and easy-to-use book that will guide its reader through various day-to-day situations. We have created 14 chapters covering the different surgical subspecialties and each chapter has been divided broadly into two: The Ward and the Emergency Department. Within each chapter the reader will find easy methods to approach the problems described, what to look for, which questions to ask, and how to cope. This is presented in as standardized a format as possible.

The book has been written *by* junior doctors committed to training in their chosen field, *for* junior doctors committed to training in different specialties. We hope you enjoy the thrill of 'on call' medicine as much as we have, yet find some comfort with this in your pocket.

Isobel Fitzgerald O'Connor
Michael Urdang
London, 2008

Acknowledgements

We are indebted to the following for their help in specific areas of the book:

Mr Richard Andrews, Mr B. M. W. Bailey, Dr Mike Barrett, Dr John Carter, Linda Cardozo, Mr Rogan Corbridge, Mr David Drake, Mr Matthew Fanshaw, Mr Khalid Ghufoor, Mr Rick Gibbs, Dr Vamsi Gullapalli, Dr Guyton, Dr Sean Henderson, Mr Simon Heppell, Dr Michael Hobbs, Dr Lucy Hudsmith, Dr Claire Maitland, Dr Maureen McCollough, Scott Mills, Professor Ed Newton, Helen Nicks, Dr Nancy Rahnama, Dr Rodney Rodrigues, Miss Seema Verma, Dr Neil Walker, and Joseph Yazbek.

We would particularly like to thank Dr Anthony Edey and Dr Dylan Lewis who have very kindly provided the radiological imaging and associated advice throughout the book.

The following people have trusted and mentored Michael, he owes them a debt of gratitude: Dr Mel Herbert, Dr Stuart Swadron, Dr Billy Mallon, Mr Norman Waterhouse, Mr Robin Touquet, Gert Truman, and Ben Urdang.

Isobel would like to specifically thank Stephen McDonnell, the Minton family, and Charing Cross and Westminster Medical School without whom this book would not have been written.

We are also grateful to those at the Oxford University Press who have been most helpful and very patient with us, and who had the foresight to publish this book, especially Catherine Barnes, Sara Chare, Bethan Lee, and Anna Winstanley.

To my parents, Alec and Angela (IFO'C)

To my mother, Diana (MU)

Contents

Reviewer

Mr R. David Rosin
Consultant Surgeon,
St Mary's Hospital,
London, UK

Contributors

A. Kate Khoo
Research Fellow,
Great Ormond Street Hospital and Child Health Institute,
London, UK

Alex Chapman
Research Registrar,
Department of Urology,
The Royal Marsden Hospital,
London, UK

Alistair Cobb
SpR in Oral and Maxillofacial Surgery,
University College Hospital and Great Ormond Street Hospital for Children,
London, UK

Anthony Edey
SpR in Radiology,
Kings College Hospital,
London, UK

Bijan Modarai
SpR in General and Vascular Surgery,
SE Thames Region, UK

Christine Johnstone
Plastic Surgery Research Registrar,
John Radcliffe Hospital,
Oxford, UK

Dylan Lewis
SpR in Radiology,
Kings College Hospital,
London, UK

James Laban,
St3 in Neurosurgery,
SW Thames Region,
London, UK

Jo Chikwe
SpR in Cardiothoracic Surgery,
Royal Brompton Hospital,
London, UK

Rachel Bright-Thomas
Consultant Breast and General Surgeon,
Worcestershire Royal Hospital,
Worcester, UK

Rob Henderson
SpR in Ophthalmology,
Moorfields Hospital,
London, UK

Rufus Cartwright
Senior Clinical Fellow,
Department of Urogynaecology,
Kings College Hospital,
London, UK

Simon Phillips
SpR in General Surgery,
NW Thames Region,
London, UK

Stephen Black
SpR in Vascular Surgery,
SW Thames Region,
London, UK

Stephen McDonnell
SpR in Orthopaedic Surgery,
Oxford, UK

Sunil Auplish
SpR in Orthopaedic Surgery,
Oxford, UK

Vikram Dhar
St3 in ENT Surgery
SE Thames Region,
London, UK

Emergency symbols

☠—A true emergency, as outlined above. Memorizing these conditions may help, rather than referring to this book when the patient is in the department! Call for immediate senior help. Try to remain calm and quickly assess the ABCs. Once the problem has been dealt with remember to re-assess—other problems may have been forgotten or missed in the heat of the moment.

✚—These patients still need to be assessed very quickly, but you do not need to drop everything and run (so long as their ABCs have been managed). These patients can quickly shift into the emergency category if not sorted soon. Consider senior advice.

ⓘ—The majority of patients will fall into this and the last category. Although they do not need to be seen straight away, make sure you assess them thoroughly—some conditions can deteriorate if not treated properly. Think carefully of potential complications that may develop, such as atrioventricular block with inferior MIs or tamponade with pericardial effusions. Liaise with specialist help, if necessary.

?—These are non urgent conditions and general points of interest. Many of these patients should not come to casualty in the first place.

Symbols and abbreviations

AAA	abdominal aortic aneurysm
ABC	Airway, Breathing and Circulation
ABG	arterial blood gas
ABPI	ankle brachial pressure index
AC	air conduction
ACE	angiotensin converting enzyme
ACE	antegrade continence enema
ACTH	adrenocorticotropic hormone
AF	atrial fibrillation
AFP	alpha-fetoprotein
AION	anterior ischaemic optic neuropathy
ALS	advanced life support
aPTR	activated partial thromboplastin time ratio
APTR	activated prothrombin time ratio
APTT	activated partial thromboplastin time
ARDS	acute respiratory distress syndrome
ASDH	acute subdural haematoma
AST	aspartate aminotransferase
ATLS	Advanced Trauma Life Support
AVR	aortic valve replacement
AXR	abdominal X-ray
β-HCG	β-human choriogonadotropin
BC	bone conduction
BG	blood glucose
BIPAP	bi-level positive airway pressure
BIPP	bismuth iodoform paraffin paste
BG	blood glucose
BPH	benign prostatic hyperplasia
BPPV	benign paroxysmal positional vertigo
BSA	body surface area
BP	blood pressure
BV	bacterial vaginosis.
CABG	coronary artery bypass grafting

CAPD	continuous abdominal peritoneal dialysis
CBD	common bile duct
CPB	cardiopulmonary bypass
CIN	cervical intraepithelial neoplasia
CNS	central nervous system
COPD	chronic obstructive pulmonary disease
CPAP	continuous positive airway pressure
CRAO	central retinal artery occlusion
CRP	C-reactive protein
CRVO	central retinal vein occlusion
CS	caesarean section
CSDH	chronic subdural haematoma
CSF	cerebrospinal fluid
CSW	cerebral salt wasting
CT	computed tomography
CVA	cardiovascular accident
CVP	central venous pressure
CVS	chorionic villus sampling
CXR	chest X-ray
DA	dopamine (receptor)
DC	direct current
DCIA	deep circumflex iliac artery
DCIS	ductal carcinoma in situ
DCDA	dichorionic diamniotic (twins)
DDH	developmental dysplasia of the hip
DAI	diffuse axonal injury
DI	diabetes insipidus
DIC	disseminated intravascular coagulation
DIEP	deep inferior epigastric perforator (flap)
DIPJ	distal interphalangeal joint
DKA	diabetic ketoacidosis
DMSA	dimercaptosuccinic acid
DO	detrusor overactivity
DP	diastolic pressure
DRE	digital rectal examination
DVT	deep vein thrombosis
EAC	external auditory canal
EAM	external auditory meatus
ECG	electrocardiogram

EDD	estimated date of delivery
EDH	extradural haematoma
EDTA	ethylene diamine tetra-acetic acid
EMD	electromechanical dissociation
ESR	erythrocyte sedimentation rate
ERCP	endoscopic retrograde cholangiopancreatography
ERPC	evacuation of retained products of conception
ESWL	extracorporeal wave lithotripsy
EUS	endoscopic ultrasonography
ET	endotracheal (tube)
EVAR	endovascular aneurysm repair
EVD	external ventricular drain
EWTD	European Working Time Directive
FB	foreign body
FBC	full blood count
FDS	flexor digitorum superficialis
FDP	flexor digitorum profundus
FESS	functional endoscopic sinus surgery
FFP	fresh frozen plasma
FiO_2	fraction of inspired oxygen
GA	general anaesthesia
GCA	giant cell arteritis
GCS	Glasgow Coma Score/Scale
GI	gastrointestinal
GIFT	gamete intrafallopian transfer
GMC	General Medical Council
G&S	group and save
GTN	glyceryl trinitrate
HCG	human chorionic gonadotropin
Hct	haematocrit
HDU	high-dependency unit
HIV	human immunodeficiency virus
HR	heart rate
HSV	herpes simplex virus
HVS	high vaginal swab
HZV	herpes zoster virus
ICH	intracerebral haematoma
ICP	intracranial pressure
ICSI	intracytoplasmic sperm injection

IMB	intermenstrual bleeding
INR	international normalized ratio
IRAAA	infrarenal abdominal aortic aneurysm
ITU	intensive treatment unit
iu	international units
IUCD/IUD	intrauterine contraceptive device
IUI	intrauterine insemination
IUP	intrauterine pregnancy
IV	intravenous
IVC	inferior vena cava
IVF	in vitro fertilization
IVU	intravenous urogram
JVP	jugular venous pressure
KUB	kidney ureter and bladder
LA	local anaesthesia
LAD	left anterior descending coronary artery
LAP	left atrial pressure
LDH	lactate dehydrogenase
LFTs	liver function tests
LIMA	left internal mammary artery
LLETZ	large loop excision of the transformation zone
LMP	last menstrual period
LMW	low molecular weight (heparin)
LP	lumbar puncture
LRTI	lower respiratory tract infection
LSV	long saphenous vein
LV	left ventricular (function)
LVS	low vaginal swab
MAO	monoamine oxidase
MAP	mean arterial pressure
MCP	metacarpophalangeal joint
MC&S	microscopy, culture and sensitivity
MI	myocardial infarction
MIDCAB	minimally invasive direct coronary artery bypass grafting
MRCP	magnetic resonance cholangiopancreatography
MRI	magnetic resonance imaging
MRS	Mental Test Score
MRSA	meticillin-resistant *Staphylococcus aureus*
MSU	midstream urine

MVA	motor vehicle accident
MVP	mitral valve prolapse
MVR	mitral valve replacement
NA	noradrenaline
NAC	nipple–areola complex
NAI	non-accidental injury
NBM	nil by mouth
NG	nasogastric
NICU	neonatal intensive care unit
NOE	naso-orbital-ethmoid
NSAID	non-steroidal anti-inflammatory drug
NT	nuchal translucency
OA	osteoarthritis
OAB(S)	overactive bladder (syndrome)
OG	orogastric
OGD	oesophagogastroduodenoscopy
OHSS	ovarian hyperstimulation syndrome
OM	occipitomental
ONCAB	on-pump CABG
OPCAB	off-pump CABG
OPG	orthopantomograph
ORIF	open reduction, internal fixation
ACS	Picture Archiving and Communication System
aO_2	arterial partial pressure of oxygen
AWP	pulmonary artery wedge pressure
CA	patient-controlled analgesia
CB	postcoital bleeding
COS	polycystic ovary syndrome
DA	patent ductus arteriosum
E	pulmonary embolism
EA	peak endocardial acceleration
EEP	positive end-expiratory pressure
ET	positron emission tomography
ID	pelvic inflammatory disease
IP	proximal interphalangeal joint
MB	post-menopausal bleeding
MS	pre-menstrual syndrome
OP	Plaster of Paris
OP	progestogen-only pill

PPIs	proton pump inhibitors
PR	per rectum
PSA	prostate-specific antigen
PTH	parathyroid hormone
RA	rheumatoid arthritis
RA	right atrium
RCA	right circumflex artery
RCOG	Royal College of Obstetricians and Gynaecologists
RIF	right iliac fossa
RR	respiratory rate
RTA	road traffic accident
RUQ	right upper quadrant
RV	right ventricular (function)
SAH	subarachnoid haemorrhage
SBO	small bowel obstruction
SCBU	special care baby unit
SHL	sudden hearing loss
SHO	senior house officer
SIADH	syndrome of inappropriate antidiuretic hormone
SMV	submentovertex
SNHL	sensorineural hearing loss
SNP	sodium nitroprusside
SP	systolic pressure
SpR	specialist registrar
STOP	suction termination of pregnancy
SUFE	slipped upper femoral epiphysis
SVC	superior vena cava
SVD	spontaneous vaginal delivery
SVR	systemic vascular resistance
TBSA	total body surface area
TCRE	transcervical resection of the endometrium
TFT	thyroid function test
THR	total hip replacement
TIA	transient ischaemic attack
TM	tympanic membrane
TOP	termination of pregnancy
TOT	trans-obturator tape
TPN	total parenteral nutrition
TRAM	transverse rectus abdominis flap

TURP	transurethral resection of prostate
TVS	transvaginal scan
TVT	tension-free vaginal tape
U&Es	urea and electrolytes
UO	urinary output
USI	urodynamic stress incontinence
USS	ultrasound scan
UTI	urinary tract infection
VATS	video-assisted thoracoscopic surgery
VF	ventricular fibrillation
VIN	vulval intraepithelial neoplasia
VP	ventriculoperitoneal (shunt)
VT	ventricular tachycardia
WCC	white cell count
WLE	wide local excision
ZIFT	zygote intrafallopian transfer

Chapter 1

Principles of surgery

Simon Phillips
Vikram Dhar
Anthony Edey
Dylan Lewis

Introduction

All medical practice is approached from a framework of sound principles. For example, during operative surgery, normal tissue planes are defined before areas of pathology are tackled. Overlooking basic principles leads to errors, yet basic principles are often overlooked when faced with more challenging clinical problems. Arguably, clinical problems seem more complex because basic principles are overlooked. If you become puzzled about the amount of pain caused to a patient when faced with a normal-looking hip joint during surgery, it is not the moment to check that the correct side has been marked.

Surgery can be simplified enormously by adhering to very broad rules. If you have a duty of care towards a patient, you have to manage the patient. In fact, every interaction with a patient is a test of correct management, from an Advanced Trauma Life Support (ATLS) scenario to a 30sec interaction on a ward round. Patient management only has two elements: confirming a diagnosis and treating the patient.

Rule

Patient management = confirming diagnosis + treatment

This might appear oversimplistic, but the process is indeed simple. Achieving the correct management may, however, be very challenging and can be arrived at only if both elements are followed. When cross-covering an unfamiliar specialty, the basic principles of assessment will resolve the majority of problems, and, for the specifics, there is always advice from senior colleagues.

Methods of assessment

Medical schools teach that a diagnosis is arrived at through history taking, physical examination and investigations (in that order). We practise this in most acute settings when meeting new patients, but in fact every interaction should reconfirm that the correct diagnosis is being treated and that no other diagnoses have cropped up in the meantime, such as a postoperative deep vein thrombosis (DVT). The best clinicians incorporate this seamlessly into their manner on ward rounds: 'Good morning, how are you? Any change since yesterday?' (a history). They observe the patient (inspection—part of physical examination) and review the charts (an investigation). Then they institute a treatment plan: 'Good, carry on. See you tomorrow.'

Another good strategy for assessing patients is for an organ system approach. In ATLS, this provides a useful method of diagnosing and treating (i.e. managing) problems systematically in the order that threatens life the soonest. Thus, A (airway) precedes B (breathing), which precedes C (circulation and haemorrhage control). For complex situations, particularly in an intensive care setting, or when meeting new patients with multiple problems (or perhaps most usefully when reassessing a known patient who is not thriving), this allows a very thorough method. In practice, simply state the organ system out loud (Table 1.1) and think of every possible means of assessing, monitoring and improving it. More simply, just consider of every part of the body you can remember from anatomy classes and think of a way to make it better.

Advice

An organ system approach to assessment can simplify complex problems.

This organ system approach is very appropriate to cross-cover. If the patient can be kept in the best general condition possible, then specific complications for a subspecialty are less common. For example, survival of tissue flaps, healing of bowel anastomoses and recovery from neurosurgery are all helped by optimizing tissue oxygenation (a byproduct of having good respiratory and circulatory systems).

Rule

Fully optimize the general condition before considering specifics.

Table 1.1 Checklist for an organ system approach to clinical assessment

System	Comments
Respiratory	
Circulatory	
Renal	
Digestive	
Hepatobiliary	
Haematological	Including sepsis, coagulation
Neurological	
Endocrine	Diabetes, corticosteroid axis
Musculoskeletal	Mobilization status
Dermatological	Pressure areas

Many patients require repeated assessment. This ensures that a working diagnosis is sound, and that the treatment is effective. In ATLS, continued reappraisal of the patient is advocated, for these very reasons. In practice, only three things happen to patients in hospital: they get better, they get worse, or they stay about the same. You can appreciate what effect your treatment has only if you see the patient twice, and you get a far more detailed knowledge of its effect by seeing them on more occasions, even if that means passing by when you are not covering that specialty. With experience, you will learn to recognize not just when a patient is failing to improve, but when they should be improving. This allows anticipation and treatment before problems develop. In good clinicians this ability can seem like psychic powers!

Rule

Reassess all management decisions to ensure they are correct.

Advice

It is easy to recognize a patient who is deteriorating. Anticipate this so that you never have to.

Lastly, when cross-covering specialties, never omit asking about and checking on past diagnoses and treatments. Senior doctors do not appreciate giving advice on chronic and stable conditions at 3am.

Advice

A chronic condition does not require emergency treatment.

Maximizing clinical experience

It cannot be stressed enough how repeated assessment of patients give direct feedback on the chosen treatment plan. This feedback allow learning to take place and ∴ improves future decision making, i.e. i maximizes the value of clinical exposure.

Rule

Experience is not simply a result of time spent with patients.

The increasing trend towards specialty cross-cover and the low emphasis placed on patient handover risks limiting clinical experience, because feedback and ∴ learning are not incorporated into the working day. Moreover, the implications of the European Working Time Directive (EWTD) minimize the osmosis of knowledge (and ∴ experience) that occurred when working hours were longer.

The handover process offers an enormous and under-rated resource for learning. It begins with a change in emphasis from simply triaging patients between teams to improving care for patients by utilizing the expertise of many individual members. Sharing expertise educates others, and a team approach can ensure consistently good care and minimize errors. Doctors are not traditionally trained to work in teams, but the changes in working patterns have made this essential and it becomes a vital skill for senior clinicians who develop management roles later in their careers.

The handover meeting

The handover of patient care has become normal practice. Your seniors will reminisce how previous clinicians knew all the details intimately of the presenting illness, operative treatment and hospital care because they were the sole doctor responsible. Handover was ∴ unnecessary, continuity of care better and the personal rewards of the job greater. They will also explain that summers were long and sunny, neighbours left their doors unlocked and ruddy-faced children smiled as they drunk cod liver oil.

The handover meeting can serve several purposes, but it is not a formalized process. In time a structured format will emerge such that a clinician may visit any hospital and contribute to an efficient handover meeting with minimal readjustment, much as the ATLS system is adhered to worldwide for the management of trauma care.

1. Handover of patient care

This remains a 1° role, and will be discussed later.

2. A forum for clinical feedback

Direct feedback about clinical management should really occur at the bedside with a more experienced clinician, when performance at history taking, examination and interpretation of investigations can be judged against those with more experience. Shift patterns should be arranged to allow overlap, and the expectation should be that the handover of care continues during a ward round following the meeting. If a ward round is possible, it clearly needs to be focused and not encompass all inpatients. The clinician handing over care may then benefit from feedback from more experienced clinician, or vice versa.

Realistically, however, the handover book may be used to review cases and direct feedback appropriately, such as operative findings or successful/unsuccessful treatment plans. This can also be seen as an appraisal of practice for others, but the leadership of the meeting needs to ensure the correct format is adopted. It is not appropriate to concentrate simply on performance that was poor.

3. A business meeting

Many administrative matters often crop up at handover meetings. For this reason it is useful for the meeting to be viewed as considerably more than the simple handover of patient care, and for as many people to attend as is practical. Simple details might be noted, such as clinical cover for people on annual leave, or collection of data for audit meetings. Rota and shift arrangements can be agreed, and theatre sessions allocated if certain cases are likely to be more beneficial to an individual's training.

4. Political and social

In many hospitals the Doctors' Mess serves few functions. Many have lost the lobbying powers for doctors' interests within the hospital and referral of patients between specialties increasingly involves anonymous cardboard forms rather than happening over a cup of coffee.

The handover meeting can serve as a forum for hospital matters to be discussed and grievances aired. Appropriate members can be charged with tasks if individuals' interests appear to be threatened, such as clarifying study leave reimbursement. In this way, the influence of junior staff can be strengthened. This becomes acutely relevant when major changes are proposed, such as changes in working patterns and reduction in pay due to pay scale rebanding.

On a lighter note, the meeting can greet new faces, discuss ideas, and arrange social gatherings.

Proposed agenda for ideal handover meeting

- Attendance register:
  - Date, time, persons present.
- Patient handover:
  - New admissions.
  - Inpatients.
  - Outpatient follow-up.
- Clinical feedback:
  - Operative findings for acute admissions.
  - Clinical status of acute admissions with non-operative treatments.
  - Other inpatients.
  - Outpatients.
- Business:
  - Including, rota, leave cover, internal politics, items to prepare (audit, meetings).
- Social.

The structure of the meeting is important. It should be respected in a similar manner to that employed by nursing staff.

- Shift times overlap (30min minimum).
- The teams:
  - An attendance register is kept.
  - At least all clinicians from preceding 24hr attend (or 48/72hr if weekend/bank holiday).
- The environment:
  - Away from immediate clinical environment, preferably in an allocated room.
  - Semi-formalized layout, such as boardroom table layout.
  - Space for all attendees to contribute equally, i.e. no economy class seats.
  - Chaired by senior, ideally consultant responsible.
  - Open and non-judgemental to allow feedback.

Handover of patient care

A simple principle exists: good handover aims to pass on knowledge to the receiving doctor, such that they might have been that doctor him or herself, i.e. nothing is lost in the process. Any loss of information may become highly significant later. This is particularly important over sequential shifts crossing weekends or long holidays.

Rule

An ideal handover loses no information about any patient details.

It is usual to have a handover book during a period of duty. This may cover all subspecialties, or a loose-leaf folder may be used, from which pages can be passed into a separate, single-specialty folder. In whatever case, a record of all patients assessed during the duty period should be kept, including those discharged from hospital care or for whom arrangements are made for outpatient follow-up. If patients are 'carried over' several shifts, then the need for careful handover is even greater. For this reason, each change of doctor should sign the sheets to acknowledge that accountability has passed over, much like an 'on-call bleep' is passed across like a baton.

Rule

An accountable trail of care needs to be kept for all patients during a period of duty.

Some hospitals employ electronic systems for handover details. This may be more versatile once the data has been entered, but cannot be faster than good paper records. The important factor is the time spent collating the necessary data prior to the handover meeting. It is not sufficient to attend the meeting with incomplete information scattered across several pieces of paper.

Rule

All meetings of importance require some degree of preparation beforehand.

The data

- Proforma for patients covering new, existing patients and referrals (Fig. 1.1). To include:
  - Patient details/demographics.
  - Location.
  - Differential diagnoses.
  - Investigations performed, date and results.
  - Proposed treatment plan (and job list).
- Signing off data by receiving teams.

Date ____________________

Patient name ____________________

Date of birth ____________________

Hospital number ____________________

Referral type A/E ☐ Inpatient ☐ Other ____________________

Specialty ____________________

Location ____________________

Differential diagnosis:

Investigation	Date/Time	Result

Proposed treatment plan:

Assessing doctor ____________ Signed ____________

Date ____________

Receiving doctor ____________ Signed ____________

Date ____________

Receiving doctor ____________ Signed ____________

Date ____________

Receiving doctor ____________ Signed ____________

Date ____________

Fig. 1.1 Example of handover sheet.

The presentation of data for handover differs from that of a standard clinical presentation. This is really for pragmatic reasons. It is not possible to assimilate information from a dozen or more different presentations particularly if the diagnoses do not fit into standard categories. An abbreviated scheme is ∴ adopted.

The presentation

- Succinct diagnosis first, then supporting information. If diagnosis unclear, admit this and discuss relevant features and differential diagnosis.
- State investigations, results and treatments so far.
- Give intended treatment plan and job-list.

Other background information given after clear understanding of patient. Difficulties can arise for cross-specialty cover from attending multiple handover meetings. No easy solution exists for changing times of meetings or for which specialty takes precedence over another. Priority will have to be given to those with either a greater volume of patients for handover or, more arguably, to those having patients with greater clinical need (acute neurosurgery trumps elective orthopaedics).

Juniors should not get tangled up in departmental arguments about where and when they should attend handover meetings. Always pass these discussions up the chain of command, as they need to be agreed upon at senior level.

Record keeping

Good record keeping is essential when covering unfamiliar specialties, and poor record keeping causes much difficulty when defending medical negligence claims. Giving evidence under oath from patchy medical notes is not an experience you will wish to experience. Although these situations are still quite rare, in reality poor record keeping reflects poor communication, for which there is no excuse. The General Medical Council (GMC) refers to record keeping in its advice, Good Medical Practice, as do most medical defence organizations.

Advice

Poor record keeping correlates with poor clinical communication between specialties.

Ensure your records are clear, concise and accurate, and remember to document the time they were written (with reference to the time of clinical assessment if written retrospectively). What you commit to paper, however, is no substitute for direct communication, ideally face to face with all team members involved in the patient's care. Use the telephone if necessary, and certainly ensure that the treatment plan is passed on at the handover meeting.

Advice

Do not assume that entries written in the notes will be (or can be) read.

Use the process of making medical entries as an opportunity to advertize your clinical acumen and precision, and make a reputation for clarity. Your entry should finish with two important components:

- Your identity:
  - Sign, and print name.
  - GMC number.
- Your contact details:
  - Bleep number, extension or mobile telephone number.

Your GMC number remains a fixed means of identification, and can be searched easily in future. It will soon allow proof of your fitness to practise. Your contact details allow others to clarify your intended management, and a mobile telephone number is particularly useful to those covering across different hospital sites. If you do not wish to write the number down in the notes, then at least add, 'Contact via switchboard', and ensure that the switchboard has your current details.

Dealing with urgent calls

When working in an unfamiliar hospital, covering an unfamiliar special unexpected calls can leave a distinctly lonely feeling. Remember th ward staff can be your allies, rather than enemies. Doctors who smile t least usually claim to have the most difficult periods of duty.

Certain categories of call are common to all specialties:

'Mrs White doesn't look right'

An assessment of priority is essential. Will it take more time to discu the patient than simply to walk up the stairs to see them? If your worki pattern allows periods of sleep, this can condense into whether mo rest will be had by seeing the patient and returning to bed, or by lying bed worrying that you didn't see the patient.

In essence, you must try to manage the patient by proxy, i.e. take a h tory, examination, perform investigations and suggest treatment over t telephone, but in reality most patients need direct assessment.

- Establish ABC (Airway, Breathing and Circulation) parameters initially
- Take the history (by proxy).
- Consider an organ-specific questioning policy for the history/ examination findings.
- Confirm the patient's details and location, then plan a visit to the war

'Professor Plum's patient has just had an … after his … procedure'

As a covering doctor, this may be a common (or uncommon) occurren for a specialty with which you are very familiar (or very unfamiliar). Co mon problems within a familiar specialty are easily managed, and you v quickly learn the common problems within unfamiliar specialties. Tho that are uncommon and from an unfamiliar specialty will always be ch lenging, and uncommon problems from a familiar specialty are interesti and 6 satisfying to manage.

When covering unfamiliar territory, revert to first principles, optimi the general aspects, and then progress to specifics. Remember that the are few specific emergencies that require immediate action—even wi bleeding beneath a thyroidectomy wound → stridor there is often tir to involve an anaesthetist, as controlled re-intubation is the preferr course of action.

- Resuscitate, establish basic parameters.
- Optimize general aspects.
- Consult experienced ward staff.
- Contact senior staff for advice.

'Reverend Green's son needs his oesophagostomy dilatation at 22:45 this evening'

On first impressions, this might seem wildly unreasonable and, although you might not really know why an oesophagostomy needs dilating, nor even what it is, you're fairly sure it will not need to happen at 22:45. Do not, however, dismiss this type of call. The staff may not be able to explain the indication for this procedure, but they may have called you correctly. Do not question the medical indications from staff who cannot explain the rationale. Resist criticism until you have established the full background to the call. In fact resist criticism entirely.

- Confirm patient details and location, then plan a visit.
- Discuss indication and how to achieve procedure with a senior.

Contacting seniors

Covering unfamiliar specialties does not require bravery. It requires self-insight into the limitations of one's clinical experience and the ability to request help with as little effort as possible from the senior colleague. Calling a senior can be the most daunting situation that a junior doctor will face, yet, if done efficiently, can make the biggest impression as to the junior doctor's competence and professionalism.

Advice

Contacting senior doctors is an opportunity to impress.

As in life, it helps to consider other people's viewpoints. As a senior clinician, not receiving any calls at night and sleeping soundly will not compensate for the surprise in finding ill patients the next morning, or the 'of piste' management decisions that have been made without consultation. The ward staff will probably know that Miss X prefers to be called about any management decisions, whereas Mr Y encourages autonomy. If in doubt, tend towards caution and inform seniors.

Rule

Seniors prefer to be told things than to find them out.

A robust scheme for calling seniors at 3am will also work at 10am or even 5pm on Friday afternoon:

- Confirm identity of senior
  - Good morning, is that Miss Scarlet, ophthalmologist on call for St Irises Hospital?
- Introduce yourself:
  - This is Dr Black, FY2 cover for surgical specialties at St Irises.
- Be humble, state purpose of call, then *pause*:
- I'm sorry to have to call you, but may I discuss the patient, Colonel Mustard, with you …?

The pause allows thoughts to recollect, and to prioritize. At 3am this is essential. Do not launch into a clinical description until invited to—it is not unusual for seniors to arrive at work having dreamt that they were called, then discovering that they had given advice by telephone. In addition, at 3am, it is often natural to be antagonistic towards the caller. Minimize this by showing courtesy and by displaying professionalism that demands respect.

- Present the case succinctly.
- Document the discussion.

Preoperative preparation

Preparation for surgery is a common area of anxiety when covering subspecialties. In essence, the needs of all the surgical team must be anticipated. Avoid any surprises for any member of the team.

Rule

Less criticism will arise from over-preparation than from under-preparation.

The surgical team involves both the theatre teams and the ward/discharge teams. When dealing with any individual, it is useful to ask, 'Is there anything further that I can do to make your life easier?'. This puts the ball firmly in their court and it is then more difficult to be criticized for lack of forethought prior to surgery.

Advice

Ask all personnel whether anything else is required to make life run smoothly.
Hospital policies exist for many things such as DVT prophylaxis, bowel preparation—adhere to them (see Guidelines on Protocols and Guidelines, 📖 p24)

In practice, consider each person's role in the proceedings.

The surgeon needs

- A patient to operate on:
  - Ensure patient has planned admission (and bed):
    —liaise with the admissions manager.
    —liaise with the bed manager.
    —telephone the patient directly, if necessary, with details.
    —check on transport for patient.
- A patient to be prepared for surgery:
  - Correctly consented by appropriate doctor.
  - Marked if required.
  - Required investigations performed *and available*:
    —imaging, blood investigations, specialty-specific tests.
  - Aspects affecting surgery considered:
    —anticoagulants, antiplatelet agents.
    —DVT prophylaxis.

Preparation for surgery involves many aspects of physical and psychological preparation, which commence before and end after the act of surgery itself. In principle, aim to keep all aspects as close to physiological normality as possible. Ensure optimal care of coexisting conditions so that the healing response is also optimized and encourage physical exercise during the waiting period for surgery (if an elective procedure is intended).

Consent for surgery is addressed fully by the GMC (http://www.gmc-uk.org/guidance/current/library/consent.asp) and by medical defence organizations. This guidance should be referred to regularly.

Prophylaxis against DVT is often determined by published hospital policy and should be referred to. Many surgical patients currently receive low molecular weight heparin and TED® antiembolism stockings. Conventionally, DVT prophylaxis is administered at 6pm, as, if surgery is anticipated the following morning, this allows sufficient time to elapse to enable placement of invasive lines such as epidural catheters without concern over prolonged coagulation times. Heparin administration is commonly delayed for 6hr *after* removal of epidural catheters, for similar reasons. In emergency patients, heparin may be administered during surgery or commenced after operation. Many variations exist, however, and it is always best to consult the surgeon conducting the procedure in advance.

Patients receiving warfarin or potent antiplatelet agents warrant special consideration. Those on both clopidogrel and aspirin are particularly susceptible to bleeding during and after surgery. In all cases, a balance between surgical urgency and medical necessity for anticoagulation needs to be made. This usually requires the consultation of a cardiologist and often that of a haematologist, if emergency surgery is required.

Advice

Do not reverse anticoagulation without careful discussion of the benefits/disadvantages, and preferably with advice from a haematologist.

The anaesthetist needs

- A patient they can anaesthetize and un-anaesthetize:
  - Ensure the patient is in optimal physiological condition:
    —Organ-specific assessment in turn to optimize.
    —Flag allergies to appropriate staff.
  - Consider nil-by-mouth policy for anaesthetist.
  - Consider medication changes.

In practice, anaesthetists vary in their requirement for ancillary investigations prior to surgery. It is always preferable to ask the specific anaesthetist of their requirements than to guess. This applies to nil-by-mouth policies, which may vary between anaesthetists. In general, the safest policy is to restrict all oral food/liquid for 6hr, although some relax this to 6hr for food and 2hr for clear liquids in moderation. It is better to ask, however, than to guess.

Similarly, alterations to medications vary. Policies will exist on the management of diabetics in the perioperative period, but in general it is prudent to maximize glycaemic control by use of an insulin sliding scale (until normal diet/metabolism is resumed) in most diabetic patients. Other medical conditions are best discussed with the anaesthetist concerned.

Advice

Telephone anaesthetist with patient details prior to list to check all is in order.

The theatre sister needs

- An accurate list of planned procedures in order to check equipment:
  - Check submitted list is accurate and additions/cancellations noted.
  - If unusual equipment is needed, contact in advance.

The ward staff need (including ITU/HDU staff)

- Advance notification if a bed is likely to be needed—this allows the correct balance of skill mixes and staff numbers to be planned for.
- An explanation of the operation, usually to the most senior nurse, to anticipate specific needs such as drain irrigation, monitoring requirements (e.g. epidural/neurological) or special measures (e.g. prone nursing). Do not rely on the operative note to transfer all requirements.

Guidelines on 'Protocols and guidelines'

Unless you are providing locum cover in an unfamiliar hospital, you will have been supplied with an induction pack, which commonly includes a handbook for junior staff. This will contain outlines of hospital policies as diverse as antibiotic and radiology guidelines to bereavement matters and complaints procedures. This handbook will not be read cover to cover, but you should make it available for reference. If you have a regular area or office for note writing, then use this.

Advice

Leave information from induction pack in an accessible area.

You *must*, however, read one section: the *major incident* policy. Learn exactly where *you* must report to and what *your* role will be. You will not regret being prepared for the uncertainty that a major incident invokes.

Guidelines for patient care serve many purposes. At their best they ensure that optimal and consistent care is given to all patients, and at their worst they limit individual management choices due to financial restraints. The hospital in which you work will have published a set of guidelines that are specific to the hospital. These are usually published on the hospital intranet, but these are often patchy in their clinical coverage and rarely conform to the standards by which national bodies construct their guidelines. They may also be out of date, but, as your direct employer, your hospital's guidelines supersede those elsewhere, at least in theory.

Advice

Check your hospital intranet for relevant hospital guidelines.

Unfortunately, many guidelines are published in similar clinical areas (such as gastrointestinal bleeding) by many organizations. National, regional and local policies often coexist, and professional bodies and societies often contribute their own. Occasionally these policies are directly contradictory, but it is probably safest to comply with local policies if they seem appropriate.

Most concerns in cross-cover relate to prescribing details. If faced with a scenario with which you are not familiar, consult a local handbook, ask the ward staff whether they are aware of a policy, or contact a senior for advice. If all else fails, then turn to the *internet*. A search for 'diabetes sliding scale' yields dozens of appropriate regimens.

And lastly...

Covering for surgical specialties is not the same as being a caretaker. There is a danger that you perceive your role as one of minding patients until their regular team takes over. Several consequences come from this strategy:

- You undervalue your role in managing patients, and ∴ perform less well. This then becomes self-fulfilling, and your role indeed devalues.
- Others undervalue your role, and you do not seek to correct their impression. They ∴ fail to teach you about their specialty, and your knowledge fails to improve. Once again, this becomes self-fulfilling.
- Eventually you personally feel undervalued, and this spills over into your regular work and often into your private life.

Most importantly, however, if you mentally see your role as a covering doctor, you do what is necessary to perform your role, and no more. This attitude cannot be switched off and on depending on what specialty you work in, and will affect your own training, and ultimately the care of your patients.

In essence, subspecialty cover should be seen as an opportunity to experience a varied diet of surgical disease. In operative surgery many technical aspects have parts transferable to other specialties, and in ward management many problems are shared between specialties and ∴ directly applicable.

Finally, do not forget that many surgical examinations test areas that are most easily picked up and remembered from direct clinical experience. In 6 years' time, you may still be asked about the complications of blood transfusions and how to manage postoperative complications in orthopaedics, endocrine or vascular surgery.

Introduction to emergency radiology

Imaging is arguably the most rapidly developing aspect of modern medicine. Modern medical imaging can localize and evaluate pathology with great accuracy, allowing more focused management of the sick patient. The radiology sections in each chapter of this book does not represent an exhaustive radiology manual, rather they aim to cover key emergencies, many of which will require involvement of specialist radiological services.

Using an out-of-hours radiology service

There are two aspects of radiology that junior doctors caring for sick patients in an out-of-hours situation should be able to use. The first is that which is interpreted by the referer (i.e. you)—essentially plain radiographs—and the second, using more sophisticated imaging modalities, is interpreted by and requested from a radiologist.

Interpreting plain radiographs requires some understanding of anatomy and the principles by which abnormalities may be picked up on radiographs. The radiology sections of this book provide some practical tips for achieving this. Radiographers are frequently helpful in both selecting the right radiographic test and assessing it: after all, they look at radiographs all day long, and this is particularly true of fractures.

In most hospitals in the UK the use of computed tomography (CT), angiography and magnetic resonance imaging (MRI) out of hours necessitates the involvement of a radiologist. What follows is stating the obvious … unfortunately the obvious is not what many of us consider at 3am, when confronted by an unfamiliar situation. Please heed it, as it will make those late night discussions with a radiology consultant with 30 years' experience, and an almost unnatural need for REM sleep, just a little bit more friendly.

All clinical tests must be understood and filtered through a thorough clinical assessment and understanding of the situation—this information should be provided by you and *shared* with the radiologist! Discussion with a radiologist should centre on the clinical scenario and you should have specific endpoints in mind when requesting a test. From both the clinician's and the radiologist's point of view, this endpoint should necessitate an alteration in the acute management of the patient.

Table 1.2 Typical values of dose to patient for particular examination

Modality	Dose (mSv)	Equivalent of back ground exposure
Chest X-ray	0.2	1 month
IVU	5	2 years
CT head	2	10 months
CT abdomen	8	3 years 4 months

Dose varies according to machine, patient and operator.

Disadvantages of imaging

Unfortunately medical imaging does have its downsides. The most important of these is that the most commonly used modalities (CT, radiography and fluoroscopy) expose patients to ionizing radiation (Table 1.2). Data suggest that each year ~15 deaths in the UK are indirectly attributable to exposure to radiation from medical imaging, usually as a result of cancer. Most of the evidence for risk of cancer induction is derived from the outcomes, since 1945, of the 90 000 survivors of the atom bomb explosions in Nagasaki and Hiroshima. Quantifying and explaining the risks to patients can be very difficult as the numbers become too abstract to apply to individual situations. A good starting point is the knowledge that, on average, each person in the UK is exposed to ~2.5 milliSiverts (mSv) of radiation a year (regional variation due to geographical factors, especially the underlying rock structures of areas, means that this varies; e.g. in Cornwall normal yearly doses are up to three times this amount).

In many radiological examinations an intravenous (or intra-arterial) contrast agent is used to visualize structures. When imaging with non-ionizing radiation, the majority of agents use iodine-based contrast agents. Modern agents are comparatively safe. However, you should be aware of certain risks when requesting tests. Anaphylaxis is the most dramatic of these, but relatively uncommon. Possible risk factors to be aware of include a history of contrast reactions and a strong history of asthma. Historically, an allergy to shellfish has been a relative contra-indication to the administration of iodinated contrast media. However, more recent guidelines published by the Royal College of Radiology state that there is no evidence for a cross-reaction and it is therefore not contra-indicated. Unfortunately it is possible to have had a previous contrast injection with no reaction on a previous occasion—at which time the patient becomes sensitized to the allergen—and subsequently to have a full-blown anaphylactic response on subsequent injection. Renal toxicity is seen most often in patients with pre-existing renal dysfunction and those on metformin; most hospitals have protocols for cut-off levels. However, in reality many would argue that if the scan is genuinely urgent (e.g. trauma) then the risk of worsening renal function is justified by the greatly increased diagnostic accuracy provided by contrast, particularly if there are local facilities for renal dialysis.

Chapter 2

General surgery

Bijan Modarai

Introduction

General surgery involves the management of a broad variety of elective and emergency conditions. Armed with knowledge of the most common of these conditions, most doctors should be able to provide safe cross-cover. It is, however, important to recognize when a patient is seriously ill, requiring urgent attention, and to communicate effectively with senior colleagues to enlist their help.

All management plans assume initial and repeated assessment of Airway, Breathing and Circulation (ABC).

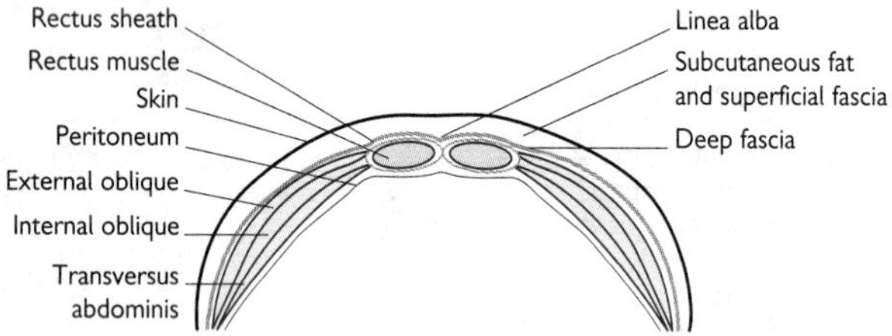

Fig. 2.1 Layers of the abdominal wall.

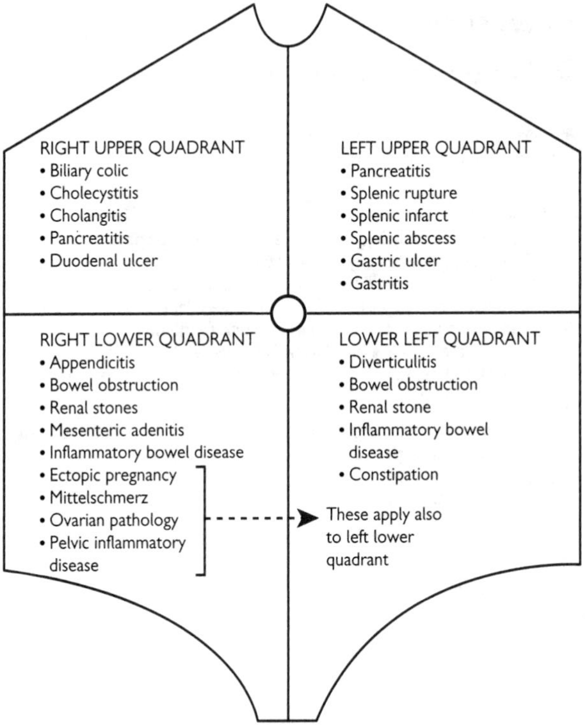

Causes of diffuse abdominal pain
- Early appendicitis
- Pancreatitis
- Bowel obstruction
- Mesenteric ischaemia
- Ruptured abdominal aortic anourysm
- Gastroenteritis
- Inflammatory bowel disease

Fig. 2.2 Common causes of abdominal pain.

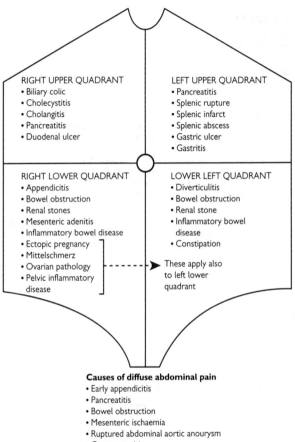

Emergency department

Abdominal trauma

- Alert senior on call immediately.
- Patients can deteriorate rapidly.

Think about

Blunt impacts commonly injure the spleen, liver and retroperitoneal organs (e.g. kidney and duodenum). Penetrating injuries (e.g. stab and bullet wounds) can affect the small bowel, colon, liver and vascular structures. It is more important to recognize the need for urgent laparotomy in the unstable patient than to diagnose the specific injury. Remember chest and pelvic injuries as a source of blood loss. Do not confuse tenderness from contusions to abdominal wall musculature with deep abdominal tenderness.

Ask about

It is important to obtain accurate information from the ambulance crew:

- Events associated with injury.
- Speed of vehicle.
- Time taken to extricate patient.
- Wearing seat belt?
- State of windscreen.
- Injuries to other car occupants.
- Characteristics of penetrating object.
- Blood lost and fluids given at scene.
- Any abdominal pain.
- Possibility that patient is pregnant.
- Medications (including those given at scene).
- When last ate and drank.

Look for

- Signs of shock: tachycardia and hypotension (systolic blood pressure (BP) <90mmHg).
- Oxygen saturation.
- Bruising to abdomen, back and flank, seatbelt sign.
- Abdominal distension.
- Generalized or focal tenderness, rebound or guarding.
- Bowel sounds may be absent.
- Examine perineum and external genitalia.
- Look for blood at urethral meatus.
- Carry out PR examination (?blood, ?high-riding prostate).

Investigations

- Bloods including full blood count (FBC) and amylase.
- Group and save (if patient haemodynamically stable) or cross-match (if haemodynamically unstable).
- Arterial blood gas (ABG): metabolic acidosis?
- Urine dipstix: to detect haematuria or pregnancy.
- Chest X-ray (CXR): to exclude haemothorax, pneumothorax, free air under diaphragm, lower rib fractures and diaphragmatic rupture.
- Pelvic X-ray: pelvic fractures?
- Ultrasound scan (USS) of abdomen, (FAST). Look for free fluid.
- CT of abdomen and pelvis, if haemodynamically stable.

Management

Adhere to Advanced Trauma Life Support (ATLS) principles for initial management of the patient:

- Prioritize attention to the airway, breathing and circulation.
- Give oxygen (15L/min) by mask.
- Obtain intravenous (IV) access (14G) in both antecubital fossae.
- Commence IV fluid resuscitation: 2L crystalloid + assess.
- Assess response to fluid: responders vs transient responders vs non-responders.
- Consider a urinary catheter.
- Some of the indications for urgent laparotomy are:
  - Persistent hypotension despite adequate resuscitation.
  - Peritonitis.
  - Evisceration.
  - Free air seen on X-ray.
- Further imaging (usually CT) to assess the abdomen may be possible in the haemodynamically stable patient, but this decision should be made by the senior surgeon.

Acute abdomen

Assessment and resuscitation of the patient should be rapid.

Think about

History and examination are of paramount importance. For the more common causes of an acute abdomen, see the appropriate chapters in this book. Aetiologies include perforated appendicitis, perforated duodenal/gastric ulcer disease, perforated colon (e.g. caused by diverticulitis, obstruction or cancer), and ischaemic bowel. Do not forget gynaecological causes, e.g. ectopic pregnancy, salpingitis and ruptured ovarian cyst. It is important to decide whether urgent surgery is required.

Remember the common medical causes of abdominal pain, e.g. pneumonia, myocardial infarction (MI).

Is this patient going to the theatre emergently or is there time for watchful waiting?

Ask about

Nature, time of onset (sudden or insidious), location, radiation, duration, what worsens pain (e.g. coughing/movement) and characteristics of abdominal pain, abdominal distension, nausea, vomiting, similar pain experienced before?, rigors, when bowels last open, passing wind?, change in bowel habit, blood/mucus PR, gynae history, urinary symptoms, chest pain, cough, previous abdominal surgery, gynae symptoms, cardiac/chest co-morbidity.

Look for

- Tachycardia, pyrexia, hypotension.
- Dehydration: reduced skin turgor, sunken eyes, dry tongue.
- Tachypnoea, chest signs.
- Lymphadenopathy.
- Abdomen: scars, distension, tenderness, ascites, bowel sounds, organomegaly, abdominal aortic aneurysm.
- Peritonitis: inflammation of peritoneal lining of abdomen, signs: guarding, rebound rigidity.
- Hernial orifices.
- Genitalia.
- Digital rectal examination.

Investigations

- Baseline bloods: FBC, urea and electrolytes (U&Es), liver function tests (LFTs), clotting, amylase, group and save (G&S), blood cultures, arterial blood gas (ABG).
- Urine dipstick ± microscopy.
- Urine β-human choriogonadotropin (β-HCG).
- Erect CXR (suspected perforated viscus—air under diaphragm, effusion, consolidation).
- Abdominal X-ray (AXR), e.g. dilated bowel, Rigler's sign, absent psoas shadows, constipation, radio-opaque stones, calcified abdominal aortic aneurysm (AAA).
- USS of abdomen, e.g. gallstones, intraperitoneal fluid, intra-abdominal collections.
- Intravenous urogram (renal tract obstruction, stones, etc.).
- Further assessment using CT abdomen/pelvis is possible if patient stable, and may allow therapeutic intervention (e.g. percutaneous drainage of abscesses/collections). For CT abdomen/pelvis: consult senior.

Management

- Analgesia: DO NOT withhold analgesia—no effect on assessment.
- Keep nil by mouth.
- Oxygen by mask.
- Aggressive IV fluid resuscitation.
- Consider urinary catheter.
- Consider nastrogastric (NG) tube (e.g. vomiting, dilated bowel loops).
- Consider IV antibiotics (e.g. cefuroxime 750mg TDS and metronidazole 500mg TDS).
- Consider central line.
- Deep vein thrombosis (DVT) prophylaxis/TED® stockings.
- Alert senior to assess re need for surgery.
- Inform anaesthetist/intensive treatment unit (ITU) early.

Perforated viscus

- Alert senior.
- Prompt surgery is usually required after appropriate resuscitation.

Think about

Perforations can occur 2° to obstruction (e.g. carcinoma), ulcer disease (e.g. gastroduodenal), inflammation (e.g. appendicitis, diverticulitis, inflammatory bowel disease) and iatrogenic cases (e.g. following colonoscopy). Note that clinical signs may be masked in elderly and immunocompromised patients.

Ask about

- Onset of pain (often sudden).
- History of any of the conditions outlined above.
- Alcohol, steroids and non-steroidal anti-inflammatory drug (NSAID) ingestion.
- See also Acute abdomen (📖 p36).

Look for

- Tachycardia, pyrexia, hypotension, dehydration.
- Signs of peritonism.
- Reduced/absent bowel sounds.
- See also Acute abdomen (📖 p36).

Investigations

- See under Acute abdomen (📖 p36).
- Show X-ray with free air under diaphragm.

Management

- Start management as per Acute abdomen (📖 p36).
- Alert senior—majority of cases will require laparotomy.
- Some cases with minimal intra-abdominal contamination (e.g. perforation after colonoscopy) may be treated conservatively.

Intestinal obstruction

Think about

Patients can present with small (85%) or large (15%) bowel obstruction. Commonest causes of acute large bowel obstruction are colorectal cancer, diverticular disease and volvulus. Causes of small bowel obstruction (SBO) include adhesions and herniae. Acute large bowel obstruction must be differentiated from acute colonic pseudo-obstruction (e.g. renal failure, MI, pneumonia, post-spinal surgery, etc.).

Ask about

- Colicky abdominal pain.
- Absence of pain may indicate pseudo-obstruction.
- Vomiting.
- Constipation.
- Absolute constipation (no stool or flatus passed).
- Proximal obstruction: more vomiting, bowels may still work, colicky pain usually periumbilical.
- Distal obstruction: less vomiting, absolute constipation, infraumbilical colicky pain.
- Recent change in bowel habit.
- Weight loss.
- Previous abdominal surgery.

Look for

- Signs of peritonitis may indicate perforation.
- Abdominal distension: less in proximal obstruction.
- Scars from previous abdominal surgery.
- Palpable bowel loops or abdominal mass.
- Visible peristalsis.
- Distension with little tenderness may indicate pseudo-obstruction.
- Abdominal wall hernia.
- Hyperactive, high-pitched bowel sounds.
- Digital rectal examination: ?tumour, ?impacted stool.
- Rectum is usually empty.

Investigations

- FBC, U&Es, amylase, LFTs, ABG, G&S.
- AXR: large bowel loops—look for haustra.
- Small bowel loops—look for valvulae conniventes. Dilatation >3cm considered abnormal.
- Valvulae conniventes seen crossing entire bowel lumen; haustra cross only half of lumen.
- Distended bowel loops may not be visible if fluid filled or if obstruction is proximal.
- Erect CXR—free air under diaphragm?

- Gastrografin® enema to delineate large bowel obstruction—consult senior.
- Gastrografin® follow-through to ascertain small bowel obstruction.
- CT abdomen in selected cases—discuss with senior.

Management

- Intravenous fluids to replace losses from vomiting and third space sequestration.
- NG tube to decompress bowel.
- Nil by mouth.
- Urinary catheter to ensure adequate replacement of fluid losses—ensure output is >0.5mL/kg/hr.
- Urgent laparotomy if signs of peritonism/bowel strangulation/perforation.
- In stable patient with none of the above signs, trial of conservative management may allow investigation with contrast studies or CT of abdomen (discuss with senior).
- Majority of SBO 2° to adhesions settle with conservative treatment.

☠ Mesenteric ischaemia

Life-threatening condition requiring early laparotomy.

Think about

Ischaemia of the bowel can develop from arterial or venous occlusion (either thrombotic or embolic) and is notoriously difficult to diagnose, requiring a high index of suspicion especially in the elderly.

Ask about

- Colicky abdominal pain (often vague and diffuse).
- Diarrhoea.
- PR bleeding.
- History of atherosclerotic disease.
- Cardiac arrhythmias.
- Recent MI.

Look for

- Pyrexia.
- Hypotension.
- Abdominal distension.
- Generalized tenderness.
- Peritonitis.
- Abdominal signs may be minimal.
- Blood PR.
- Cardiac arrhythmias.

Investigations

- See investigations for Acute abdomen (📖 p36).
- ABG (metabolic acidosis, ↑ lactate).
- AXR (thick walled and separated dilated small bowel loops).

Management

- See management of Acute abdomen (📖 p36).
- Urgent laparotomy.

Gastrointestinal haemorrhage

Hypotensive patients have usually had substantial blood loss and need urgent review.

Think about

Δ for upper gastrointestinal (GI) bleeding are duodenal/gastric ulcers, gastric erosions, oesophageal varices and Mallory–Weiss tears. Δ for lower GI bleeding are diverticular disease, angiodysplasia, polyps, colitis (infective, ischaemic, inflammatory bowel disease), haemorrhoids, anal fissures and cancer. Some 10% of patients with apparent lower GI bleeding have a gastroduodenal source.

Ask about

- Upper GI: frequency and colour of vomit, volume of blood lost (unreliable).
- Lower GI: colour of stool, bright red or altered blood, blood mixed in or on surface of stool, estimated amount lost.
- Previous episodes.
- Weight loss.
- Change in bowel habit.
- History of gastroduodenal ulcers, liver disease, haemorrhoids, cancer, previous AAA surgery (e.g. aortoduodenal fistula).
- Ingestion of anticoagulants, NSAIDs, steroids, iron, alcohol.

Look for

- Tachycardia.
- Hypotension.
- Postural drop in BP.
- Oxygen saturations.
- Inspect stool/vomit.
- Stigmata of liver disease.
- Abdominal tenderness/abdominal masses.
- PR: colour and amount of blood, melaena, rectal mass, haemorrhoids.
- Rigid sigmoidoscopy/proctoscopy for lower GI bleed if you have expertise.

Investigations

- Bloods: see Acute abdomen (📖 p36).
- For further investigations involve seniors.
- Urgent oesophagogastroduodenoscopy (OGD) if shocked.
- Colonoscopy once lower GI bleeding settles.
- Mesenteric angiography ± embolization of bleeding vessel.
- Red cell scan.

Management

- For larger bleeds or concerning co-morbidity: IV access (14G) both antecubital fossae, resuscitation with crystalloid, colloid or blood as necessary.
- Oxygen by mask.
- Keep nil by mouth.
- Consider urinary catheter.
- Drug therapies:
  - IV proton pump inhibitors (PPIs).
  - Octreotide for bleeding varices: 25–50mcg/hr IV infusion.
  - Terlipressin for bleeding varices: 2mg every 4–6hr.
- Correct clotting abnormalities with fresh frozen plasma (FFP), vitamin K, platelets as indicated.
- Urgent OGD for upper GI bleeding.
- Consider Sengstaken (or Linton) tube for bleeding varices—alert senior.
- High-dependency unit (HDU) admission if ongoing bleed and haemodynamically unstable.
- Majority of lower GI bleeds will stop with expectant therapy.
- Surgery may be required if uncontrolled or recurrent bleeding.

☠ Acute pancreatitis

Patients can deteriorate rapidly.

Think about

Severity is graded from mild to severe. The majority of cases are due to gallstones and alcohol, but hyperlipidaemia, mumps, trauma, steroids and post-endoscopic retrograde cholangiopancreatography (ERCP) are some of the other causes. Chronic pancreatitics may have little pancreatic tissue left and may not have a raised serum amylase level. Δ includes cholecystitis, peptic ulcer, ischaemic bowel and MI.

Ask about

- Epigastric/right upper quadrant (RUQ) pain radiating to back.
- Previous attacks: similar pain?
- Nausea/vomiting.
- Risk factors for pancreatitis: gallstones, alcohol intake, family history, viral causes/prodromal symptoms.

Look for

- Pyrexia, tachycardia, hypotension.
- Dehydration.
- Jaundice.
- Stigmata of alcoholic liver disease.
- Cullen's (bruising around umbilicus) and Grey–Turner's (bruising to flanks) signs of retroperitoneal haemorrhage.
- Abdominal distension.
- Tender epigastrium ± peritonitis.
- Chest signs: ?pleural effusion, ?consolidation.

Investigations

- FBC, U&Es, LFTs, lactate dehydrogenase (LDH), calcium, amylase, glucose, C-reactive protein (CRP) (>150mg/mL at 48hr indicates severity), ABG.
- AXR: pancreatic calcification (usually suggestive of chronic pancreatitis), loss of psoas shadow, 'sentinel' dilated jejunal loop adjacent to pancreas.
- CXR: consolidation, pleural effusions.
- USS: to ascertain presence of gallstones and dilated extrahepatic biliary tree.
- CT for diagnosis or to delineate pancreatic necrosis, haemorrhage, pseudocysts.

Modified Glasgow criteria (>3 suggest severe pancreatitis)

- White cell count (WCC) >15 x 10^9/L.
- Arterial partial pressure of oxygen (PaO_2) <8kPa.
- Age >55yr.
- Ca^{2+} <2mmol/L.
- Urea >16mmol/L.
- LDH >600iu/L.
- Aspartate aminotransferase (AST) >200iu/L.
- Albumin <32g/L.
- Glucose >10mmol/L.

Management

- Oxygen by mask.
- IV access and consider central venous pressure (CVP) line to guide fluid resuscitation.
- Adequate (urine output >0.5mL/kg) prompt fluid resuscitation may prevent systemic complications.
- NG tube.
- Nil by mouth.
- Analgesia.
- Urinary catheter.
- No consensus on benefit of IV antibiotics.
- Monitor WCC, blood sugar, U&Es, calcium, CRP and ABG regularly.
- Calcium gluconate if ↓ Ca.
- Admit to HDU/ITU if severe.
- Known complications include pancreatic necrosis, renal failure, respiratory problems, disseminated intravascular coagulation (DIC), haemorrhage, pancreatic pseudocyst and abscess formation.
- Consider urgent ERCP for associated cholangitis or severe gallstone-associated acute pancreatitis.

Diverticulitis

Think about

Diverticulae are mucosal protrusions that commonly affect the distal colon. The most common complications of diverticular disease are diverticulitis, pericolic abscess formation, fistulation, stricturing presenting as large bowel obstruction and perforation.

Ask about

- Abdominal pain.
- Localized to left iliac fossa?
- Anorexia.
- Nausea.
- Rigors.
- Suspected colovesical fistula: urinary frequency, dysuria, pneumaturia.
- Known to have diverticular disease on previous investigations?

Look for

- Pyrexia.
- Tachycardia.
- Localized tenderness in left iliac fossa with rebound/guarding.
- Generalized peritonitis if advanced/perforated.
- Palpable mass (diverticular abscess).

Investigations

- FBC, U&Es, LFTs, amylase.
- Erect CXR (free air seen in only 50% of perforations).
- AXR (dilated bowel, ?obstruction).
- CT of abdomen and pelvis to delineate pericolic/pelvic abscess.
- Water-soluble enema if large bowel obstruction.

Management

Initially treatment is conservative in localized cases with IV fluids and broad-spectrum IV antibiotics (e.g. cefuroxime 750mg TDS and metronidazole 500mg TDS). The indications for surgical resection of the affected colon include a free perforation causing generalized peritonitis (purulent or faeculant) or diverticulitis not settling with conservative treatment. Pelvic and pericolic abscess may be drained under CT guidance.

Biliary colic and cholecystitis

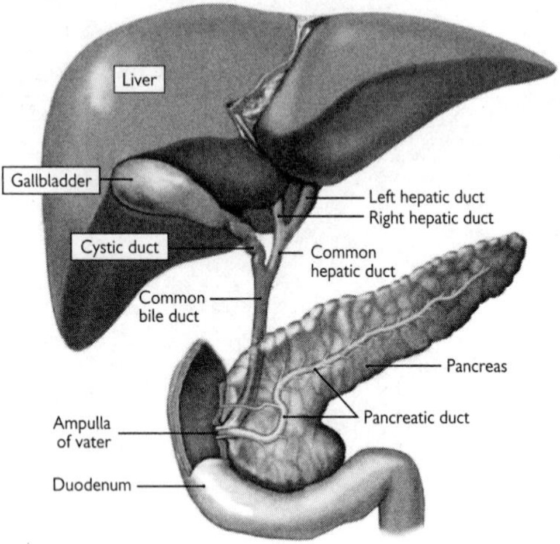

Fig. 2.3 Anatomy of hepatic and pancreatic ducts.

Think about

Impaction of a stone in the neck of the gallbladder causes 'colicky' pain in the upper abdomen. Cholecystitis develops when the contents of the gallbladder become secondarily infected. Gallstones can pass into the common bile duct (CBD) and cause pancreatitis, obstructive jaundice or cholangitis. ~10% of patients have CBD stones at presentation. Consider peptic ulcer, liver disease and right lower lobe lung conditions as ΔΔ. Gallstones can also pass into the duodenum to cause SBO.

Ask about

- RUQ/epigastric pain.
- Pain after eating?
- Duration of pain.
- Worse with fatty foods.
- Vomiting.
- Rigors.
- Shoulder-tip pain.
- Pale stools/dark urine.

Look for

- Cholangitis: fever, Jaundice and RUQ pain.
- Biliary colic: afebrile, tender RUQ/epigastrium.
- Cholecystitis: as biliary colic with ↑ temperature, tenderness over gallbladder worsening on inspiration (Murphy's sign).
- Jaundice: signals gallstone impacted in CBD.
- PR: ?pale stool.

Investigations

- FBC (↑ WCC: cholecystitis/cholangitis), LFTs, amylase, CRP.
- AXR: 10% gallstones radio-opaque, air in biliary tree?
- CXR: ?consolidation, ?effusion.
- USS: ?gallstones, ?dilated biliary tree, ?free fluid.

Management

- IV fluids.
- Oral sips only.
- Analgesia.
- Treat cholecystitis with ciprofloxacin 500mg/12hr IV/PO.
- Surgical management may include early cholecystectomy (48hr from diagnosis).
- Magnetic resonance cholangiopancreatography (MRCP)/ERCP can be used to diagnose CBD stones. Endoscopic ultrasonography (EUS).
- ERCP can be therapeutic, especially in cholangitis/obstructive jaundice.
- Cholangitis requires prompt ERCP to relieve obstruction.

Appendicitis

Think about

Appendicitis is the commonest surgical emergency. It may occur at any age, but the highest incidence is in 10–30-year-olds. Δ include non-specific abdominal pain (up to 40% of cases), mesenteric adenitis, urinary tract infection (UTI), gastroenteritis, inflammatory bowel disease and gynaecological causes including ectopic pregnancy, fibroids, ruptured ovarian cyst and pelvic inflammatory disease. Clinical presentation of appendicitis varies widely. If in doubt about diagnosis, observe patient overnight.

Ask about

- Onset and character of pain: classically diffuse central abdominal pain localizing to right iliac fossa (RIF).
- Pain worse on coughing/movement?
- Similar pain before?
- Nausea and vomiting.
- Feels hungry?
- Diarrhoea.
- Rigors.
- Urinary symptoms.
- Gynae history.
- Pregnant? Possibly pregnant?

Look for

- Flushed.
- Pyrexia.
- Tachycardia.
- Hypotension.
- Coated tongue.
- RIF guarding/rebound/tenderness maximal at McBurney's point.
- Be vigilant for an appendiceal mass.
- Tenderness on PR examination.
- Gynae cause likely if adnexal tenderness/cervical excitation on PV examination.

Investigations

- FBC (↑ WCC), U&Es, ↑ CRP, amylase, G&S.
- Appendicitis unlikely if WCC and CRP normal.
- Urinalysis: ?β-HCG, ?leukocytes.
- USS/CT abdomen: may show mass or abscess.

Management

- Keep nil by mouth.
- IV fluids.
- Analgesia.
- IV antibiotics (cefuroxime 750mg/8hr and metronidazole 500mg/8hr) if decision made to operate.
- Withhold antibiotics if uncertain of diagnosis.
- If signs of systemic toxicity expedite surgery.
- If diagnosis uncertain, admit and carry out serial examinations with regular observations. Appendicitis less likely if FBC and CRP not raised.
- Initial treatment of an appendix mass is with IV antibiotics and USS or CT.
- Consider laparoscopy in difficult cases, especially young female with RIF pain.

Alvarado scoring

One point each for:
- Migration of pain to RIF.
- Anorexia.
- Nausea/vomiting.
- RIF tenderness.
- Rebound tenderness.
- Pyrexia (>37.5°C).
- WCC $>10^9 \times 10^9$/L.
- Left shift (>75% neutrophils).

Score:
- <5: appendicitis unlikely.
- 5–6: possible.
- 7–8: probable.
- >8: very likely.

Abdominal wall herniae

Think about

Is it reducible?—irreducible hernia may need urgent surgery. An irreducible hernia may contain obstructed or strangulated bowel. Irreducible herniae can be strangulated or obstructed.

Think about lipoma, lymphadenopathy, undescended testes, hydrocele, saphena varix, aneurysm and psoas abscess as Δ for a possible groin hernia.

Ask about

- Longstanding lump?
- Suddenly enlarged or appeared suddenly?
- Able to reduce lump?
- Pain? Dragging sensation?
- Abdominal pain or distension.
- Vomiting.
- Constipation.
- Passing flatus?

Look for

- Patient systemically unwell—tachycardia, dehydrated, pyrexia.
- Location of lump:
  - Inguinal hernia—lump above and medial to pubic tubercle.
  - Femoral hernia—lump below and lateral to pubic tubercle.
  - Paraumbilical hernia—lump through weakness in linea alba above/below umbilicus.
  - Epigastric hernia—hernia in midline through defect in linea alba above umbilicus.
  - Incisional hernia—lump protruding near scar from previous wound closure.
- Tender lump?
- Reducible lump?
- Abdominal distension?
- Obstructed bowel sounds?

Investigations

- FBC, U&Es, G&S.
- AXR: distended bowel loops?

Management

- IV fluids.
- Analgesia—incarcerated herniae may reduce spontaneously with adequate analgesia. Get senior help for this. Use gentle pressure only.
- A patient with a reducible hernia can be seen as an outpatient to arrange elective repair.
- An irreducible hernia needs urgent repair, especially if there is suspicion of obstructed or strangulated bowel.
- Patients with an incarcerated hernia that reduces spontaneously will normally be admitted for hernia repair on the next available elective list.

Anorectal emergencies

Think about

The most common emergencies are anorectal abscesses, pilonidal abscesses, thrombosed haemorrhoids and perianal haematomas.

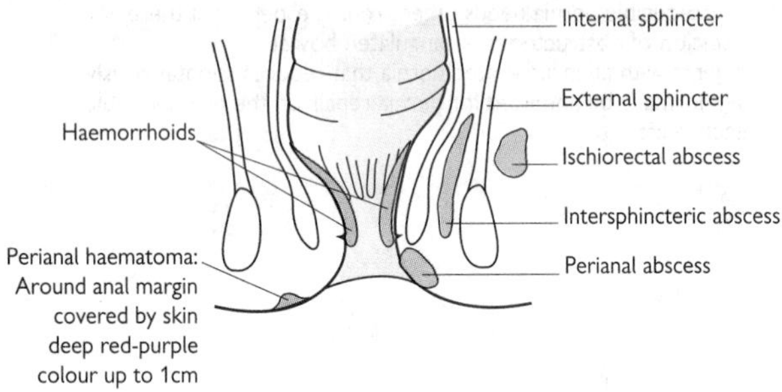

Fig. 2.4 Anorectal area.

Ask about

- Pain—associated with a lump appearing after difficult defaecation?
- Fever.
- Inability to sit or pain on defaecation.
- Any discharge of pus or bloody material PR.
- Previous abscesses.
- History of haemorrhoids.
- Predisposing conditions for anorectal abscesses—inflammatory bowel disease, diabetes, immunocompromise (human immunodeficiency virus, drugs), underlying anorectal cancer.

Look for

- Perianal abscesses: tachycardia, pyrexia, painful perianal swelling, surrounding cellulitis.
- Pilonidal abscess: painful swelling in midline close to natal cleft, pits in natal cleft?
- Perianal haematoma: tender lump, red–purple in colour, up to 1cm and close to anal verge.
- Thrombosed haemorrhoids: obvious prolapsed haemorhoids ± necrosis of overlying mucosa; exquisitely tender.
- Do not attempt PR if very tender. A thorough examination may require general anaesthetic.

Investigations

- FBC, glucose.

Management

- Anorectal and pilonidal abscesses should be drained promptly.
- Send sample of pus at operation.
- Consider sending sample of perianal skin at operation.
- Thrombosed haemorrhoids: treat conservatively with analgesia, topical lidocaine jelly, ice, and reassure patient that pain will settle in 4–5 days. Prescribe laxatives to keep stool soft. Surgery may be required if these measures fail.
- Perianal haematoma is a subcutaneous ecchymosis and may respond to early drainage.

On the wards

Postoperative abdominal pain

Think about

Causes of postoperative abdominal pain include inadequate analgesia, urinary retention, constipation, intra-abdominal sepsis (p62), intestinal obstruction/ileus, anastomotic leak, pseudomembranous colitis and ischaemic bowel.

Ask about

- Location and nature of pain.
- Using patient-controlled analgesia (PCA)? Epidural?
- Fluid/food intake.
- Nausea/vomiting.
- Passing urine?
- Desire to micturate?
- Bowels open? Diarrhoea?
- Passing wind?
- Straining at stool?
- Rigors?

Look for

- Pyrexia, swinging temperature.
- Tachycardia.
- Abdominal distension.
- Abdominal tenderness, peritonism.
- Palpable bladder?
- Digital rectal exam: ?faecal loading, ?tender.

Investigations

- FBC, U&Es, LFT, ABG.
- Urinalysis.
- Stool sample.
- AXR: dilated loops?, faecal loading?
- USS/CT abdomen: collection?
- Gastrografin® studies: leak?

Management

- Ensure adequate analgesia.
- Pass a urinary catheter in suspected retention (usually 500mL residual volume).
- Constipated patients should be given oral aperients and PR enemas (caution after low rectal surgery).
- Management of other Δ is discussed elsewhere.

Postoperative haemorrhage

Think about

Postoperative haemorrhage can be divided into 1° and 2°. 1°, within 24hr of operation, occurs when vasospasm of vessels relaxes or when 1° clots are dislodged with rise in BP. 2° occurs 7–14 days after operation, due to infection.

Ask about

- Assess patient's level of consciousness.
- Ask about blood soaking any dressings and drains.
- Is patient anticoagulated?

Look for

- Signs of shock.
- Pallor, cold, clammy.
- Tachycardia.
- Low-volume pulse.
- Hypotension.
- Jugular venous pressure (JVP)/central venous pressure (CVP).
- Blood loss into drains.
- External bleeding (e.g. from wound).
- Abdominal distension—intra-abdominal haemorrhage.

Investigations

- FBC, clotting.
- Cross-match blood.

Management

- Adhere to ABC principles.
- Oxygen.
- Alert senior: if blood loss is rapid, patient will need to return to theatre for laparotomy/wound exploration.
- Large-bore IV access.
- Resuscitate with crystalloid, then blood.
- Raise the legs.
- Correct any coagulation problems.
- Consider a pressure dressing for minor bleeding from the incision.

Table 2.1 Classification of haemorrhagic shock

	Class I	Class II	Class III	Class IV
Blood loss (mL)	<750	750–1500	1500–2000	>2000
Volume (%)	<15	15–30	30–40	>40
Heart rate (bpm)	<100	>100	>120	>140
BP	Normal	Postural drop	Markedly low	Profoundly low
Capillary refill	Normal	May be delayed	Usually delayed	Always delayed
Respiration	Normal	Mild increase	Moderate tachypnoea	Marked tachypnoea
Urine output (mL/hr)	>30	20–30	5–15	<5
Mental state	Normal or agitated	Agitated	Confused	Obtunded

Intra-abdominal sepsis

Think about

Pus can collect after generalized peritonitis (e.g. after appendicitis, diverticulitis or perforated viscus), and an abscess can also develop from infected haematomas. Common sites for collections include the subphrenic spaces, paracolic gutters, pelvis or between loops of small bowel—typically 4–20 days after operation.

Ask about

- Pain.
- Radiation to shoulder-tip (subphrenic abscess).
- Breathlessness (pleural effusion associated with subphrenic abscess).
- Discharge from rectum/vagina (pelvic abscess).
- Diarrhoea.
- Vomiting.

Look for

- Systemically unwell.
- Swinging pyrexia.
- Tachycardia.
- Abdominal tenderness.
- Signs of pleural effusion/lung collapse (subphrenic abscess).
- Digital rectal examination (DRE): boggy swelling anteriorly with pelvic abscess.

Investigations

- FBC, LFTs, U&Es, CRP, blood culture.
- CXR: pleural effusion, atelectasis, raised hemidiaphragm.
- AXR: dilated loops of bowel (ileus), air/fluid level (abscess cavity).
- USS of abdomen.
- CT of abdomen and pelvis.

Management

- Resuscitate patient with IV fluids, oxygen.
- Commence broad-spectrum intravenous antibiotics (e.g. cefuroxime 750mg IV TDS and metronidazole 500mg TDS).
- Inform seniors and consider HDU/ITU admission.
- Well localized abscess may be drained under USS or CT guidance.
- Multiple, loculated abscesses may need drainage by laparotomy.

☉ Wound infections

Think about

Surgical incisions complicated by superficial infections and superficial/deep collections. Skin infections are commonly caused by staphylococci, whereas deep collections may contain bowel flora (e.g. *E. coli/Bacteroides*).

Ask about

- Painful wound?
- Redness.
- Discharge (colour and amount).
- Have wound edges come apart?

Look for

- Pyrexia.
- Swinging pyrexia (collection).
- Erythema around wound.
- Localized wound tenderness.
- Purulent exudate?
- Deep fluctuant collection.
- Sloughy, necrotic wound.

Investigations

- FBC.
- Wound swab.
- USS to delineate deep collection.

Management

Pus must be released, ensuring that there is adequate drainage, and any necrotic material must be debrided. Consider opening superficial layer of wound and probing gently to allow drainage of a superficial collection; aspiration with needle/syringe may reveal superficial wound collection. Deeper collections can be drained using USS/CT guidance. Infected wounds can be irrigated with saline and dressed with hydrocolloid dressing. Never resuture an infected wound. Use broad-spectrum antibiotics if signs of cellulitis/systemic toxicity. Once microbiology results are available, tailor antibiotics accordingly.

☠ Wound dehiscence

Think about

Dehiscence of laparotomy wounds usually occurs 5–10 days after operation. In partial dehiscence the skin closure holds but breakdown of the deep fascial layer means an incisional hernia will develop. Complete dehiscence results from the skin and fascial layer 'bursts', exposing underlying bowel/omentum into the wound. Predisposing factors include poor closure technique, obesity, wound infection and haematoma, and raised intra-abdominal pressure.

Ask about

- ↑ wound pain.
- A feeling of 'give' in the wound.
- Discharge (colour and amount).
- Wound redness.

Look for

- Serosanguineous (pink coloured) discharge from wound.
- Pus discharge from the wound.
- Distinguish superficial dehiscence of skin closure from dehiscence of deeper sutured layers by gentle probing with the gloved finger.
- Swinging pyrexia.
- Protruding loops of bowel/omentum in abdominal wound.

Investigations

- FBC.
- G&S.

Management

For laparotomy wound dehiscence: lie patient flat, cover wound with sterile saline-soaked gauze, give analgesia, establish IV access and commence fluid resuscitation; alert senior for urgent resuture of wound in theatre.

For superficial skin dehiscence: leave wound open and dress with, for example, Kaltostat®, allowing wound to granulate; close by 2° intention.

ⓘ Post-laparotomy patient care

Think about

Patient may have had a laparotomy for trauma, small/large bowel resection (e.g. cancer, ischaemic bowel, diverticular disease), gastric/hepatobiliary surgery, etc. Specific complications include haemorrhage, anastomotic dehiscence, infection (wound and intra-abdominal) and postoperative ileus. Also remember cardiorespiratory complications and urinary tract infections.

Ask about

- Abdominal pain.
- Passing wind?
- Bowels open?
- Diarrhoea? (Consider *Clostridium difficile*).
- Constipation?
- Fluid/food intake.
- Pain well controlled?
- Cough?

Look for

- Pyrexia.
- Tachycardia.
- Dehydration.
- Abdominal distension.
- Abdominal tenderness.
- Bowel sounds.
- Erythema/discharge from wound.
- Urine output.
- Auscultate the chest.
- Drainage.

Investigations

- FBC, U&Es, LFTs (biliary surgery).
- Urine sample.
- Stool sample.
- CXR (If indicated).
- Check swab culture results.

Management

Consider the following points when you review the patient:

- Analgesia: PCA/epidural? When to convert to oral analgesia.
- Oral intake: practice changing to more aggressive introduction of oral intake (start with free fluids then to light diet) and early removal of NG tube.
- Removal of NG tube.
- Removal of urinary catheter.
- Need for antibiotics.
- Chest physiotherapy.
- Look for postoperative complications.

ⓘ Stomas

Think about

An ileostomy has a spout (usually located right iliac fossa) and produces a semi-liquid output. Colostomies are fashioned flush with the skin (usually located in the left iliac fossa) and generally produce a more solid output than an ileostomy. Stomas can also be brought out as a loop or double barrelled (e.g. Paul Mikulicz type, loop transverse colostomy).

Ask about

- Output from stoma?
- How recently was bag changed?
- Stopped working?
- Bleeding into stoma bag?
- Retraction or prolapse of stoma through skin?
- Change in colour of stoma?
- Any lumps felt next to stoma?
- Irritation of skin around stoma.

Look for

- Contents of stoma bag—liquid? formed? blood?
- Check for signs of dehydration and electrolyte imbalance 2° to high-output stoma.
- Any bleeding from bowel edges?
- Retraction/prolapse of stoma.
- Use a torch to illuminate the stoma: dusky/dark colour (remember colon looks dark with melanosis coli) may signal an ischaemic stoma—patient may be systemically unwell.
- Parastomal hernias?
- Excoriation and dermatitis around stoma site.
- Gently pass a gloved finger into the stoma: is there any obstruction or faecal loading?

Investigations

- AXR: obstructed bowel loops?
- U&Es—stoma output can cause large metabolic losses.

Management

Postoperative bleeding from bowel edge is usually self-limiting; ischaemic stomas need prompt revision; obstruction can be 2° to intra-abdominal adhesions or faecal loading. Passing a glycerine suppository into the stoma may relieve the latter condition. Ensure that high output from ileostomy does not lead to ↓ K. Irritation of surrounding skin can occur from bowel contents or adhesive from bowel bag.

ⓘ Drains

Think about

Drains are used to evacuate pus, blood, bile, faeces, urine or lymph. Open drains drain into a dressing or bag (e.g. Yates' drain—consisting of a series of polyethylene capillary tubes joined side to side). Closed drains consist of an airtight tube that drains into a container. The latter type of drain can be left on free drainage or on suction (e.g. Redivac drain). T-tube drains are inserted after bile duct surgery. Drains are also placed in the rectum/sigmoid to decompress the bowel (e.g. pseudo-obstruction, sigmoid volvulus) or after surgery (e.g. anterior resection).

Look for

- Operation note: ?position of drain, ?any specific instructions.
- Colour and consistency of fluid in drain: ?blood, ?serous, ?pus, ?bowel contents, ?urine.
- Amount of drainage.

Investigations

Analysis of drain fluid for amylase, urea and creatinine, etc. may give clues as to the type of fluid drained. T-tube cholangiography is performed to ensure patency of distal CBD before removing the drain.

Management

Consult with senior before removing.

Use the drainage over past 12–24hr as a guide to whether the drain can be removed. Left in for too long, drains can introduce infection. Drains that are continuing to drain >30mL/hr should generally be left in, although individual preferences vary. Drains inserted to monitor postoperative bleeding and haematoma formation can be removed after 48hr. Drains used to prevent serous collections may be removed after 3–5 days. T-tubes are normally removed after 6–10 days, but do not remove these before consulting with seniors.

Remember to cut the sutures holding the drain and to release any suction before removal.

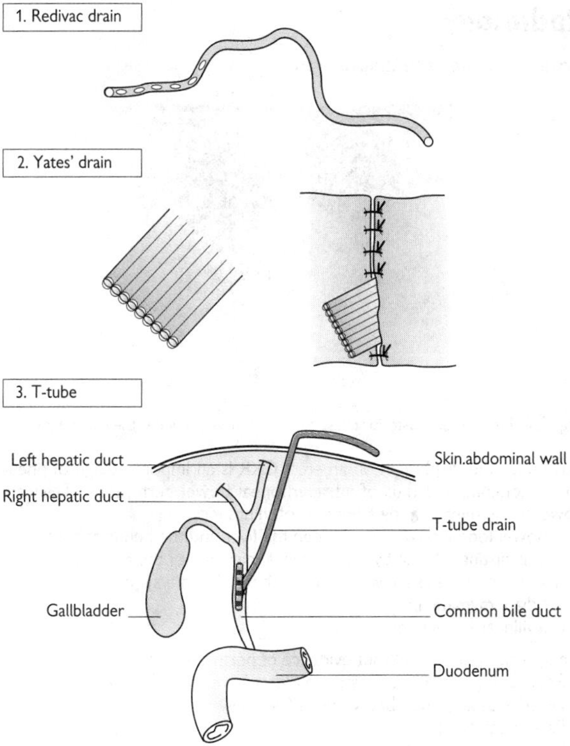

Fig. 2.5 Types of surgical drain.

Radiology

Free gas under the diaphragm

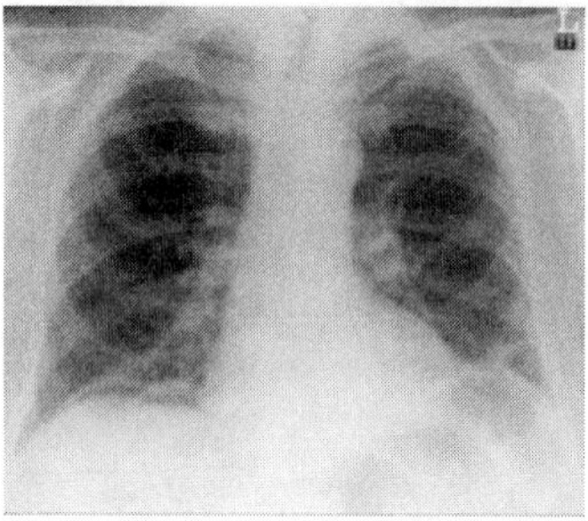

Fig. 2.6 Erect anteroposterior chest X-ray with free gas under the diaphragm.

Gas under the diaphragm on an *erect* CXR is an important sign of pneumoperitoneum, and thus of intraperitoneal bowel perforation. This can, however, be mimicked by a number of things including:

- A bowel loop interposed between the liver and the hemidiaphragm. This is distinguishable by the apparent thickness of the diaphragm, which should be as shown crisp and thin (Chilaiditi syndrome).
- Subdiaphragmatic fat.
- Curvilinear lung atelectasis.

It may also be found without evidence of perforation in:

- Recent surgery: 60% of postop. patients have intra-abdominal gas, which is usually absorbed within a few days.
- Peritoneal dialysis.
- Silent perforation of an intra-abdominal viscus.

Unsure?

This can be a misleading sign and, if in doubt, a lateral decubitus plain X-ray will be very useful. Remember that free air will lie in the most superior (i.e. non-dependant) part of the abdomen.

Free intra-abdominal gas

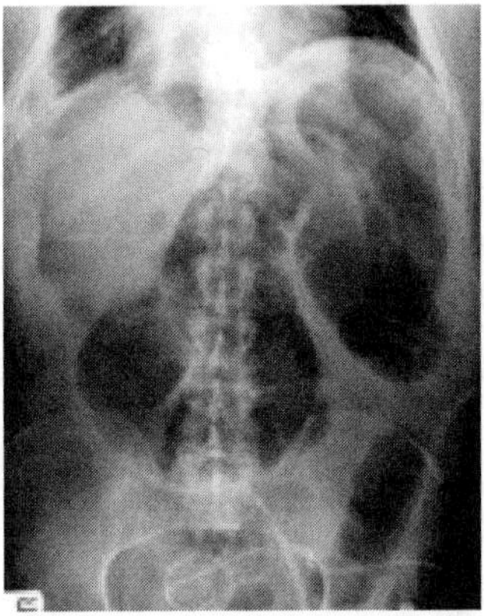

Fig. 2.7 Abdominal X-ray (supine) showing free intra-abdominal gas.

On this supine AXR there is gaseous distension of large bowel, with gas seen in the sigmoid colon. Free intra-abdominal air is shown by the lucency overlying and outlining the superior and lateral aspects of the liver. Furthermore, it illustrates Rigler's sign—the ability to visualize both the inner and outer bowel wall when free gas lies adjacent to a loop of bowel. This sign can be difficult to detect and may be mimicked by loops of bowel overlying one another. There is a continuous abdominal peritoneal dialysis (CAPD) catheter in the pelvis. The patient has a large bowel ileus due to an electrolyte imbalance and no evidence of peritonism—the free air is a consequence of dialysis.

Retroperitoneal gas

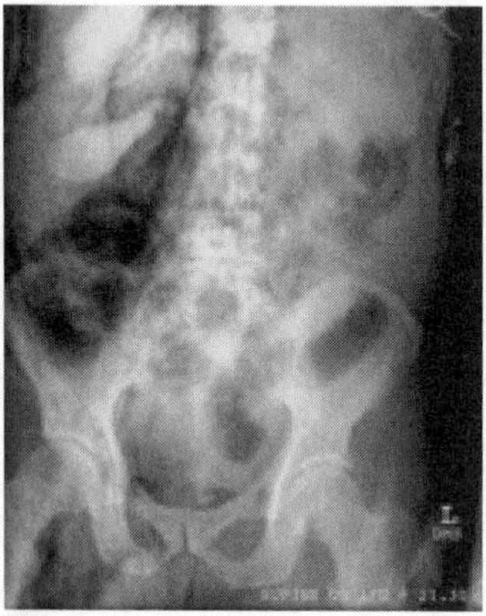

Fig. 2.8 Abdominal X-ray (supine) showing retroperitoneal gas.

Extensive retroperitoneal air is seen tracking predominantly up the right side of the abdomen. Note how crisp the retroperitoneal structures such as the right psoas muscle and right kidney are due to the presence of air immediately adjacent to them. There is also extensive subcutaneous (surgical) emphysema. Note that the gallbladder is filled with contrast and that a biliary drain has been sited—the perforation resulted from ERCP.

Retroperitoneal gas has a very different appearance to free intra-abdominal gas, as it is contained.

Total small bowel obstruction

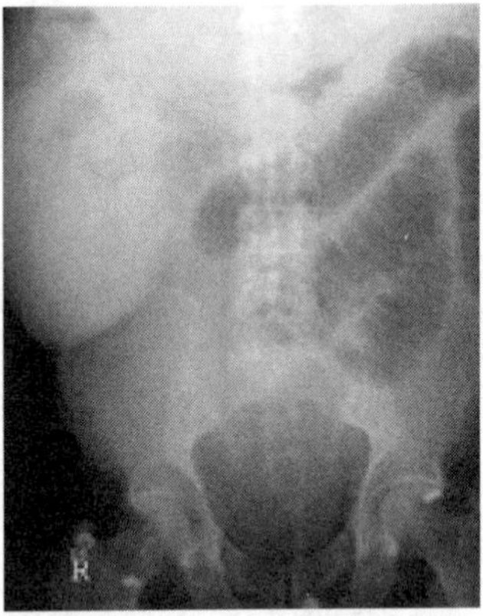

Fig. 2.9 Abdominal X-ray (supine) showing total small bowel obstruction due to a large incisional hernia (shown over the right side of the abdomen).

Note the presence of valvulae conniventes, the central location of the loops and the diameter, which is 4cm. There is no evidence of perforation.

Partial large bowel obstruction

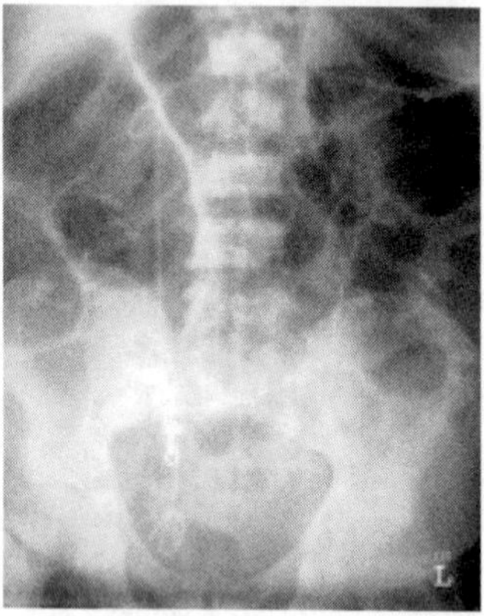

Fig. 2.10 Abdominal X-ray (supine) showing low partial large bowel obstruction to the level of the rectum (proven by Gastrografin® enema).

The transverse colon measures 8cm. Note that the lumbar vertebral bodies and pelvic bones are sclerotic and there is a right JJ ureteric stent. The obstruction was a result of T4 prostatic carcinoma extending into the rectum with extensive bony metastases.

Table 2.2 Differentiating large from small bowel dilatation

	Small bowel	Large bowel
Valvulae conniventes (circumferential opaque bands across bowel loops)	Seen in jejunum	Not seen
Diameter	>3cm	Transverse colon: >6cm Caecum: >9cm
Haustral folds (thick incomplete bands across colonic shadows)	Not seen	May be identified
Distribution of loops	Central	Peripheral
Formed faeces	Absent	Present

Watch out!

- If the ileocaecal valve is incompetent, large bowel obstruction may be manifested by dilated loops of both large and small bowel.
- In early small bowel obstruction there may be gas-filled loops of bowel distal to the point of obstruction; however, these will clear with time.
- Pseudo-obstruction may mimic bowel obstruction—clinical assessment is vital. Further imaging with either CT or a contrast study is often of use to differentiate this from mechanical obstruction.

Chapter 3

Trauma and orthopaedics

Stephen McDonnell
Sunil Auplish

Introduction

Trauma and orthopaedics is one of the surgical specialties you are most likely to encounter. There are 'T&O' departments in all district general hospitals, with busy emergency and ward workloads. It is very likely that, if you are involved in the care of surgical patients or admissions, you will have to cover some orthopaedic patients. You will not be expected to know what operation these patients will require or any detailed anatomy; however, some orthopaedic problems are more urgent than others. This is by no means a complete guide to all fractures, but should be a guide to their general management,

List of operations and glossary of orthopaedic terminology

General terms

- Arthrodesis—fusion of a joint.
- Arthroscopy—looking into a joint.
- Arthroplasty—joint replacement.
- Osteotomy—cutting a bone.
- MUA—manipulation under anaesthetic.
- K-wire—a Kirschner wire fixation: a thin, rigid wire that can be used to stabilize bone fragments. These wires can be drilled through the bone to hold the fragments in place. They are placed percutaneously. In other cases, K-wires are used after an operation to hold bone fragments in place.
- Hemi-arthroplasty—half joint replacement.
- DHS—dynamic hip screw.
- External fixators/circular frame.
- THR and TKR—total hip replacement and total knee replacement.
- ORIF—open reduction internal fixation with plates and screws of any bone.
- Tendon repair.
- Long bone nail—tibial, femoral, and humeral, radial.
- Nancy—flexible intermedullary nail.

Anatomy of a long bone

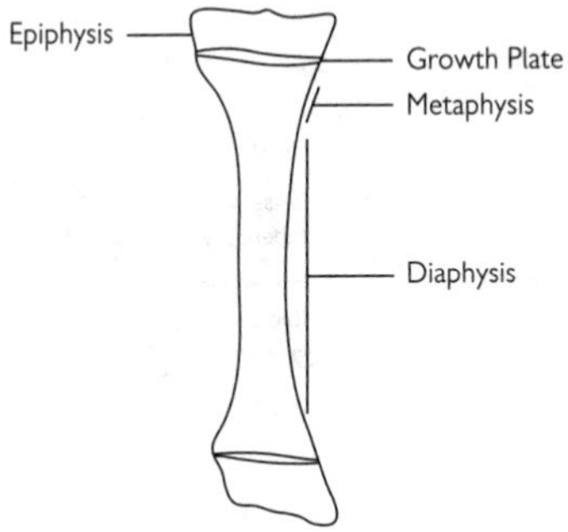

Fig. 3.1 Anatomy of a bone.

Any long bone may also be subdivided into specific sections:
- Epiphysis—the end of a long bone.
- Physis (growth plate)—the region in a long bone between the epiphysis and diaphysis where growth in length occurs; seen only in the immature skeleton.
- Metaphysis—the transitional zone at which the diaphysis and epiphysis of a bone come together.
- Diaphysis—the shaft of a long bone.

Overview of the skeletal system

It is essential that you have the correct anatomical description of the bones involved.

The upper limb

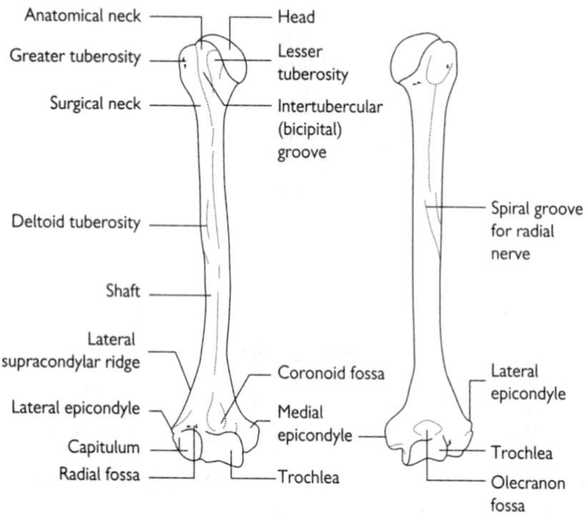

Fig. 3.2 The humerus.

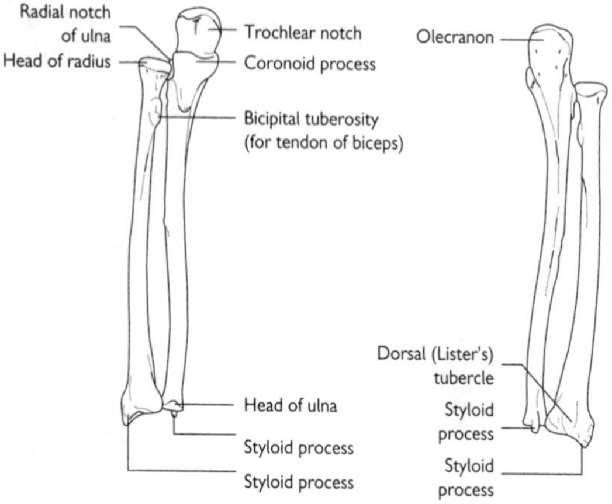

Fig. 3.3 The radius and ulna.

The lower limb

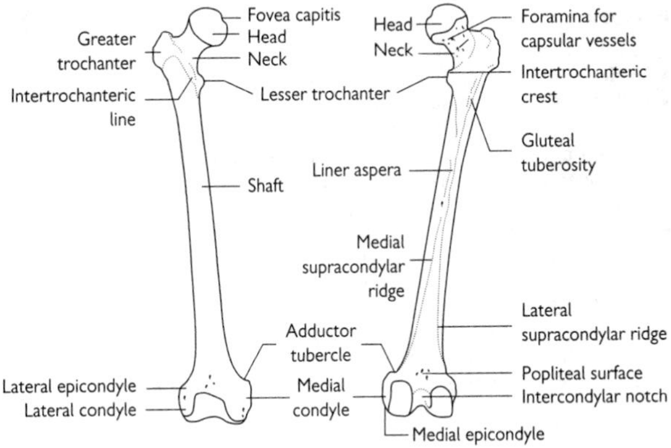

Fig. 3.4 The femur.

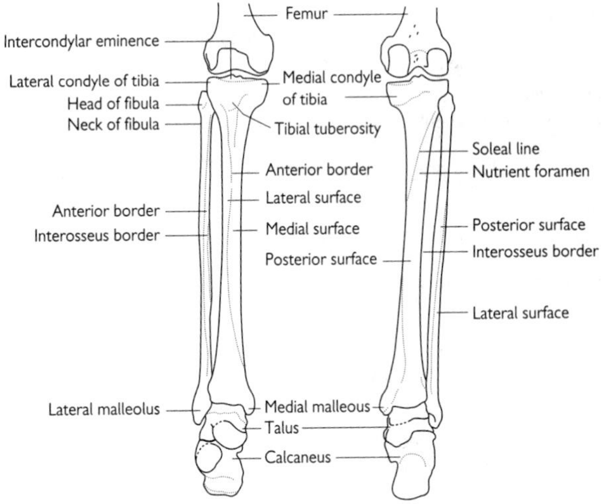

Fig. 3.5 Tibia and fibula.

History and examination

History

- What is their occupation?
- Which side is affected?
- Left- or right-handed dominance?
- How did the accident happen?
- Pre-morbid activities of daily living (washing, dressing, cooking, shopping). Use this to plan appropriate discharge.
- Was there a medical reason for the fall?
- Do they smoke or drink alcohol?
- Hobbies, do they play a musical instrument?

Examination

- Full examination of cardiovascular and respiratory system.
- Examination of limb or site of injury.
- Detailed neurovascular examination—comment on named individual vessels and nerves.
- Baseline Mental Test Score (MTS) (see 📖 p128).

Mark patient

- Use a permanent marker to mark the affected limb—put your initials by the arrow, the date and the planned operation (e.g. → SM dd/mm L-DHS).

X-rays

- Ensure that you have the affected bone in two views.
- Also include the joint above and below.

Urine dip

- Urine dipstick should be noted to exclude a urinary tract infection (UTI).
- In young ♀ do a pregnancy test—will affect X-ray use in theatre.

Drug chart

- Write up the patient's normal medications.
- Write up appropriate PO and IM analgesia.
- Write up antiemetic PO, IM, IV.
- Write up PRN lactulose and senna.
- Write up thromboprophylaxis as per local protocol.
- Write up allergies on the front of the drug chart.
- Write up fluids if patient to be kept nil by mouth.

Things to think about

- Does the patient need a medical review?
- Do they need an orthopaedic registrar review?
- Do they need to go to theatre tonight?
- Do they have an infection that could threaten implanted metalwork?
- Have I missed any other injuries?

Radiology

Radiology is an essential part of trauma and orthopaedic practice. A clear description of the fracture is essential when discussing a fracture and its radiograph. The person to whom you are describing the fracture has to have a clear idea of exactly what the radiograph and clinical examination look like. It is ∴ essential that you use accurate and precise language.

The orthopaedic language

First, check the NAME and DATE. Do this every time to save a lot of embarassment and potentially more serious consequences. When describing a fracture, it is helpful to use the following template:

'There is an *open/closed pattern* fracture of the *part of bone name of bone*.'

e.g. 'There is a closed spiral fracture of the distal shaft of the humerus.'

Orthopaedic terms

- *Open/closed*—not a radiographic description, but, if the skin is broken, it is important to mention this early.
- *Pattern*—the fracture can be transverse/oblique/spiral. It may be in lots of pieces, i.e. comminuted (multifragmentary).
- *Part of bone*—can use the diaphysis/metaphysis description as given above. The fracture may be at the 'junction of the proximal and middle thirds of the diaphysis'. A fracture than goes into the joint is intra-articular.

Afterwards, describe the displacement of the fracture. These are length, angulation, rotation and displacement:

- *Length*—measured in centimetres (cm), e.g. 'This fracture is shortened by 3cm', if there is a 3cm overlap of the bones.
- *Angulation*—measured in degrees (°), e.g. 'The fracture is angulated 30°'.
- *Rotation*—usually assessed clinically. However, if an X-ray of a tibial fracture shows an anteroposterior (AP) appearance of the knee and a lateral appearance of the ankle, there is likely to be a 90° rotation at the fracture. ∴ include the joint above and below the fracture.
- *Displacement*—given as %, e.g. 'The distal part has displaced 20% in a lateral direction'. When the fracture has displaced 100% then the bones are no longer in contact and the fracture is 'off-ended' and can shorten (see length).

Other useful terms

- Dislocation—total loss of congruity between articular surfaces.
- Subluxation—partial loss of congruity between articular surfaces.
- Crush or compression—loss of bone volume. Occurs in cancellous bone that is compressed beyond the limits of its tolerance. Common sites for these fractures are the vertebral bodies and calcaneum.
- Butterfly or wedge—a smaller but significant third fragment in conjunction with the two main fragments in a long bone fracture.
- Burst—a burst fracture is a descriptive term for an injury to the spine in which the vertebral body is severely compressed. The vertebra is seen to 'burst' out in all directions.
- Segmental—a bone that has two fractures and a piece between them, i.e. one bone that has two or more breaks along its shaft.
- Torus—a knuckle or bump greenstick fracture; a term used for this appearance in the distal radius. Occurs only in children.
- Impacted—occurs when one fracture fragment is driven into another.
- Avulsion—a piece of bone that is usually small and has been pulled away from the main bone by a ligament when a joint is stretched violently in one direction.
- Undisplaced—no loss of position of the fracture, i.e. a break where the bone has not moved.
- Greenstick—the break starts at one side of the bone but does not go all the way through the bone, and the bone bends. Occurs in children.
- Pathological—a break through abnormal bone, e.g. through a tumour.

'The rule of 2s'

Ignore this rule at your peril!

When looking at X-rays there should be two views (e.g. AP and lateral) with two joints (the joint above and below the fracture). If in doubt, X-ray two sides (i.e. the normal side) on two occasions.

ATLS and a 'trauma call'

If you are regularly present at trauma calls then you need to be trained on a recognized Advanced Trauma Life Support (ATLS®) course (http://www.rcseng.ac.uk/education/courses/trauma_life_support_advanced.html).

You will be attending with other doctors from emergency medicine, anaesthetics, and other surgical specialties.

A trauma call is put out when a multiply injured trauma patient is on their way to or has arrived at hospital. It is important that all of the appropriate specialties are present to ensure the best chance of survival for the patient. Most hospitals have criteria for trauma call and the people who attend are fast-bleeped via switchboard. You must make your way to the emergency department as soon as possible.

Trauma calls and ATLS® have a very strict structure to follow. These principles are directed to treat the greatest risk to life first:

- 1° survey and resuscitation (all being assessed concurrently):
  - A = Airway and cervical spine control.
  - B = Breathing.
  - C = Circulation and haemorrhage control.
  - D = Dysfunction of the central nervous system.
  - E = Exposure.
  - 1° survey X-rays.
  - 1° survey bloods.
- Treatment instigated and treated as the problems are found.
- 2° survey.
- Definitive treatment.
- Re-assessment of patient at any change in their status.

Airway (and cervical spine control)

The patient must be considered to have a C-spine injury until this has been cleared clinically and radiologically. They ∴ require immobilization with a hard collar and three-point immobilization with blocks and tape.

- Airway—this will usually be managed by the anaesthetist. Simple jaw thrust manoeuvre and airway adjuncts, oropharyngeal, nasopharyngeal tubes can be used. However, a definitive airway is an endotracheal tube with the cuff inflated.
- Don't forget to put any trauma patient on high-flow oxygen (>10L/min) through a re-breath bag.

Breathing

Assessment of the chest. Ensure good air entry through both sides of the chest. What is the respiratory rate?

Causes of breathing problems that need to be addressed are:

- Airway obstruction.
- Tension pneumothorax.
- Large haemothorax.
- Sucking chest wound.
- Flail chest.
- Cardiac tamponade.

Circulation

- First gain IV access with two large bore cannulas (14G)—grey is good, brown is better.
- Take routine trauma bloods: FBC, U&Es, LFTs, amylase (including cross-match).
- Start fluids—2L warmed Ringer's lactate immediately; catheterize the patient when time allows.

Assess the patient's haemodynamic state. Are they pink and warm? What is the capillary refill? Put on monitoring and measure pulse rate, blood pressure, urine output.

Common places for haemorrhage are intra-abdominal, intra-thoracic, long bone fractures, pelvic fractures and external haemorrhage.

Dysfunction

This is an assessment of the patient's neurological status. It is assessed with the AVPU scale:

- A = Alert.
- V = Responds to vocal stimulus.
- P = Responds to painful stimuli.
- U = Unresponsive.

It is best to use the Glasgow Coma Scale, which should be on the trauma sheet.

Primary survey X-rays

These should be undertaken in all trauma patients. They include lateral cervical spine, AP chest and AP pelvis. It must be ensured that you can see the whole of the C7–T1 junction.

Log roll

The patient is normally brought in immobilized on a spinal board. Four people (three body, one at the head) are needed to roll them and another to do the physical examination of the spine. A digital rectal examination should also be performed at this stage to assess for any signs of PR blood and anal tone, for bowel, prostatic or neurological spinal injuries. The spinal board will cause pressure sores and should be removed as part of the log roll, even in the presence of a spinal injury.

An AMPLE history

In the trauma situation an accurate focused history is essential. Pictures form the accident scene and the paramedics are a valuable resource. The mnemonic AMPLE contains all of the key facts that need to be obtained:

- A = Allergies.
- M = Medications.
- P = Past medical history.
- L = Last ate or drank.
- E = Events that led up to the accident and following the accident.

Secondary survey

This is a complete physical examination of the patient, from head to toe. Once initial resuscitation of the patient has occurred, a thorough examination to identify the presence of non-life-threatening injuries can be performed. Long-term morbidity and litigation is often associated with minor injuries that have been missed in the 2° survey. The 2° survey may often not occur until all of the major life-threatening problems have been treated. This may be a few days following admission. It is good practice to go back and repeat the 2° survey 24hr after admission on the ward to ensure that nothing has been missed.

Think about:

- Look in the mouth, eyes and ears.
- If anything changes in the patient's condition, go back and re-assess, starting at ABC.
- Make sure that bloods are sent, including cross-match, and not just left on the side.
- Is the patient pregnant?
- Be aware of neurological changes from a progressive head injury.
- If patient becomes unstable when admitted to the ward, review and call for an urgent senior review.

Common fractures and dislocations

Each bone can be broken in a variety of ways. This chapter aims to highlight the essential features of the fractures that are common or have important clinical signs that you should be looking out for. You should consult a more detailed textbook or ask for senior review if unsure. There will be a fracture clinic in your Trust; arrange follow-up for any fracture patients you see out-of-hours according to local protocols.

You should always look for and document neurovascular status, the presence of an open fracture, and signs of compartment syndrome. Anything that looks unusual, alarming or very displaced needs to be checked with your seniors.

Upper limb

Shoulder dislocation

99% will be *anterior* dislocations. The diagnosis is usually obvious from the history and X-rays. Always look at the X-rays for any fractures. It is vital to look at the neurovascular status, especially the distal pulse and the *axillary nerve*. This is intact if there is normal sensation over the deltoid muscle on that side. You must document this *before* reduction as it can be damaged by both dislocation and reduction. Obtain X-rays before and after reduction, and always get *at least two views*.

There are many techniques of reduction. The Kocher method is commonly used and involves traction to the elbow with external rotation of the humerus and adduction of the elbow toward the chest. Reduction should be attempted only by an experienced person to avoid humeral fractures in the elderly and neurovascular damage.

Posterior dislocation

Less frequent dislocations, however, are often missed! These injuries often occur after a fall on to an internally rotated hand or from a direct blow from the front. Classically they may be seen following a fit or after an electric shock. They are very difficult to see on AP radiographs so it is essential that another view is also obtained.

Clavicular fractures

Rest in sling or collar and cuff for 2 weeks. Needs to be brought in for fixation only if the skin is tented, there is an open injury or neurovascular injury. Otherwise, send the patient home and see them in the fracture clinic.

Humerus—surgical neck

Always look for dislocation. Can be difficult to assess and may require AP, Y and axial view X-rays. Usually a fracture in the elderly and treated by hanging cast and clinic review. Ask senior opinion if the fracture looks very displaced, or if the tuberosities have fractured and sit away from the humeral head. Pre-morbid state is crucial in decision making about whether to operate.

Humeral shaft

Up to 30° angulation in any plane is treated in a brace or hanging cast. Look for radial nerve injury (wrist drop)—if present, provide a wrist splint and await recovery.

Humerus—paediatric supracondylar fractures

Look for skin puckering by fracture. Beware of neurovascular injury: it is very important to feel for the pulse. Ask about pins and needles, and assess nerve injury carefully. For the anterior interosseous nerve (branch of the median nerve), ask the child to make a circle shape with their fingers by pinching the tips of their thumb and index finger together. May be easier to do all this in POP backslab. Beware compartment syndrome, both before and after surgery. Must discuss with senior if fracture displaced—this may well need to go the theatre as an emergency.

Other paediatric elbow fractures

Beware the painful paediatric elbow post-injury. The X-ray may show that the medial epicondyle has avulsed and is sitting in the joint (often seen as a blob on the lateral). A fracture of the 'lateral mass' (the distal humerus on the lateral side of the elbow) looks like a very minor injury but often needs an operation. X-ray signs are subtle—taking a radiograph of the normal side and comparing may be helpful. Look for anterior fat pad.

Olecranon

Undisplaced fractures need immobilization in right-angled arm plaster.

Displaced and comminuted fractures require admission and internal fixation.

Dislocated elbow

Ensure neurovascular status in the hand. Obtain pre-reduction X-rays. Reduce in the emergency department. Place arm and elbow in a backslab and see in fracture clinic. Take post-reduction films. If, however, there is any fracture of the radial head, humerus, coronoid or olecranon, a senior opinion should be obtained as operative intervention may be necessary.

Radius—radial head

If minimal displacement, place in collar and cuff for 3 weeks. If displaced or severely comminuted, the patient may need admission and radial head fixation, excision or replacement.

Forearm fractures

Mid-shaft fractures do not tolerate deformity, and loss of pro/supination will occur. Adults with displaced fractures require operative fixation. Admit, put on a backslab, elevate in a Bradford sling, and beware compartment syndrome. Children over the age of 12yr should be considered as adults. Measure the angle of deformity—although there is no consensus, children over the age of 10yr with greater than 10° deformity will not remodel (grow straight) and will need to go to theatre. If there is any visible deformity, it is often better to admit for theatre. Discuss with your registrar—they will need to know the age of the child and the angle of deformity.

The forearm bones are joined at the top and bottom, and form a rigid ring. A break in one bone means that you should see a break somewhere in the other. If you do not, you should look for the following two injuries:

- Galeazzi fracture—a fracture of the distal one-third of the radius with dislocation of the distal radioulnar joint.
- Monteggia fracture—a fracture of the ulna (usually proximal one-third) with dislocation of the radial head.
- **Remember the 'rule of 2s'.**

Scaphoid

Be suspicious of anyone who has a good mechanism of injury and has tenderness in the anatomical snuff box and pain on ulna deviation of the wrist. Scaphoid fractures are not always seen on the first set of X-rays. If this is the case, apply a scaphoid cast/backslab/Fenturi splint and send to next fracture clinic for review. Treatment for fractures may be immobilization in a scaphoid cast until the fracture has united. If there is delayed union, consider ORIF with a Herbert screw.

Wrist fractures

Colles' fracture

This is a transverse fracture of the distal radius within 2.5cm of the wrist, with a characteristic 'dinner fork' deformity of dorsal displacement and dorsal angulation. The distal radius can be fractured in many patterns—this is only one. ∴ say 'distal radius #' and not 'Colles' #' when describing it, unless you are absolutely sure. This is a very common fracture seen in postmenopausal ♀. These fractures are usually manipulated in the emergency department and put into a backslab. They are then followed up at fracture clinic. You will be called to admit if this has not worked.

Smith's fracture

This is often referred to as a reverse Colles' fracture. Instead of the fracture displacing in a dorsal direction, it displaces in a volar (opposite) direction. This fracture is commonly unstable and will require surgery.

Barton's fracture

This is an intra-articular fracture of the distal radius that will be seen on the lateral X-ray. The anterior (volar) part of the radius is fractured and displaced. Closed reduction is often difficult, so these fractures are usually treated with ORIF.

Carpal dislocations

If the wrist is painful and swollen, but you are unable to see an obvious problem on the radiograph, consider a carpal dislocation. Follow the distal radius on the lateral X-ray. It should lead directly to the crescent-shaped lunate and then to the long and slender capitate. If you can't see this, call for help.

Fractures in the hand

These are covered in the chapter on Plastic surgery (see 🕮 p402).

Lower limb

Femur—shaft

Operative reduction and surgical fixation is usually required (usually by means of an intermedullary nail, rarely plate and screws or external fixator). Before surgery the patient may be managed in traction or with a Thomas splint. Admission and a full preoperative workup are required. As these are high-energy injuries, 2 units of blood can be lost at the fracture site into the thigh. 4 units of blood *must* be cross-matched. Look carefully for other injuries.

Femoral fractures is children

These are high-energy injuries.

Management:

Children aged <2yr are commonly treated by *gallows traction* (both the fractured and the intact femur are placed in skin traction and the infant is suspended by these from a special frame). If aged 2–6yr, the child can be treated by traction alone. Some will place in a hip spica instead (plaster that goes around pelvis and down the leg). If older than 6yr then admit in a *Thomas splint* (leg splint consisting of two rigid rods attached to an ovoid ring that fits around the thigh; it can be combined with other apparatus to provide traction), usually applied by paediatric nurses. Some will treat non-operatively, but others will pass flexible nails, so if in doubt prepare for theatre.

Femoral neck

See Hip fractures. Rare in the young, but due to high-energy injury. ∴ look carefully for other injuries. Call your registrar—the patient may need surgery that night.

Patella

Undisplaced fractures should be protected in a full leg cast for 3 weeks. Displaced fractures require internal fixation with screw or tension band wire. Document whether the patient is able to straight leg raise.

Dislocation of the patella

This typically occurs laterally and may be recurrent. Reduction can be performed under Entonox analgesia. The patient should have a backslab or cricket pad splint, and be seen in the next fracture clinic. Patients who have recurrent dislocations may need to consider operative management to prevent future dislocations, but will not need admission for this.

Tibial plateau

These need anatomical reduction, with an ORIF or external fixation. Admit with full-length backslab. Arrange CT scan of the knee.

Tibial shaft fractures

Beware compartment syndrome, even in undisplaced fractures. You will not be criticized for admission of fracture for analgesia, and observation. If displaced, an intramedullary nail is likely to be needed. If the fracture pattern is transverse, manipulation and plaster may suffice. Either way, prepare for theatre if the fracture is displaced.

Fibula—shaft

Just like the forearm, the fibula forms a rigid ring with the tibia. ALWAYS look for tibial fractures. If not, then it is very possible that the inferior tibiofibular joint is disrupted (Maissoneuve injury), so X-ray the ankle to see whether these two bones are splayed apart from each other. If OK, look at the proximal tibiofibular joint. If the proximal fibula is fractured then examine for a foot-drop (common peroneal nerve injury).

Golden rule in all orthopaedics

Forget the X-ray at first and EXAMINE the patient to see whether they are actually tender at the area of concern.

Foot

Ankle fractures

See Ankle injuries below.

Calcaneum fractures

Often sustained after a fall from a height. Suspect thoracolumbar spine injuries in anyone with a calcaneal fracture. There is variation amongst orthopaedic surgeons on whether these fractures are fixed with ORIF or treated in a POP. All patients should be admitted for elevation. Likely to need a CT scan.

Talus fractures

Patients need admission and elevation. You must call your registrar if the fracture is displaced—the patient may need surgery that night. ORIF is performed, depending on the degree of displacement.

Lisfranc injuries

This describes disruption between the tarsal bones and the metatarsals in the midfoot. This is a very important injury that is often missed. If the foot is very painful and swollen but has a 'normal' looking X-ray then be very suspicious. Look at a normal foot X-ray and see how the bones are arranged around the base (proximal) second metatarsal. Any change to this should ring alarm bells.

Base of fifth metatarsal fractures

Put in plaster and send to fracture clinic.

Metatarsal shaft fractures

Treated in plaster, but consider bringing in for surgery if multiple fractures.

Toe fractures

Very rarely operated on unless impressive displacement. Can give a ring block to the toe with local anaesthetic, pull straight and buddy strap to its neighbour.

Open fractures

Inform orthopaedic senior on call.

An open fracture is one where the bone is sticking out or has stuck, through the muscle and skin. Any bone with a wound over it should be treated as an open fracture. As the bone is open to the air there is a high risk of infection, so appropriate management is essential. Open fractures of the tibia are common due to the thin layer of skin and subcutaneous tissue over its anterior border.

It is usually obvious if the bone is sticking out but you must be suspicious if there is a wound anywhere near the fracture site or there is tenting of the skin.

Think about
- This is an orthopaedic emergency and the fracture will need to be reduced and stabilized by internal or external fixation. Current best practice is to operate within 6hr from the time of injury to prevent infection.
- Open fractures are usually high-energy factures and cause a large amount of associated soft tissue damage.

Ask about
- Immunosuppression risk factors.

Look for
- Pain, deformity, a wound over the fracture site.
- Any puncture wound, no matter how small.
- Clearly document the neurovascular status of the limb. Individually name pulses and nerve function.

Management
- ATLS—forget the bone sticking out of the leg and treat the tension pneumothorax.
- Analgesia.
- Assess the degree of open injury (see classification in Table 3.1) and neurovascular status.

In emergency department

Soft tissue
- Photograph/Betadine® dressing.
- Tetanus.
- Intravenous antibiotics (local protocol).
- Get ready for theatre TONIGHT.

Bone
- Gentle correction of deformity if very marked.
- Splint in POP backslab.

Table 3.1 Gustillo classification of open fractures

Type 1	Open fracture where the wound is <1cm long and appears clean
Type 2	Open fractures where the wound is >1cm long
Type 3A	Open fracture with adequate soft tissue coverage of bone despite extensive soft tissue damage, flap laceration. This should include any high-energy injury independent of soft tissue damage
Type 3B	Open fracture with soft tissue loss, periosteal stripping and exposure of bone
Type 3C	Open fracture with a vascular injury requiring repair

Low-energy fractures are usually type 1 or 2 (e.g. sports injuries). High-energy open fractures (e.g. from road traffic accidents) are type 3.

In theatre

Soft tissue

- Debride, i.e. remove foreign bodies/dead tissue.
- Thorough irrigation with a minimum of 6L saline.

Bone

- Stabilize bone by appropriate means, e.g. ORIF/Ex-Fix.

If you have any suspicion that a fracture may be open, you should discuss it with the registrar on call.

Pelvic fractures

These are orthopaedic emergencies and are often as a result of high-energy injuries and severe trauma. Patients can lose a large amount of blood very quickly, mostly from the pelvic veins. Pelvic fractures should be managed through the ATLS® protocols with other members of a trauma team. Open pelvic fractures have a 50% mortality rate.

Think about
- How did the injury happen? Mechanism of injury?
- Was it a lateral impact injury, e.g. side on road traffic accident (RTA)?
- Did the patient fall astride something?
- Is there any evidence of an intra-abdominal problem? Bone fragments from fractures of the pelvis can perforate intra-abdominal viscera.

Look for
- Blood PR.
- Blood at the urethral meatus.
- Feel for high-riding prostate—suggestive of urethral damage.

The urogenital diaphragm is attached to the pubic rami, and fractures of the pelvis may damage the membranous urethra that pierces it, or the bladder that lies behind it; ∴ look for blood at the urethral meatus. Digital rectal examination (DRE) is essential. The patient may have a high-riding prostate suggestive of urethral damage, or blood on DRE caused by a bowel perforation.

Caution is needed when catheterizing someone with a possible pelvic fracture and urethral damage. Discuss with the urologists on call if there is any suspicion, as a suprapubic catheter may be preferred.

Management
- Follow the ATLS® protocol .
- When examining for circulatory problems the pelvis should be felt ONCE by the most experienced orthopaedic person at the trauma call.
- Basic management is to resuscitate the patient.
- A pelvic sling or sheet can be used to stabilize the pelvis if the patient is hypotensive because of bleeding from an unstable pelvis. This is slid under the pelvis and then tied or closed anteriorly.
- An external fixator may be used to stabilize the pelvis if the patient is hypotensive because of bleeding from an unstable pelvis. This attempts to tamponade the pelvis.
- The only invasive operative option is to pack the pelvis. Veins are exceedingly difficult to repair.

Once the patient is haemodynamically stable, they will often require a CT scan to assess the injury fully. Patients needing fracture fixation are usually sent to specialist centres for surgery.

Hip fractures

If young patient

A fracture of the proximal neck of femur is the most common cause for an acute orthopaedic admission in patients over the age of 70yr. Some 60 000 hip fractures occur each year in the UK. The mean age of patients is 80yr. Incidence increases exponentially above the age of 65yr. The main risk factors are ♀ sex and osteoporosis.

Think about

- Knee pain can often be referred from a fractured neck of femur.
- Why did this patient fall?
- Was it mechanical or is there another cause?
- Was it witnessed?
- Any history of chest pain?
- Any history of blackout or collapse?
- Does the patient have any history of a UTI?
- What is the patient's social situation at home?
- Whom do they live with?
- How do they normally mobilize? Stick, frame?
- What is their abbreviated MTS?

Ask about

- Other medical conditions.

Many people have been caught out taking X-rays of a patient's knee and missing a fractured neck of femur. There may be foreshortening of the leg and it may be held in external rotation. Be suspicious of any elderly patient with a sudden inability to weight-bear. Do a thorough examination, as the patient may have other injuries sustained during the fall.

If the patient lives in a nursing home, obtain as much information from family and nursing home staff as possible.

Management

- Admit/ATLS.
- X-rays—AP pelvis and lateral hip.
- Bloods–FBC, U&Es, liver function tests, coagulation screen, cross-match 2 units.
- Consider a medical review early if concurrent medical problems.
- TEDS and thromboprophylaxis.
- IV access and IV fluids.
- Electrocardiography (ECG).
- Chest X-ray (if indicated).
- Urine dipstick to check for evidence of UTI.
- Catheter if required.
- Mark hip with permanent marker (with date and initials).
- Drug chart—analgesia oral and IV/IM (as will be nil by mouth).

Differential diagnosis

Be suspicious if there is a fracture with a very minimal history of trauma.

- Is there a pathological lesion?
- Is there a pubic ramus fracture?

General points

Fractured neck of femur can be separated into intracapsular and extra-capsular fractures. Intracapsular fractures reduce the blood supply to the femoral head, which is then at high risk of delayed union, non-union or avascular necrosis. If there is no displacement of the femoral head (Garden 1 or 2), the head can be held in place with cannulated screws. If there is displacement of the femoral head on the proximal femur, the patient will normally undergo a hemi-arthroplasty.

Extracapsular fractures do not interfere with the femoral head blood supply. Patients undergo fixation with a dynamic hip screw.

Garden classification for intracapsular fractures of the neck of femur

- Grade 1—incomplete or impacted fracture.
- Grade 2—complete fracture with no displacement.
- Grade 3—complete fracture with partial displacement.
- Grade 4—complete fracture with full displacement.

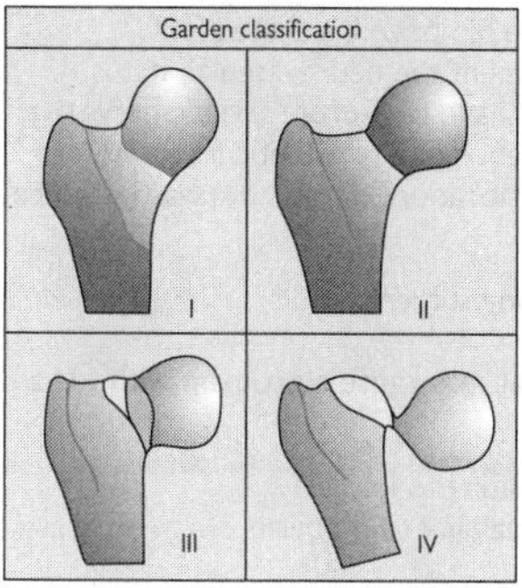

Fig. 3.6 The Garden classification.

Prognosis

- 40% of patients with a hip fracture die within a year.
- 50% of survivors are less independent than before the injury.
- Most morbidity is related to coexisting medical conditions.

Special cases

Is there a fracture? In some elderly patients, the pain may be due to bruising, a pubic ramus fracture or osteoarthritis. Other patients can actually walk on a fracture if it is undisplaced and impacted. If in doubt, the patient should have an MRI scan to determine whether a fracture is present. Some hospitals admit under the care of the elderly team.

In a young patient, some believe that the operation to fix the fracture should take place within 6hr of injury. Although the evidence is controversial, you should treat these patients differently and always inform your registrar.

☠ Dislocated total hip replacement

This is a complication of total hip replacement (THR) seen in 1–4% of 1° total hip replacements and in up to 16% in revisions.

Patients may give a history of overexertion and a sensation of the hip popping out. Usually occurs in the early postoperative period. Patients must avoid hip flexion greater than 90° (shoes and socks must be put on with adaptive equipment) and any hip adduction (no crossing of legs). Dislocation is occasionally seen in patients with excessive alcohol intake. More common in patients who have THR for neurological or developmental dysplasia of the hip.

- Posterior dislocation—caused by flexion, adduction, internal rotation.
- Anterior dislocation—caused by extension, adduction, external rotation.

Anatomy

The sciatic nerve supplies all motor functions of the lower leg except adduction and flexion of the thigh and extension of the knee. It supplies sensation to the lower leg and foot. Sciatic nerve lesions cause foot-drop.

Think about

- How long has the hip been dislocated for?
- Check and document the neurovascular status.
- Does the patient have foot-drop? (sciatic nerve).
- Is there any evidence of a prosthetic fracture?
- Is this the first dislocation? If not, how was it reduced?

Ask about

- Problems following surgery.
- Past revisions.
- Co-morbidity that may cause a problem with the anaesthetic.

Look for

- Pain in groin radiating to knee.
- Deformity, and inability to mobilize.

Management

- ABC.
- IV access.
- Bloods for general anaesthetic.
- Analgesia—IM opioid analgesia as appropriate.
- X-rays of the hip (AP and lateral).
- Nil by mouth.
- Consent for closed ± open reduction.
- Book for MUA in theatre/discuss with anaesthetist regarding the patient's fitness for a general anaesthetic or regional block.
- Relocation is an emergency if neurovascular compromise. Otherwise OK to wait until the next day.

Differential diagnosis

Peri-prosthetic fracture of the femur. Severe injury requiring a revision.

General points

The patient may need a revision procedure if having recurrent problems with dislocation.

Spinal fractures and injuries

'Spinal injury should be suspected in any major trauma.'

Background

The major concern in any spinal injury is not with the bony structures of the spinal column but with the closely related neurological elements. If there is no neurological complication at the time of injury then risk of later neurological complications must be assessed. If there are any possibilities of damage to the spinal cord then *all precautions must be taken at all stages to avoid this.*

Anatomy

There are 7 cervical vertebrae, 12 thoracic, 5 lumbar and 5 fused sacral vertebra. The spinal cord is shorter than the spinal canal. The cord ends at the interspace between the L1 and L2 vertebrae. Below the termination of the cord, the nerve roots form the cauda equina. Within the cervical spine, segmental levels of cord correspond to bony landmarks. Below this level there is increasing disparity between levels. Spinal pathology below L1 presents with root signs only.

Aetiology

Fractures at different levels of the spine are caused by different mechanisms of injury. It is important to determine what structures have been damaged and the stability of the spine. Spinal stability is formed by the complex interaction of spinal ligaments.

The spine may be considered to have three columns: anterior, middle and posterior. Unstable injuries occur when damage to the middle column is combined with damage to either the anterior or the posterior column. Damage to more than one column is considered to be unstable, as described below.

Patterns of spinal fracture

Spinal injuries are subdivided into minor and major. Minor injuries are represented by fractures of transverse processes, facets, pars interarticularis and spinous process. Major spinal injuries are classified into four different categories: compression fractures, burst fractures, seatbelt-type injuries and fracture dislocations.

Compression or wedge

Simple compression fractures are common and often only the anterior column. They are caused by hyperflexion of the spine around an axis. There is a loss of height of the anterior portion of the vertebra. The posterior portion of the column is maintained. Wedging >15–20° indicates damage to more than one column,

Burst
Axial loading of the spine may cause failure of the anterior and middle column; one or both of the vertebral body endplates may be involved and bone fragments may extrude into the spinal canal causing cord damage.

Seatbelt-type injuries (flexion distraction injuries of the spine)
Rapid deceleration of the neck and spine as caused by a seatbelt in an RTA can cause failure of the posterior and middle columns. These fractures can occur through the bone, through ligaments, or a combination of both patterns.

Fracture dislocations
This is a failure of all three columns. There is loss of the normal constraints of the column so that dislocation and subluxation may occur. This may be suspected if there are multiple rib or transverse process fractures.

Think about
- All but the simple single-column fractures should be discussed with the orthopaedic registrar on call.

Ask about
- Mechanism of the accident.
- Alterations in sensation.
- Sudden or gradual loss of function.
- Bowel and bladder function.

In managing a patient with spinal injuries it is important to determine what structures have been involved. Do a full neurological examination, DRE (see Chapter 6, 📖 p212). Also consider CT and MRI scans.

Management
Lie the patient flat and keep immobilized. Use a hard collar, sandbags and tape for cervical spine injuries. Discuss with senior.

General points
Spinal patients, when being nursed, are susceptible to a number of medical problems, acutely and during their usually prolonged admission. Things to think about are:
- Deep vein thrombosis.
- Chest infections.
- Pressure sores.
- Depression.
- Maintain IV fluids as at risk of 'spinal shock', which is seen in patients who have a loss of autonomic control and are ∴ unable to maintain normal vascular tone.
- Gastrointestinal prophylaxis, as at risk of stress ulcers.
- Urological review.

Septic arthritis

'Can you have a look at this hot, red, swollen, painful joint?'

The acute infected joint is an orthopaedic emergency. When patients have a red, hot, swollen painful joint, with no history of trauma, you should consider it to be infected until proven otherwise.

It may be a result of haematological seeding from a concurrent illness or a puncture wound causing infection in the joint. Septic arthritis usually affects only one joint.

Think about

- Has the patient had any recent foreign travel?
- Are there any suspicions of IV drug abuse, as this can often lead to abnormal presentation of septic arthritis?
- Tuberculosis.
- Foreign travel.
- Reiter's syndrome.
- Ask for any history of gout,
- Is the patient at risk of sexually transmitted infections?

Ask about

- Other joints that may be involved.
- Any of the risk factors mentioned above.

Look for

- A hot, red, swollen, painful joint—the joint is held in the most comfortable position and the patient will not let you near the joint, let alone move it.
- Is the patient unwell? Systemic signs of sepsis: fever, tachycardia, shock, rigors.

Investigations

- X-ray—AP and lateral of the affected joint.
- Bloods—FBC looking for ↑ WCC, CRP, ESR, blood cultures.
- *Joint aspiration* sent for urgent microbiology is the most important investigation. Send the sample for Gram stain, crystal examination and cell count.
- Analgesia.
- Nil by mouth.
- Mark the line of any cellulitis, and date and time.
- Start IV antibiotics when all the joint aspiration samples and bloods have been taken.
- Check the local hospital protocol for recommended antibiotics.

Differential diagnosis

- Is there a pathological fracture?
- Gout.
- Pseudo-gout.
- Perthes' disease.
- Rheumatic fever.
- Gonococcal arthritis.
- Viral arthritis.

General points

Discuss with the orthopaedic registrar on call as the patient may need to go to theatre for a *joint washout*. Sepsis within a joint can destroy the cartilage within 24hr. Organisms responsible include:

- *Staphylococcus aureus.*
- *Streptococcus pyogenes.*
- *Haemophilus influenzae.*
- Gram-negative organisms.
- Salmonella—often seen in patients with sickle cell anaemia.

Important summary points

- Red, hot, swollen joint = septic arthritis until proved otherwise.
- Joint must be aspirated and fluid sent for urgent Gram stain. If this shows organisms, the patient must go to theatre for an urgent joint washout.

Ankle injuries

There is a great variation in the severity of ankle fractures. Ankle injuries are a common problem and account for a high number of emergency department attendances. Most of these are ankle sprains or minor fractures, but some are more severe. A fracture dislocation of the ankle is an orthopaedic emergency and needs urgent reduction before the patient is sent for an X-ray.

Anatomy

The interaction of the fibula, tibia and talus make up the ankle. The bony landmarks of the ankle are the medial and lateral malleoli. The talus acts as the central portion, which is supported by the two malleoli. The lateral malleolus is firmly attached to the talus by strong talofibular ligaments. On the medial side, the strong deltoid ligament attaches the medial malleolus to the talus. The syndesmosis is the attachment of the distal fibula to the tibia.

The mechanism of ankle injury is usually inversion or eversion. Inversion is when the foot is forced inwards (medial) and the lateral aspect of the foot is against the floor. Eversion is when foot is turned outwards (laterally).

Think about

For obvious fracture dislocation, the ankle should be reduced before an X-ray is taken; this prevents tension on the overlying skin. Assess vascular supply (capillary refill time). If the foot points the wrong way, then put it back straight and into a plaster *before* X-ray.

If you are the first person to assess the patient, use the Ottawa ankle rules to decide whether an X-ray is indicated. These are:

Ottawa ankle rules

- Bone tenderness at posterior edge of distal 6cm, or tip of medial or lateral malleolus.
- Unable both to weight-bear immediately after injury and to walk four steps in A&E department.

Ask about

- Mechanism of injury.

Look for

- Pain and swelling of the ankle.
- Point tenderness over medial or lateral maleoli.
- Neurovascular status.

When to admit and operate

The ankle is a very precise joint. As a rule of thumb, any patient whose X-ray looks as if the bones have moved probably needs an operation and should ∴ be discussed for admission.

Differential diagnosis

- Ankle sprains—these are treated with RICE advice (Rest, Ice and Elevation; C was for compression but is now considered unlikely to be of benefit). Patients able to mobilize within the limits of pain should wear supportive shoes/boots and refrain from extreme exercise and uneven ground for 4–6 weeks.
- Weight-bearing—if there is a fracture the patient should be kept non-weight-bearing (NWB) until they have been seen in the fracture clinic. Anyone who has an operation is likely to be advised not to weight-bear on that side for 6 weeks.

Weber classification of ankle fractures

This refers to the fibula fracture only:

- Weber A—fracture below the level of the syndesmosis. Treat in plaster.
- Weber B—fracture at the level of the syndesmosis. Operate if unstable.
- Weber C—fracture above the level of the syndesmosis. Needs an operation.

Pathological fractures

'Fractures where there has been no history of trauma.'

Think about

- Metabolic bone disease.
- Paget's disease.
- Neoplasia/metastases.
- Osteoporosis.

Ask about

Tumours that most commonly metastasize to bone are:

- Breast.
- Renal.
- Thyroid.
- Prostate.
- Lung.
- Colon (to a lesser degree).

Look for

- Any physical signs of malignancy.
- Signs of hypercalcaemia.
- Back pain caused by vertebral crush fractures.

Investigations

- Full history and physical examination.
- X-rays of the area involved.
- Chest radiography.
- Bloods—FBC, U&Es, bone profile, Ca^{2+}, phosphate , G&S, serum electrophoresis, ESR, coag., CRP.
- Urine—send urine for Bence Jones protein 24hr collection.
- Serum immunoglobulins.
- ECG.

Take an X-ray of the WHOLE bone and not just the fracture—there may be lesions all along the bone.

Other accident & emergency department problems

Peri-prosthetic fractures

This is a fracture that occurs around an implant, usually a joint replacement. These patients usually need admission and workup for surgery.

Patients who can feel their metalwork

Some patients attend A&E following recent surgery, saying that they can feel the screws and plate under the skin. It is not unusual to be able to feel the metalwork, especially if it is in an area with little soft tissue cover.

- Have things changed? Get a new X-ray and compare with the last one. Look at the bone, soft tissue, spaces between the implant and bone. Are their new spaces or larger spaces?
- Is there any pain associated with the screw or plate?
- What does the overlying skin look like?
- Are there any signs of pain, infection or skin compromise. If so, the patient need admission and review by senior.
- If you are happy that this is not an acute problem needing admission, arrange a fracture clinic appointment within the next few days.
- If in doubt, discuss with registrar.

Irreducible dislocation

If the joint cannot be reduced in the emergency department, to have the best chance of a successful reduction:

- Review the radiographs and dislocation.
- Re-assess the neurovascular status.
- Check that the patient has enough analgesia.
- Check that the patient is relaxed.
- Always get a post-reduction film.

If you still can't reduce the joint, the patient should be admitted and the joint reduced under general anaesthetic, with image intensifier assistance. Consent for open reduction.

On-call decision making

You have decided that the patient needs surgery. When? Read the following as a set of guidelines to be taken into consideration with the injury and characteristics of each individual patient.

If the patient needs an operation, find out when they last ate or drank. If there is space in theatre then they may be able to have the operation immediately and will not have to wait until the next day.

Emergency: will go to theatre that night

- Open fractures.
- Vascular injury.
- Bony or joint deformity with pins and needles/neurodeficit.
- Compartment syndrome.
- Septic arthritis.
- Traumatic hip dislocation (patient's own hip, not THR).

May not go to theatre that night: likely to, and treat as if they will

- Cauda equina syndrome.
- Joint dislocations.
- Paediatric supracondylar fractures.
- Polytrauma (i.e. multiple fractures—needs careful anaesthetic review).
- Young patient with fractured neck of femur.

Admit for surgery and prepare for the next day

- Femoral/tibial fractures.
- Ankle fractures (elevate—can't operate until the swelling goes down).
- Forearm and distal radius fractures.

Knee injuries

You may be called to see a patient with a swollen knee and normal X-ray post-injury. Consider cruciate, collateral and meniscal injuries. These patients can be seen in the fracture clinic. Local guidelines vary for the 'locked knee', in which the knee cannot fully extend but can flex. Some will receive an arthroscopy the next day, but others will order an MRI scan via the fracture clinic.

Back pain

Don't miss ***cauda equina syndrome***—a disc that presses on the S2, S3 and S4 nerve roots, which supply the bowel and bladder. The patient will complain of *back pain associated with bowel and bladder symptoms* (which may include incontinence). They may have 'saddle' anaesthesia in the perianal region, and have a reduced anal tone on PR. Missing this will produce permanent incontinence.

- Decompression is an emergency. Let your registrar decide whether to get an MRI scan that night or the next morning.
- Look for history of infection and tumour—unwell, fevers, bad night pain, X-ray changes, intravenous drug use.
- Most patients with back pain in the absence of the above are discharged on analgesia (codeine, NSAIDs and diazepam). Occasionally you will have to admit people who are immobile or in severe pain.

Paediatric fractures

Fractures in children are different to those in adults in many ways. The unique anatomy of children's bones leads to fracture patterns not seen in adulthood. The first difference between paediatric and adult bones is the presence of epiphyseal growth plates. Children's bones are surrounded by thick periosteum, which provides extra support. The arrangement of the protein making up a child's bone allows the bone to be more plastic, so that it can bend before it breaks. This also allows for the different types of fracture seen in children and not adults. Even in dramatic paediatric fractures, a MUA and plaster may be all that is required.

Think about

- Is the fracture through the growth plate? If so, what is its Salter–Harris classification?
- Is there any evidence of non-accidental injury (NAI)—does the story fit?
- If no history of trauma, is there any evidence for a septic joint?
- Applying EMLA® cream, as the child will need venous access.

Ask about

- Mechanism of injury.
- Past injury and fractures.

Look for

- Check the neurovascular status of the limb.
- Check for any other injuries.

Investigations

- X-rays of the limb, AP and lateral.

Table 3.2 Salter Harris Classification of fractures through the epiphyseal growth plate in the immature skeleton

I	Fracture through physis
II	Fracture up into metaphysic (Most common)
III	Fracture down joint
IV	Combination of II + III
V	Compression of epiphyseal plate. Not seen on X-ray. Uncommon. Suspect if persistent pain/compression mechanism and negative film. These fractures are difficult diagnose and can result in limb shortening

Management

It is very unlikely for children to make up injuries, so be suspicious in all children who have stopped using a limb. It may be difficult to get an exact mechanism of injury from children.

Always be on the lookout for suspicious fractures in children and NAI.

The limping child and painful hips

Children very rarely make up symptoms. If a child is not walking for some reason, be suspicious that there is a pathological process going on.

Children who are limping are often referred from A&E. They have no real history of trauma, they have no obvious fracture on their radiographs, and unfortunately they often are unable (because of their age) to tell us where the pain is or why they are unable to walk.

Think about

- Septic arthritis until proved otherwise.

Ask about

- Any problems with their footwear—stone in shoe?
- Any history of trauma.
- For how long have they not been walking properly?
- Have they been unwell? Viral illness? Systemic illness?
- Any family history of joint problems—developmental dysplasia of the hip (DDH), slipped upper femoral epiphysis (SUFE)?
- During the examination try to localize the specific area/joint involved.

Management

- Full history including other illness in the family, history of any other orthopaedic problem, any systemic upset, fevers, rigors and foreign travel.
- AP and lateral X-rays of the limb (frog lateral X-ray of the hip).
- Bloods—FBC, ESR and CRP; WBC or inflammatory markers will be raised in septic arthritis.
- Blood cultures.
- Discuss with registrar on call.
- Ultrasound scan (USS)—put local anaesthetic cream over the hip (anteriorly) so that, if there is an effusion present, the radiologist may be able to aspirate it. This is not available in some hospitals.

Differential diagnosis

- Perthes' disease.
- SUFE.
- Juvenile-onset arthritis.
- Septic arthritis.
- Osteomyelitis.
- Rheumatic fever.
- Unseen fracture.

Table 3.3 Common childhood hip problems and ages at which they occur.

Birth	Congenital dislocation
0–5yr	Perthes' disease (osteochondrosis) DDH (late presentation)
5–10yr	Perthes' disease Irritable hip
10–15yr	Irritable hip SUFE Juvenile-onset rheumatoid arthritis
Any age	Septic arthritis Transient synovitis

Infection can occur at any time and at any age!

☠ Non-accidental injury

Those working in orthopaedics and radiology need always to have the possibility of NAI in the back of their mind. Be suspicious if the story does not fit the injury or if the story changes.

If you have any concerns, discuss the case with a senior colleague and the paediatric registrar on call.

Compartment syndrome

An ↑ pressure within a musculofascial compartment. This ↑ pressure causes ↓ perfusion of the muscle. This usually occurs within the limbs, but can be within any body compartment, and is seen most commonly within the first 48hr of an injury.

Possible causes

- Trauma:
  - Tibial fractures (especially comminuted fractures).
  - Long bone fractures.
  - Forearm fractures.
- Soft-tissue injury or crush injury.
- Vascular injuries:
  - Ischaemia–reperfusion injury.
  - Patients with haemorrhage on anticoagulation.
- Intravenous or intra-arterial drug injection.
- Dressings applied too tightly (POP).
- Prolonged limb compression.
- Burns.
- Iatrogenic (poor positioning during general anaesthesia or on ITU).

Think about

The forearm has two compartments, the thigh has three and the lower limb four.

Ask about

- Mechanism of trauma or insult.
- For how long these signs and symptoms have been progressing.
- Drug chart and analgesia required.

Look for

- Pain that is greater than would be expected for the type and severity of injury.
- Pain that is not relieved with opioid analgesia.
- Pain on passive movement of muscles from within the compartment.
- Tense and swollen compartments.
- Pulses *are* present in developing compartment syndrome.
- If the patient has an absent pulse they are in the late stages of compartment syndrome.

If you think a patient may have a compartment syndrome, they need URGENT senior review.

Investigations

It is possible to measure the pressure in a compartment with a monitor, or using arterial line apparatus from ITU or recovery. Your seniors should make the decision to do so.

Management

- Split plaster to SKIN/remove constricting dressings.
- Elevate limb.
- If patient is unconscious (ITU), intercompartmental pressure monitoring may be considered.
- Nil by mouth.
- Call registrar **NOW**—if you leave the patient, it may be too late and they will lose the limb.

Deep vein thrombosis

DVT occurs where there is a thrombus in a deep vein, usually of the lower limb.

Look for

A DVT is often first noticed as an insidious, progressive, annoying, 'pulling' sensation at the insertion of the lower calf muscle into the posterior portion of the lower leg. This feeling can than become more pronounced and accompanied by warmth, swelling and erythema. Tenderness may be present along the course of the involved veins. 'Homans' sign', an ↑ resistance or pain during dorsiflexion of the foot, is unreliable and non-specific. Signs may be very soft.

Differential diagnosis

- Cellulitis.
- Ruptured Baker's cyst.
- Muscle rupture.

Management

- Take a full history and examination of the leg swelling. Review the patient's drug chart to ensure they are written up for the correct thromboprophylaxis (as per your hospital protocol).
- Review observation chart.
- Organize a venous duplex or USS—have a low threshold for these.
- Take blood for FBC, coag. If there is a possibility of cellulites take blood cultures.
- D-dimer—if negative and low, clinical suspicion for DVT; then you do not need to do a Doppler USS.

General points

Ensure that all patients are written up for prophylactic heparin and TED stockings on admission or at the pre-assessment clinic (as per protocol in your hospital). Consider this if you have a high clinical suspicion.

Table 3.4 Risk factors for DVT

Congenital factors	Acquired risk factors
Mutation in Factor V gene	Age >60yr
Mutation in Protein C gene	Extensive surgery
Protein S deficiency	Marked immobility, long flight
Antithrombin III deficiency	Pre or postoperative
Antiphospholipid antibodies	Major orthopaedic surgery
Raised concentration of Factor VIII	Fracture of pelvis, femur or tibia
	Malignancy
	Hypercoagulable state
	Obesity
	Pregnancy
	Oestrogen use, oral contraceptive pill
	Postoperative sepsis
	Heart failure
	Inflammatory bowel disease
	Sepsis

Fat embolism syndrome

'This patient is not quite right 2 hours post tibial nailing.'

Fat droplets form following a fracture or manipulation of long bone marrow and enter the venous circulation. Chylomicrons may also aggregate due to lipase release. Fat embolism syndrome is has a broad spectrum of severity. The mortality rate in severe cases can be as high as 15%. Fat embolism syndrome is a relatively rare diagnosis, but should be considered in all patients, irrespective of age, following long bone surgery. Involve the intensive care team early.

Think about

- Patients who have had a long bone fracture and had an intermedullary procedure.
- Usually occurs 24–48hr after the initial insult.

Look for

- This is often a diagnosis of exclusion and may have an indolent clinical course.
- It may present with pyrexia, tachycardia, tachypnoea, reduced consciousness.
- A petechial rash is sometimes seen.
- Clotting may be deranged with features of disseminated intravascular coagulopathy (DIC).
- Severe cases may develop respiratory distress and acute respiratory distress syndrome (ARDS).

Think about

- Is this a pulmonary embolism (PE)? Sepsis or haemorrhage?

Differential diagnosis

- PE.
- Chest infection.

Management

- Treatment is supportive.
- Check bloods, FBC, U&Es, clotting profile.
- Arterial blood gases.
- Supportive treatments include oxygen, IV fluids and close monitoring of haemodynamic status and urine output.
- Ensure the patient has IV fluids up and running.
- Catheterize the patient.
- Close monitoring of fluid balance; consider transfer to HDU.
- In severe cases involve ITU early. Transfer to ITU may be needed for supportive treatment and ventilation.

Wound infections

'You are called to see someone who had an ankle "ORIF" 5 days ago. The wound is red and inflamed.'

Wound infections in orthopaedics are different to those in other surgical specialties. If the surface skin wound is in close proximity to metalwork following an ORIF then there is the potential for a deep-seated infection to occur.

Think about

- What operation has the person had?
- When did they have the operation?
- What metalwork do they have in?
- Have they had any wound swabs taken (check the computer) previously?

Ask about

- Fevers, sweats.
- Other sites of infection (e.g. UTI, upper respiratory tract infection).

Management

- Mark the area of cellulitis with a waterproof pen.
- Discuss with senior orthopaedic surgeon and microbiologists.
- **Do not** start antibiotics until senior discussion.
- To treat this wound infection appropriately, microbiology and antibiotic sensitivities are required. This may require a washout of the wound and the taking of some superficial and deep samples.
- By starting antibiotics inappropriately the superficial wound infection may clear, but the deep infection may persist.
- If there are signs of systemic illness, antibiotics should be started after blood and wound cultures.

Plaster problems

Plasters are used to stabilize fractures, thereby reducing pain and promoting healing. The aim is to immobilize the fracture and the joint local to the fracture. The plaster can also be used to maintain position of the fracture.

- Plaster of Paris (POP) is the most commonly used plaster.
- Back slab—this is where the limb is has plaster on only one side and is then wrapped in a bandage. It is a temporary dressing and allows degree of swelling to occur. It should not be used as a definitive long-term dressing.
- Resin casts are lighter and more durable than POP. They are more difficult to apply. Always use gloves when applying.
- The plaster is not applied directly to the skin. A soft (Velband) layer is used as the first layer to reduce the risk of pressure points occurring. Pressure points are most likely to occur over bony presences such as the medial or lateral malleoli in the leg, or ulna or radial styloid processes in the forearm.
- Painful plasters—if a plaster is painful you must assess the neurovascular status of the limb.

Think about

- The neurovascular status of the limb. Individually identify and record the motor and sensory function of the peripheral nerves.
- Is the patient complaining of ↑ pain or paraesthesia?
- What is the capillary refill (normal <2sec).
- Is the plaster too tight or too loose? Review the patient drug chart for ↑ analgesia requirements.

Management

- Elevate the limb.
- Use a plaster cutter to split the plaster.
- Cut the soft layers of the plaster dressing all the way to the skin, as it may be these that are causing the problem.

If the plaster is too loose and clearly movable over the limb, it may need to be removed and redone. If you are unhappy with your plastering skills, ask the nurses from A&E or the orthopaedic wards for help, or, if during the day, send the patient to the plaster room.

Summary of complications of fractures

Table 3.5 Complications can be subdivided into those that occur early or late

	Early	Late
Local	Muscle and tendon injuries	Avascular necrosis
	Nerve injuries	Malunion
	Vascular injuries	Delayed or non-union
	Visceral injuries	Myositis ossificans
	Compartment syndrome	Stiffness and instability
		Volkmann's ischaemic contracture (unable to work/do sport)
General	Haemorrhage/shock	Pain
	Fat embolism/ARDS	Dysfunction
	DVT/PE	

Abbreviated Mental Test Score

1. Age	☐
2. Time to nearest hour	☐
3. An address—for example 42 West Street—to be repeated by patient at end of test	☐
4. Year	☐
5. Name of hospital, residential institution or home address, depending on where patient is situated	☐
6. Recognition of two persons—for example doctor, nurse, home help	☐
7. Date of birth	☐
8. Year First World War started	☐
9. Name of present monarch	☐
10. Count backwards from 20 to 1	☐
Total score	
A score <6 suggests dementia.	

Table 3.6 Mini mental test score.

Chapter 4
Vascular surgery

Stephen Black

Introduction

For most doctors who have not spent time in a vascular unit, the thought of dealing with vascular problems or emergencies is daunting. Most vascular problems are easily dealt with by simple and logical assessment of the patient.

Location of leg and foot pulses

Femoral

Located in the line of the mid-inguinal point (midway between the symphisis pubis and anterior superior iliac crest). In difficult cases (i.e. obese or muscular patients), externally rotate the hips; the pulse should be palpable ~2 finger-breadths lateral to the pubic tubercle.

Popliteal

This is difficult to feel. If it is easy, consider popliteal aneurysm. Hold the patient's partially flexed knee, hook the tendons across the joint with fingers of one hand, and palpate the middle of the popliteal space with the fingers of the other. If the pulse cannot be palpated in this manner, hyperextending the straight leg with the fingertips of the examining hand in the midline of the popliteal fossa may be successful; alternatively palpate the popliteal fossa with the patient prone.

Dorsalis pedis

This is palpable on the dorsum of the foot between the first and second metatarsal bones.

Posterior tibial

Most easily palpable in the hollow behind the medial maleolus but may be palpable ~ one-third of the way along a line from the medial maleolus to the point of the heel.

Describing pulses over the phone

It is most easily understood if pulses are described as being ipsilateral (i.e. the affected side) and contralateral (the unaffected side) e.g.: in a patient with an ischaemic foot: on the ipsilateral side they have a palpable femoral but absent popliteal and distal pulses; on the contralateral side all pulses are present.

Risk factors for vascular disease

This should be asked about and included in the presentation of any patient presenting with possible vascular disease. The single most important factor is smoking. In addition all patients should be asked about diabetes, hypertension, hypercholesterolaemia and family history of vascular disease (including myocardial infarction; MI). Past medical history includes a history of MI or stroke and any clotting disorders, e.g. Factor V Lieden deficiency.

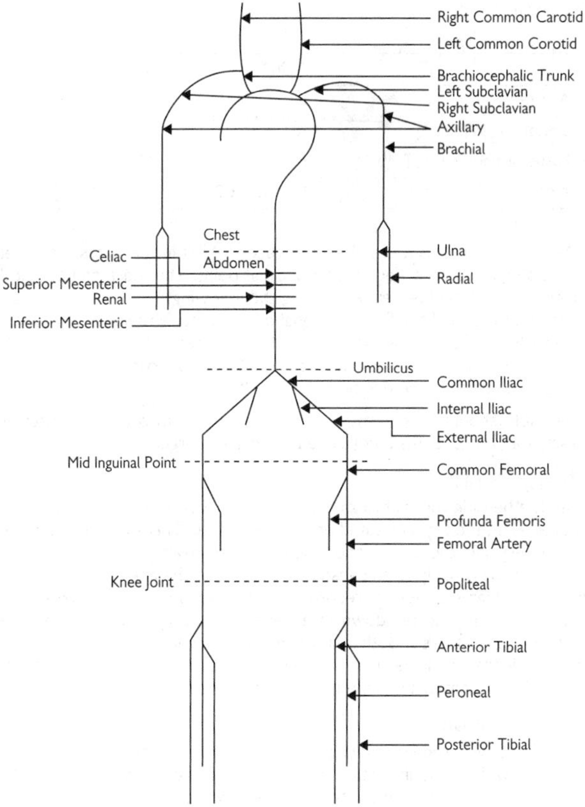

Fig. 4.1 Vascular anatomy of major arteries.

Ankle Brachial Pressure Index (ABPI)

This is a measure of the pressure of the blood supply in the ankle compared with the arm, which in a normal patient should be ~ equal (i.e. 1 or >0.8); <0.8 implies disease and <0.5 severe disease. The ABPI is not used as part of the definition of critical leg ischaemia. It is calculated by using a hand-held Doppler probe to record the systolic pressure at the brachial, and the highest reading from the posterior tibial and dorsalis pedis in both feet in turn.

For example:

	Right	Left
Arm (mmHg)	140	
Dorsalis pedis (mmHg)	100	90
Posterior tibial (mmHg)	80	105
ABPI	100/140 = 0.7	105/140 = 0.8

The above format is a useful way to record ABPI in the notes. The final value should be recorded to one decimal point. There are some typical findings that should be recorded using the following:

- Incompressible if the Doppler signal does not go. This applies to heavily calcified arteries and is typical of diabetes.
- 'No signal'; if the pulse is absent completely, as opposed to 0 if the signal disappears immediately.

The ABPI should be determined in any patient with presumed vascular disease and on patients before and after bypass surgery.

Buerger's test

This is a bedside clinical test of arterial insufficiency. It is performed in two stages. First, the leg is elevated until it goes white. This angle between the raised leg and the examination table is known as *Buerger's angle* and corresponds roughly to the absolute pressure at the ankle; however, it is not particularly useful to record this. The second stage involves the patient hanging the leg down in a dependant position and observing a colour change to red. Both changes need to occur for Buerger's test to be considered positive. It is a useful test to suggest whether arterial disease is present in a patient in whom the clinical picture is not clear.

Heparin infusion

In patients who require anticoagulation, heparin may be started simultaneously with warfarin until the international normalized ratio (INR) reaches a therapeutic range (typically 2–3), or alone in patients in whom anticoagulation may need to be reversed rapidly (i.e. before surgery).

Typically, unfractionated heparin is given via an infusion pump and the dose adjusted up or down until anticoagulation is optimized. A loading dose of 5000units followed by an infusion of 24 000units in 24hr adjusted to achieve an aPTR of 1.5–2.5 is usually adequate. The aPTR (activated partial thromboplastin time ratio) should be checked 6hr after commencing heparin and 6hr after any adjustment. Most units/hospitals have a protocol for heparin administration that should be consulted and followed.

☠ Acute leg ischaemia

- Alert senior on call immediately.
- Intervention is required within 6hr to save the affected limb.

Think about

In a patient presenting with sudden onset of paralysis, think about vascular causes. Always check the pulses in the affected limb(s).

Ask about

Try to determine the cause. The majority are 2° to embolic occlusion or thrombosis of pre-existing disease.

- History of MI or valvular heart disease.
- Atrial myxoma.
- Arrhythmias (esp. atrial fibrillation; AF).
- Aneurysmal disease (abdomen, popliteal).
- Previous history of claudication (acute on chronic ischaemia).
- Previous bypass grafts (bypass graft occlusion).
- Recent coronary or radiological interventional procedures.

Look for

- '5 Ps'—palor, pulseless, paralysis, paraesthesia, perishing cold.
- If the last are present, situation critical.
- Viable limb—no neurology, audible Doppler at ankle.
- Critical limb—sensory loss, tense calf, no audible Doppler.
- Dead limb—fixed mottling, complete neurological deficit.
- Examine the abdomen for aneurysmal disease.
- Assess which pulses are present and whether there is aneurysmal disease.

Investigations

Investigations are aimed at finding a cause of the ischaemia and preparing the patient for reperfusion.

Finding a cause

- Echocardiogram (look for valve abnormalities, atrial myxoma, etc.).
- Electrocardiogram (look for AF and other arrhythmias).

Intervention

- FBC, clotting, G&S.
- Chest X-ray (CXR).

Management

- Resuscitate the patient.
- Adequate analgesia.
- Heparin.
- Once senior review has taken place, the patient may be managed either in theatre, with thrombolysis or conservatively.

Critical leg ischaemia

This can be managed overnight with senior review on the morning round.

Definition

Rest pain for more than 2 weeks requiring analgaesia and/or tissue loss and/or gangrene and/or absolute pressure at the ankle <50mmHg.

Think about

Ensure that this is not acute limb ischaemic. Check that the patient has not gone into cardiac failure, which may be the cause of the ischaemia.

Ask about

Usually patients develop critical leg ischaemia as a result of deterioration of their underlying vascular disease.

- Previous history of claudication.
- Previous vascular surgery (especially bypass surgery).

Look for

- Signs of cardiac insufficiency.
- Anaemia (may precipitate ischaemia).
- Pulses: supra- and infra-inguinal.
- 'Sunset limb': the patient's foot is brick red and they are hanging their legs over the edge of the bed.
- Determine the ABPI.
- Perform Buerger's test.

Investigations

- Baseline bloods: FBC, U&Es, G&S.
- ECG and cardiology review (can be done during the course of an inpatient admission or as an outpatient referral).
- CXR.
- Angiography.

Management

- Analgesia and heparin infusion.
- The aim of treatment is to improve blood supply to the affected limb.
- Treatment is directed by extent of disease and may include interventional radiological procedures or bypass surgery.
- If reconstruction is not an option it may be necessary to offer amputation.
- In some cases leg ischaemia is an end-of-life event and palliation may be most appropriate.

ⓘ Leg ulcers

Think about:

Ensure that the ulcer is not the presenting feature of an acutely or critically ischaemic limb. There are three main types of ulcer you are likely to see: venous, arterial and neuropathic (diabetic):

- *Venous*—shallow base, weepy ulcer in the gaiter area. Surrounding skin shows evidence of lipodermatosclerosis and oedema.
- *Arterial*—Punched-out deep ulcers, often located over pressure points. There are absent foot pulses and the surrounding skin is ischaemic.
- *Neuropathic*—located over pressure areas, deep, evidence of infection. Often the surrounding skin is healthy or inflamed.

Ask about

- Concomitant medical conditions, especially diabetes.
- History of leg ischaemia or previous bypass surgery.
- History of varicose veins, previous deep vein thrombosis (DVT).
- Pain.

Look for

- Foot pulses and signs of leg ischaemia.
- Varicose veins and skin changes associated with venous disease.
- Examine for peripheral neuropathy.
- Note the site, shape and depth of the ulcer.
- Note the condition of the skin surrounding the ulcer.

Investigations

- Swab the ulcer.
- Determine the ABPI.
- Duplex scan of the venous system.
- Arteriogram.

Management

- Management is directed at the cause.
- Venous ulcers: if ABPI is normal, compression and elevation are the mainstays.
- Arterial ulcers: improve blood supply.
- Neuropathic ulcers: treat infection, diabetic control, foot care.
- If there is no sign of acute leg ischaemia, outpatient clinic review at the earliest opportunity may be appropriate.

Diabetic foot

Think about:

May need debridement to gain control of infection. Check the patient's glucose and ensure adequate control (sliding scale).

Ask about

- History of neuropathy.
- Any obvious precipitating injury.
- History of claudication or arterial insufficiency.

Look for

- Painless deeply penetrating ulcers, usually located over the 4th/5th meta-tarsal heads. Infection spreads deep in the planter spaces.
- Chronic ulceration with otherwise adequate skin perfusion.
- Extensive infection originating from an ulcer.
- Necrosis of an individual digit.
- Check for forefoot oedema. This is often a subtle sign of underlying infection that is tracking deep along tendon sheaths and planter spaces.

Investigations

- Swabs of the ulcers.
- X-ray of the foot to look for osteomyelitis.
- Mark the border of the infected area with a marker pen.
- FBC, U&Es, glucose—look for signs of systemic infection.

Management

- All patients with signs of systemic sepsis, spreading infection or extensive initial infection should be admitted. Involvement of the medical team is appropriate for medical complications of diabetes.
- IV antibiotics according to local treatment protocols.
- Surgery to remove necrotic/infected material and to drain pus.
- Diabetic feet require aggressive and attentive management.

Ruptured infrarenal abdominal aortic aneurysm (IRAAA)

- Inform senior immediately you suspect this diagnosis.
- Your role is to get everything ready for theatre and the patient there as soon as possible.

Think about

Suspect an aneurysm in any older patient presenting with pain and collapse. Only 50% of patients with a rupture will have a palpable aneurysm due to a combination of low blood pressure (BP) and abdominal wall fat. Beware the diagnosis of renal colic or hip pain or back pain blamed on arthritis—always palpate for an aneurysm.

If you find an aneurysm, it is the cause of pain until proven otherwise.

Ask about

- Onset and timing of pain.
- Whether there was collapse or not.
- Co-morbid problems.
- Any previous aneurysm repair.

Look for

- Palpate the abdomen—feel for an aneurysm.
- Look for any scars of previous surgery.
- Examine the groins—look for scars, feel pulses; assess suitability for endovascular aneurysm repair (EVAR).

Investigations

- Gain venous access—large 14G needles should be sited in both arms.
- Send blood for cross-match and inform the on-call haematologist. Many centers have a massive blood transfusion protocol. This should be activated. Ask for fresh frozen plasma (FFP) and platelets in addition to 10units blood.
- Inform the anaesthetic team and theatres that you have or are expecting a patient with a ruptured aneurysm.
- Inform the ITU team to arrange for a postoperative bed.
- Traditionally computed tomography (CT) prior to theatre was not a consideration; however, if the patient is stable and the unit in which you work provides an EVAR service, then, after senior review, this may be indicated.

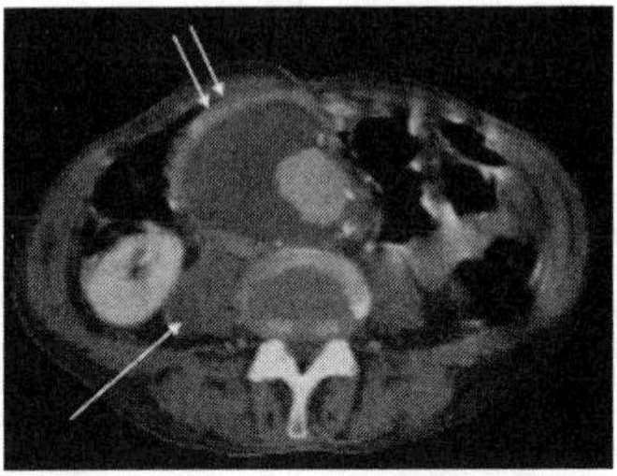

Fig. 4.2 CT scan of ruptured abdominal aortic aneurysm. Double arrow indicates aneurysm; single arrow shows retroperitoneal bleed.

Management

- *Do not resuscitate the patient aggressively.*
- Permissive hypotension—maintain systolic pressure at 100mmHg or less. Aggressive fluid can overcome natural tamponade mechanisms and lead to further deterioration.
- The standard repair is still an open repair; however, in patients who have severe co-morbidity or who are stable enough for CT, EVAR may be considered.

Table 4.1 Approximate rupture risk and rate of expansion per year for IRAAA

Aneurysm diameter (cm)	Risk of rupture (%)	Expansion rate (cm/yr)
<4	<0.5	<0.3
4–4.9	0.5–5	0.4
5–5.9	5–10	0.5
6–6.9	10–20	>0.5
7–7.9	20–40	>0.5
≥8	>40	>0.5

For any given size of IRAAA, risk of rupture is increased by ♀ sex, hypertension, chronic obstructive pulmonary disease (COPD) and current smoking.

☠ Symptomatic IRAAA

Inform senior on call and allow decision on timing of intervention.

Think about

In any middle-aged to elderly patient who has vascular risk factors, look for an aneurysm when presenting with abdominal, groin, back or hip pain. Also consider this in patients who present with sudden onset of paralysis.

Ask about

- Onset of pain, radiation site.
- Vascular risk factors.
- Previous vascular surgery.
- Cardiac history.
- Respiratory history.

Look for

- Abdominal and back pain with radiation to groin or thigh (impending rupture, expansion or intramural bleed)—no episode of hypotension/collapse.
- Distal embolization (trash foot/lower limb paralysis due to trashing of spinal cord).
- Caval obstruction.
- 1° aortoenteric fistulae (PR bleed or haemoptysis or haematemesis).
- Inflammatory—abdominal pain, malaise, weight loss, high erythrocyte sedimentation rate (ESR), periaortic fibrosis causing duodenal, left renal vein or ureteric obstruction.

Investigations

- FBC, U&Es, G&S.
- CXR.
- ECG.
- Arterial blood gas (ABG)>
- Radiological investigations pending senior review—CT first line.

Management

- As for rupture, but may be delayed to next-day list as semielective repair.
- Delay allows for optimization of cardiac and respiratory function.

Aortic dissection

Some 93% present with pain, often described as the worst pain ever felt, tearing in nature and in most cases abrupt in onset, but may present with stroke or ischaemia of viscera or limbs.

Classification

- Stanford type A—affects ascending aorta; patient typically presents with anterior chest pain. URGENT CARDIOTHORACIC REFERRAL. Mortality rate may exceed 1% per hr.
- Stanford type B—affects descending aorta; patient typically presents with interscapular pain.

Think about

URGENT SENIOR REVIEW.

In any patient who presents with sudden pain, centrally or interscapular, consider dissection in the differential diagnosis.

Ask about

- Onset of pain (patients can often give exact time).
- Site and radiation of pain.
- History of hypertension and vascular disease.

Look for

- Any suggestion of visceral or limb ischaemia.

Investigations

- CT of aorta (thoracic and abdominal).
- CXR—may have widening of the mediastinum.
- ECG.
- Bloods: FBC, U&Es, cross-match. ABG.

Management

- Initially medical.
- If hypertensive—rapid and aggressive BP control using intravenous agents: combination of β-blocker (e.g. labetalol) and peripheral vasodilator (e.g. glyceryl trinitrate [GTN] or sodium nitroprusside [SNP]) Start β-blocker first and introduce vasodilators once β-blockade achieved.
- Labetalol is administered at an initial dose of 20mg IV over 2min, followed by further doses of 40–80mg every 10–15min until adequate blockade achieved—usually evidenced by a pulse of 60–80 bpm (max. dose 300mg).

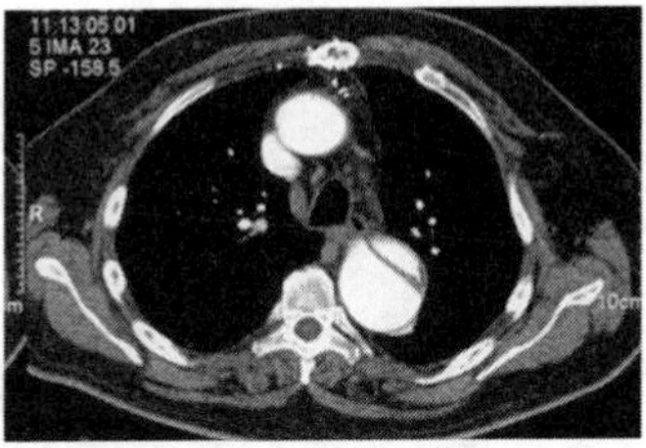

Fig. 4.3 CT scan showing acute aortic dissection.

- GTN or SNP may then be used as vasodilators to achieve adequate BP control (systolic <120–140mmHg). Doses should be governed by local guidelines and the ITU team is always a good starting point to check doses. The following serve as a guide:
  - GTN infusions are started from 10mcg/min and titrated up to 200mcg/min to achieve control. Patients may develop tolerance to long-term GTN.
  - SNP is started at a dose of 20mcg/min and may be titrated to 800mcg/min to achieve a systolic pressure reduction. SNP may cause cyanide toxicity, which may manifest as worsening acid–base status, mental changes and hyperreflexia.
- Adequate analgesia.
- Central venous access and arterial line.
- Surgical intervention indicated if there is:
  - Evidence of visceral ischaemia.
  - Evidence of limb ischaemia.
  - Persistent pain despite BP control and analgesia.
  - Suggestion of rupture.

☠ Vascular trauma

A senior should review all patients with a high suspicion of vascular injury.

A large majority of patients with vascular trauma do not reach hospital alive and die either at the scene of injury or during transport. In those that reach hospital it is useful to consider the injuries by region.

☠ Vascular injuries in the neck

The incidence of major vascular trauma following penetrating neck injury is ~1 in 5.

Think about

The neck is divided into three zones:

- **Zone 1**—extends from the sternal notch to 1cm above the clavicular head.
- **Zone 2**—extends from 1cm above the clavicular head to the angle of the mandible.
- **Zone 3**—extends from the angle of the mandible to the base of the skull.

Look for

- *Hard signs*—shock, active bleeding, expanding haematoma; these require urgent surgical intervention (8–25% of patients).
- *Soft signs*—pulsatile bleeding, small stable haematoma, cranial nerve injury, unexplained neurological deficit.
- Proximity injury—none of the above but an injury in the area.
- Platysma muscle breach.

Investigations

- Basic bloods, CXR, neurological assessment.
- Diagnostic angiography—some centres may explore zone 2 injuries without angiography.
- Diagnostic ultrasound—may be useful if experienced technicians are available.
- CT angiography—has shown excellent results in zones 2 and 3. In zone 1 artefact from the shoulder may reduce efficacy.
- Investigations should be guided by discussion with senior on call.

Management

- Traditional management involves mandatory exploratory surgery for any patients presenting with hard signs or zone 2 injuries.
- Zone 1 and 3 injuries have selective intervention following diagnostic angiography.
- Exploration should be considered for patients with platysma breach in any zone.
- If soft or no signs are present, serial clinical evaluation and conservative management may be considered.
- Endovascular options may be considered in centres with experience of carotid stenting especially in zone 1 and 3 injuries.

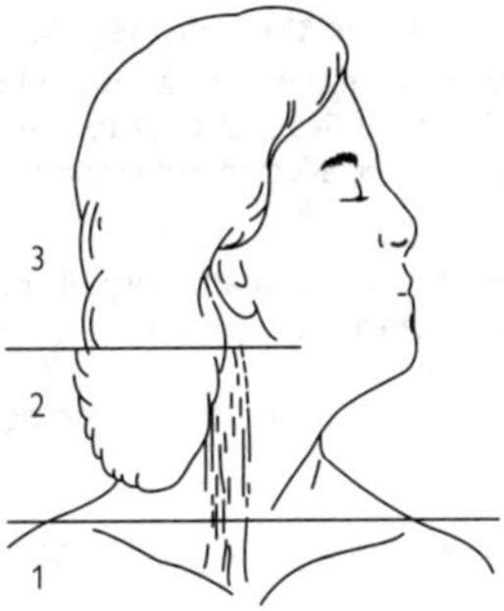

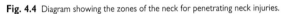

Fig. 4.4 Diagram showing the zones of the neck for penetrating neck injuries.

Vascular injuries in the thoracic segment

Most injuries to the thoracic segment are a result of blunt occur following abrupt deceleration. Most injuries are distal to the left subclavian artery (65%), although any site may be affected and in some cases may be multiple.

Think about

Any patient presenting to A&E with a history of trauma causes by rapid deceleration may have thoracic aortic injury:

- Steering wheel impact on chest.
- High-speed motor vehicle accident (MVA) with significant vehicle damage.
- Fall from a height.
- Ejection from a vehicle or death of any passengers.

Ask about

- Pain.
- Neurological symptoms.

Look for

- Evidence of cardiac tamponade (see Ch. 5).
- Patients who appear unusually agitated—suspicious of major vascular injury.
- Neurological deficit in the lower limbs.
- Absent pulses or evidence of lower limb/body ischaemia.
- *It is vital to document both neurological and vascular deficit on presentation and prior to surgery.*

Investigations

- CXR—look for widened mediastinum, loss or double shadow of the aortic knob, deviation of nasogastric tube or trachea, loss of aortopulmonary window, fracture of the sternum, apical haematoma, massive haemothorax, and blunt diaphragmatic injury.
- CT aorta—to look for mediastinal haematoma or aortic intimal flap. CT scan may be difficult to interpret.
- Angiography.
- Transoesophageal echocardiography.

Management

- Urgent surgical intervention has been the mainstay via thoracotomy or thoracolaparotomy.
- Endovascular interventions have the potential dramatically to alter management of aortic transactions in suitable patients and should be considered if available.

Vascular trauma to the limbs

Subclavian and *axillary* artery injuries generally occur following penetrating trauma and rarely after blunt trauma. The mortality rate for both is extre mely high and few patients reach hospital. Injuries to the *brachial, radial* and *ulnar* artery are commonly iatrogenic, following penetrating trauma or associated with fractures of the humerus, radius or ulna.

External iliac and *femoral* artery injuries have a high mortality rate—as high as 50% if associated with an aortic or iliac venous injury.

Popliteal injury may occur following either blunt or penetrating injury in the proximity of the knee and carries a significant risk of limb loss.

Think about

- In any patients with trauma blunt or otherwise, all pulses should be identified and their presence or absence recorded.
- Dislocations of the knee or elbow require repeated vascular assessment before and after reduction.

Look for

- *Hard signs*—observed pulsatile bleeding, arterial thrill on manual palpation bruits in the vicinity of the injury, absent pulse distal to the site of injury, visible expanding haematoma.
- *Soft signs*—a history of significant haemorrhage, neurological abnormality and diminished pulse compared with the contralateral extremity, proximity to a bony or penetrating injury.
- Most extremity injuries are not apparent at first assessment and ∴ all patients with suspicious history or proximity injuries should have regular and repeated reassessment.

Investigations

- If the patient has hard signs of vascular injury, intraoperative angiography may be used at time of exploration.
- Serial ABPIs using unaffected limb as a baseline. Arm pressure can also be followed in this way. ABPI <0.9 showed 95% sensitivity and 97% specificity for arterial injury in one study.
- If ABPI is below normal or soft signs of vascular injury are present, arteriography may be indicated.

Management

- Any patient with hard signs of trauma should be explored in theatre.
- Patients with an abnormal ABPI and soft clinical signs with angiographic evidence of major arterial injury need exploration.
- Patients with minimal angiographic signs of injury may be observed with or without serial angiography. Exploration may be necessary.
- Normal angiograms or normal ABPIs, or patients with no clinical signs and proximity injury alone, can be observed.
- Patients with isolated radial or ulnar artery injuries do not require intervention unless the palmar arch is incomplete or both are injured. The ulnar should be repaired in preference to the radial artery.

Vascular trauma to the abdomen

Most injuries (90–95%) are caused by penetrating mechanisms and are associated with a significant mortality rate.

Think about

- Blunt abdominal trauma may cause vascular trauma by one of three mechanisms: rapid deceleration (high-speed MVA and falls), direct anteroposterior crushing, direct laceration to major vessels from bone fragments (e.g. pelvic fracture).

Look for

- Penetrating injury associated with hypotension and abdominal distens is highly suspicious.
- Unequal femoral pulses—may indicate iliac artery injury.
- Vascular injuries of the abdomen can often be missed if the patient is haemodynamically stable, as signs may be absent; ∴ a high index of suspicion is needed if the history is highly suggestive.

Investigations

- Few patients with vascular abdominal injury require investigation as they invariably require urgent laparotomy.
- CXR only in gunshot wounds where the patient is haemodynamically stable.
- CT is not useful in penetrating vascular trauma but may have a role in blunt trauma where a vascular injury is not clearly evident.

Management

- **Urgent transportation to theatre for surgery in most cases.**
- Resuscitation in the emergency department should be limited to patients who are in cardiac arrest or imminent arrest, and may involve thoracotomy for aortic cross-clamping and cardiac massage.
- Large-bore venflons sited in the upper extremities or thoracic inlet—not the lower limbs in case of iliac or inferior vena cava injury.
- Controlled hypotension.
- Intubation in A&E should be avoided as it may precipitate cardiovascular decompression.

Infrarenal aneurysm repair

Improvements in both surgical technique and modern intensive care support have reduced the risks from aneurysm repair; however, significant postoperative complications are still common.

Cardiac

- Postoperative myocardial infarction (MI) is the most common cause of death following aneurysm repair. Risk is reduced by ensuring the patient is adequately filled, with a stable haematocrit and adequate analgesia. If the patient does have MI or acute coronary syndrome, discuss with senior and have a full cardiac review. Beware full ACS protocol of heparin, aspirin and clopidogrel in postoperative patients. The risk of MI needs to be weighed against bleeding risk.

Haemorrhage

- These patients often require large amounts of fluid after surgery.
- Along with fluid, blood and clotting products should be replaced.
- Monitor clotting profile and attempt to correct towards normal.
- Replace platelets—aim for a minimum count of 100×10^3 per μL.
- If, despite correction of clotting abnormalities and adequate fluid resuscitation, the patient remains hypotensive and tachycardic, discuss with senior—may require intervention.

Renal failure

- If the patient is not producing adequate urine after surgery (0.5–1ml/kg/hr), ensure that they have been adequately fluid resuscitated.
- If, despite adequate fluid, oliguria/anuria persists, furosemide can be considered, but this should be discussed first as it makes assessment of subsequent fluid balance difficult.

Gastrointestinal complications

- The inferior mesenteric artery is frequently sacrificed in IRAAA repair and there is ∴ a risk of colonic ischaemia and necrosis.
- Recognition of colonic ischaemia is difficult:
  - Bloody diarrhoea within 24–48hr of operation is the presenting feature in one-third of cases and should prompt urgent flexible sigmoidoscopy.
  - Other signs include ↑ abdominal pain, distension, fever, leucocytosis and thrombocytopenia, but are equally common in the recovering patient.
- Blood gas may be useful in demonstrating ↑ acidosis, and lactate levels may be raised.

Lower limb ischaemia

- Femoral and distal pulses should be assessed regularly after surgery.
- If the pulses are absent postoperatively this should prompt further senior assessment, as surgical intervention may be required (e.g. embolectomy).
- Assess the calves for evidence of compartment syndrome. Increasingly tense calves associated with stiff ankles on passive dorsi and plantar flexion should prompt senior review. Often patients do not complain of pain because they have an epidural anaesthetic in place.

Bypass surgery

In most bypass surgery, patients do not lose as much blood as in aneurysm repair as control is usually easier to achieve.

Complications may be as for aneurysm repair, as these patients have generalized vascular disease. Be aware for signs of MI.

- Assess pulses distal to the bypass graft and the graft itself, if it is palpable. If the signal on Doppler disappears or palpable pulses can no longer be felt, senior review should be sought as the patient may require graft embolectomy.
- ABPI should be determined once the patient is established on the ward—usually at 12hr after surgery.
- Check the calves for signs of compartment syndrome.
- Observe the proximal and distal anastomotic areas for expanding haematoma, which may suggest anastomotic leak.

Carotid surgery

- Monitor the patient for any neurological symptoms including assessment of the cranial nerves.
- Monitor the wound for any evidence of expanding haematoma which may require re-exploration.

Endovascular procedures

- In endovascular repair of aneurysms the groin wound should be closely monitored for evidence of bleeding or expanding haematoma that may indicate a false aneurysm.
- Despite the minimally invasive approach, EVAR can result in surprising blood loss as wires, catheters and devices are exchanged. Do not neglect basic principles of fluid resuscitation and replacement as for open repair. The complications may still be the same.
- Ensure patients receive adequate fluid replacement before and after any procedure in which they have received intravenous contrast to prevent renal impairment.

Radiological and coronary interventional procedures

- The most common complication is false aneurysm in the groin access site. This can usually be observed. If it continues to expand and the patient is unstable, surgical repair may be necessary and a senior should be informed.
- Occasional arterial occlusion at the site of the puncture can occur and requires urgent embolectomy and repair of the damaged artery. Always check distal pulses in patients who have had any interventional procedure.
- If a patient presents with haemorrhage, haemodynamic instability or peripheral ischaemia, consider the possibility of aortic dissection or perforation from guidewires—**urgent senior review is needed**.
- Ensure patients receive adequate fluid replacement before and after any procedure in which they have received intravenous contrast to prevent renal impairment.

Chapter 5

Cardiothoracic surgery

Jo Chikwe

Introduction

Covering the cardiothoracic surgery unit can be daunting for those who have not had any exposure. Although most of the surgery is routine, the patients have significant co-morbidity and can deteriorate rapidly. There will always be a registrar or intensive care cover close by, but you may be the first to see the patient and initiate treatment. You need to be able to think surgery *and* medicine.

Glossary of terms

Cardiac ITU

- Instead of using systolic and diastolic blood pressure (BP), arterial pressure can be described as a single figure: the *mean arterial pressure* (MAP):
  - MAP is calculated by adding one-third of the difference between diastolic (DP) and systolic (SP) pressures to the DP.
  - Only one-third (not one-half) of the difference is added to reflect the fact that diastole is longer than systole.
  - MAP on its own does not adequately describe cardiac function—a number of other parameters are frequently used.
- *Cardiac output (CO)*—the volume of blood ejected by the heart per minute.
- *Stroke volume*—the volume of blood ejected by the heart per beat.
- CO = heart rate × stroke volume.
- *Cardiac index* is CO adjusted to take into account the size of the patient, and is a more accurate reflection of cardiac function.

Preload

- Stroke volume depends on *preload, afterload* and *contractility*.
- *Preload* is a measure of the wall tension in the left ventricle at the end of diastole, but is difficult to quantify directly.
- *Central venous pressure (CVP), pulmonary artery wedge pressure (PAWP) and left atrial pressure (LAP)* are indirect measures of preload; they are sometimes referred to as *filling pressures*.

Afterload

- *Afterload* is the wall tension of the left ventricle during systole.
- It is determined by preload, which determines the maximum 'stretch', and by the resistance against which the heart must eject, which is a function of *systemic vascular resistance (SVR)*, which usually reflects the amount of peripheral vasoconstriction and MAP.

Contractility and compliance

- *Contractility* is a measure of the strength of myocardial contraction at a given preload and afterload.
- MAP and CO are commonly used indirect measures of contractility.
- *Compliance* is a measure of the distensibility of the left ventricle in diastole; stiff, hypertrophied ventricles have low compliance.
- Compliance is difficult to quantify in the clinical setting.

Important haemodynamic formulae and normal values

- CVP
- Cardiac output (CO) = SV x HR (4.5–8L/min)
- Cardiac index = CO/body surface area (BSA) (2.0–4.0L/min/m^2)
- MAP = DP + (SP − DP)/3 (70–100mmHg)
- SVR = [(MAP − CVP)/CO) x 80
- Systemic vascular resistance index = SVR/BSA (80–1200dyne-sec/cm^3)

Cardiac surgery

- *CABG (coronary artery bypass grafting):* in this operation for ischaemic heart disease, the *left internal mammary artery (LIMA)* is anastomosed to the *left anterior descending coronary artery (LAD)* and the *long saphenous vein (LSV)*, and rarely the left radial artery, is anastomosed to the coronary arteries (bottom ends) and aorta (top ends), usually via a *median sternotomy*. The operation can be done on-pump or off-pump:
  - *On-pump CABG (ONCAB)* is the conventional method—the heart is arrested and venous blood drained fom the right atrium into a cardiopulmonary bypass (CPB) circuit, where it is oxygenated, cooled and filtered, and returned to the aorta.
  - *Off-pump CABG (OPCAB)* is a newer method—the heart is not arrested, so cardiopulmonary bypass is not required. A variety of suction stabilizers are used to facilitate grafting on the beating heart.
- *Minimally invasive direct coronary artery bypass grafting (MIDCAB)* is LIMA to LAD, performed off-pump through an anterior mini-thoracotomy incision.
- *Aortic valve replacement (AVR)* is replacement of the aortic valve, invariably with cardiopulmonary bypass, with either a mechanical or a tissue (porcine or bovine) replacement.
- *Mitral valve replacement (MVR)* is replacement of the mitral valve, invariably with cardiopulmonary bypass, usually with a mechanical valve, where it is impossible for successful mitral valve repair.
- *A redo sternotomy* is more hazardous than a first-time sternotomy, as the heart, great vessels and patent grafts may be stuck to the sternum and at risk of damage from the sternal saw.

Thoracic surgery

- *Thoracotomy* is the conventional incision for lung surgery; it is usually posterolateral, but may be anterior.
- *Video-assisted thoracoscopic surgery (VATS)* involves insertion of two or more ports and collapse of the ipsilateral lung, and is a less invasive approach than a conventional thoracotomy.
- *Lobectomy* is resection of a single lobe of lung, usually through a posterolateral thoracotomy, and normally for suspected malignancy.
- *Pneumonectomy* is resection of an entire lung, usually through a posterolateral thoracotomy, and normally for suspected malignancy.

- *Pleuradhesis* is a procedure performed, usually by keyhole surgery, for recurrent pneumothorax or pleural adhesion, where dense adhesions are deliberately encouraged between visceral and parietal plera, obliterating the pleural space, either chemically (talc, gentamicin) or mechanically (abrasion).
- *Pleurectomy* is a procedure performed, usually by keyhole surgery, for recurrent pneumothorax, where the parietal pleura is stripped from apex to diaphragm.
- *Mediastinoscopy* involves blunt dissection down the front of the trachea from a small transverse collar incision at the suprasternal notch to biopsy paratracheal lymph nodes, usually to stage lung malignancy.

Basic principles

Anatomy

The mediastinum is the space between the pleural sacs. It is divided by a line drawn horizontally from the sternal angle to the lower border of T4, into the superior (bounded by the thoracic inlet above) and inferior mediastinum (bounded by the diaphragm below). The inferior mediastinum is further divided by the pericardial sac into anterior, middle and posterior.

Contents of the mediastinum

- *Superior mediastinum*—great vessels, trachea, oesophagus, phrenic nerve and vagus nerve, thoracic duct.
- *Anterior mediastinum*—pericardial ligaments, thymus, lymph nodes.
- *Middle mediastinum*—pericardial cavity, heart, great vessels, phrenic nerve.
- *Posterior* mediastinum—oesophagus, descending aorta, azygous veins, thoracic duct, lymph nodes.

Cardiopulmonary bypass (CPB)

Any operation that involves interrupting the blood supply to the head (valve surgery, surgery on septal defects, ascending and arch aortic dissection and aneurysm surgery, resection of some tumours invading great vessels, e.g. renal cell) requires CPB to maintain blood flow. This involves:

- *Heparinizing* the patient so that blood does not clot in the CPB circuit.
- Securing a 24Fr *aortic cannula* in the ascending aorta.
- Securing a 32Fr *venous cannula* in the right atrium (RA), or in the superior vena cava (SVC) and inferior vena cava (IVC).
- Connecting both cannulae to the bypass circuit.
- The venous return from the body is siphoned into the bypass circuit.
- The venous blood is *oxygenated, filtered and can be cooled or warmed*, and is pumped back to the patient via the aortic cannula.
- At the end of bypass, heparinization is reversed with protamine.

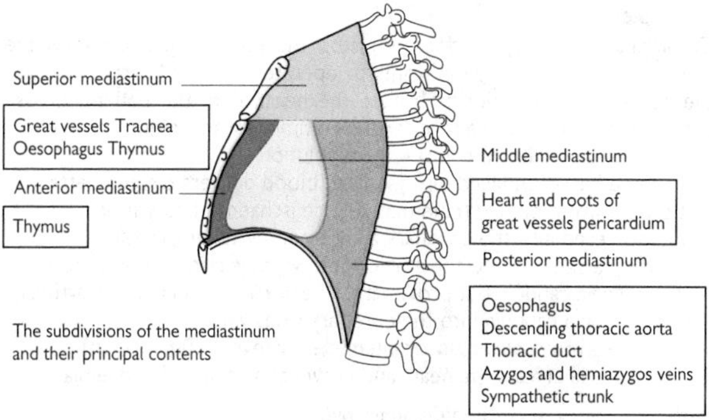

Fig. 5.1 Anatomical divisions of the mediastinum.

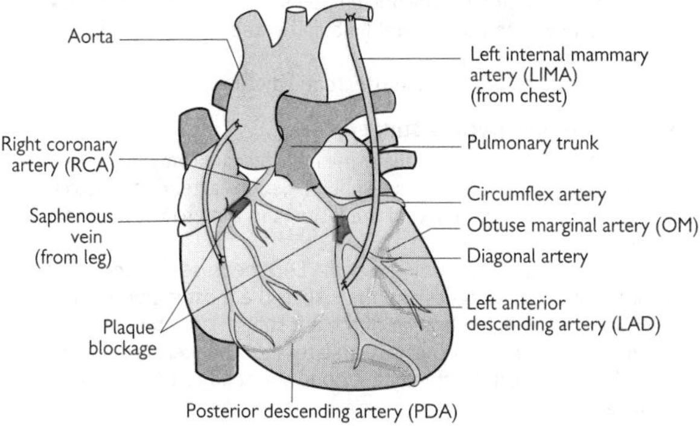

Fig. 5.2 Coronary artery anatomy post CABG.

Cardioplegia

Cardiopulmonary bypass does not stop the heart, it just bypasses the beating heart. If the surgeon wants to operate on a still heart, CPB gives the surgeon three options: fibrillate the heart, cool the patient, or use cardioplegia. Cardioplegia is by far the commonest technique.

- Cardioplegia utilizes a *potassium-rich* solution.
- It can be based on *blood* or *crystalloid* (blood delivers oxygen better).
- It can be *warm* or *cold* (cold may reduce ischaemic injury more).
- It is delivered into the coronary arteries either *anterogradely* by inserting a cannula into the aortic root, which is clamped distal to the cardioplegia cannula but proximal to the aortic cannula, or *retrogradely* by inserting a cannula into the coronary sinus vein.
- It can be given *continuously* or *intermittently* (every 20min or so).
- Cardioplegia arrests the heart and prevents myocardial ischaemia.

Pathophysiology of cardiopulmonary bypass

CPB is unavoidable for many operations. It has a major impact on nearly every organ system. Problems associated with bypass include:

- Activation of coagulation and complement cascades.
- Consumption of platelets and clotting factors causing coagulopathy.
- Microemboli and atherosclerotic emboli from aortic cannulation, which can cause stroke and peripheral limb and end-organ ischaemia.
- ↑ capillary permeability.
- Renal, pulmonary, hepatic and pancreatic dysfunction.

Coronary artery bypass surgery

- Median sternotomy. Occasionally mini left thoracotomy (📖 p159).
- A piece of *conduit* (saphenous vein, LIMA, radial artery) is anastomosed to the coronary artery beyond the lesion and then to the ascending aorta.
- The *LIMA is usually anastomosed to the LAD*, because this combination remains patent for decades and the LAD is the most important stenosis to treat. The LIMA is a branch of the left subclavian artery and runs down the inside of the rib cage 2cm lateral to the sternum. The origin from the subclavian is left intact: it does not need to be anastomosed to the aorta.
- Coronary artery bypass is mostly performed *on-pump* (with CPB), but can be performed on the beating heart without CPB (*off-pump*).

Principles of valve surgery

- Median sternotomy incision. Occasionally right thoracotomy for mitral valve.
- Valve surgery must be carried out with CPB (📖 p162).
- Once the heart is arrested on bypass, the valve is inspected and removed via an aortotomy for the aortic valve, and via a left atriotomy for the mitral valve.
- Once valve is in sewn into place, incisions are closed and air is removed from the heart, which is then weaned from bypass.
- Transoesophageal echo is used to assess the valve, particularly in mitral valve repair.

Chest trauma

Basic principles of trauma management follow ATLS guidelines:

Primary survey

This is aimed at identifying immediately life-threatening injuries (see below) and consists of:

- A—Airway maintenance and cervical spine care.
- B—Breathing and ventilation.
- C—Circulation and control of haemorrhage.
- D—Disability and neurological state.
- E—Exposure.

If you are cross-covering cardiothoracics you may not be called as part of the initial trauma call, but later if thoracic injuries have been identified.

Think about

- Does the patient have immediately life-threatening injuries?

Immediately life-threatening injuries

- Tension pneumothorax: ↓blood pressure (BP), ↑heart rate (HR), ↑jugular venous pressure (JVP), ↓sats, ↑respiratory rate (RR), mediastinal shift, ↓breath sounds.
- Massive haemothorax: ↓BP, ↑HR, ↓JVP, 2° sats, dull to percussion, ↓breath sounds.
- Open pneumothorax: sucking chest wound, ↓sats, surgical emphysema.
- Cardiac tamponade (📖 p168).
- Flail chest.

- Is the patient likely to need an emergency thoracotomy?

Indications for emergency thoracotomy

- Cardiac arrest or imminent cardiac arrest after penetrating trauma.
- Cardiac tamponade in setting of penetrating trauma.
- Limited role in cardiac arrest in setting of blunt trauma.

- Is the patient likely to need an urgent thoracotomy?

Indications for urgent thoracotomy

- Definitive treatment for bleeding >1L after insertion of chest drain for haemothorax.
- Definitive treatment of injury to heart, great vessels or lungs that is not immediately life threatening.

Ask about

- Mechanism of injury:
  - Knife—length of blade, location and number of wounds.
  - Road traffic accident (RTA)—speed of collision, collateral damage, restraints worn.
  - Gunshot—number of shots, range , location and number of exit and entry wounds.
  - Crush—amount of material, duration of injury.
- Chest pain, dyspnoea, dizziness.

Look for

- Evidence of haemodynamic compromise:
  - Hypotension, tachycardia.
  - Cool, clammy peripheries.
  - Absent peripheral pulses.
  - Altered consciousness.
  - Cardiac tamponade (↑JVP or CVP, hypotension, tachycardia; see 🕮 p168).
  - Oliguria if catheterized,
- Evidence of respiratory compromise:
  - Tachypnoea.
  - Hypoxia.
  - Absent or reduced breath sounds unilaterally (haemothorax or peumothorax).
  - Open chest wounds, surgical emphysema.

Investigations

- If the patient is unstable call for senior help.
- If the patient is stable:
  - CXR.
  - C-spine for RTA, falls, crush injuries.
  - ECHO if you suspect cardiac tamponade or cardiac injury.
  - Computed tomograph (CT) of chest if injury to other great vessels is suspected.
- Cross-match 6 units blood, FBC, U&Es. ABGs.

Management

Cardiac tamponade

- If stable, transfer directly to theatre for urgent thoracotomy.
- If unstable, emergency thoracotomy in A&E:
  - Call senior cover and anaesthetist if not already present.
  - Ask for thoracotomy trolley.
  - Ask for alcoholic skin prep, disposable scalpel, and sterile suction, all of which are vital and none of which is usually on the trolley.
  - If there is no cardiothoracic senior cover available, the A&E registrar or consultant may be able to perform a thoracotomy.
  - Pericardiocentesis is of value where there is no expertise in thoracotomy: with the patient on continuous ECG monitoring and aspirating continuously, pass a 16G needle on 50mL syringe between the xiphisternum and the left costal margin pointing towards the left shoulder until blood can be aspirated, stopping if ectopics appear.

Tension pneumothorax

- 14G cannula, 2nd intercostal space, mid-clavicular line.
- Convert to formal chest drain in 4th intercostals space mid axillary line

Haemothorax, simple pneumothorax

- Convert to formal chest drain in 4th intercostal space, mid-axillary line.

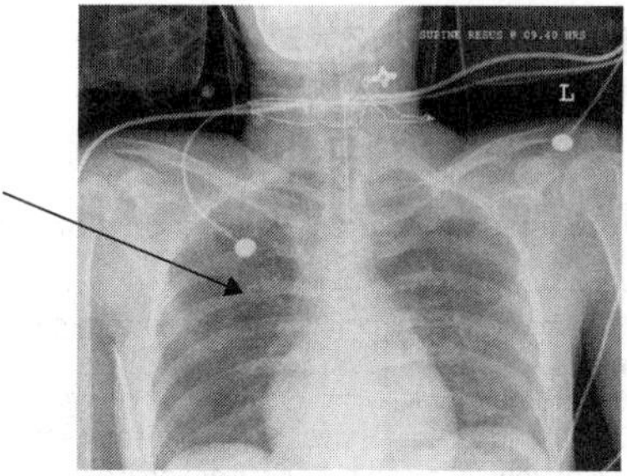

Fig. 5.3 Pneumothorax.

This patient is clearly not well. The information is there: ETT (Endotracheal tube), Rhesus and supine film.

At first glance no intrathoracic abnormality is visible. Reviewing the image, with the history of trauma, alerts you to think of rib fractures, haemothorax and pneumothorax.

There is a moderately sized right pneumothorax (arrow), which on supine films can be tricky to identify. Look for differences in the transradiancy of the left and right, lack of lung markings, the deep sulcus sign (see below) and the traditional line of the lung edge. Turning the film 90° can make this easier.

In a patient who is intubated this can easily become a tension pneumothorax. Look for mediastinal shift, diaphragmatic flattening/depression.

Five commonest calls to cardiothoracic ITU

Managing the five commonest calls to cardiothoracic ICU

Atrial fibrillation (📖 p198)
- Give 10—20mmol K^+ via central line to obtain serum K^+ 4.5–5.0mmol/L.
- Give empirical 20mmol Mg^+ via central line if none given postop.
- Give of 300mg amiodarone IV over 1hr in patients with good left ventricular function, followed by 900mg amiodarone IV over 23hr.
- In patients with poor left ventricular function, give digoxin in 125mcg increments IV every 20min until rate control is obtained, up to a maximum of 1500mcg in 24hr.
- Synchronized direct current (DC) cardioversion for unstable patients (📖 p198).

Bleeding (📖 p180)
- Get immediate help if bleeding is >400mL in 30min.
- Give Gelofusine® to achieve CVP of 10–14mmHg and systolic BP 80–100mmHg.
- Order further 4 units blood, 2 units FFP and 2 pools of platelets.
- Send clotting and FBC; request chest X-ray (CXR).
- Transfuse to achieve Hb >8.0g/dL, platelets >100 x 10^9/L, activated partial thromboplastin time (APTT) <40sec.
- Give empirical protamine 25mg IV; consider aprotinin.
- Emergency re-exploration is indicated for excessive bleeding.

Profound hypotension (📖 p184)
- Get help immediately.
- Quickly assess pulse, rhythm, rate, CVP, oxygen saturation and bleeding.
- Defibrillate ventricular fibrillation (VF) or pulseless VT; treat atrial fibrillation (AF) as above.
- Treat bradycardia with atropine 0.3mg IV or pace (📖 p198).
- Give Gelofusine® to raise CVP to 12–16mmHg; place bed head down.
- If you suspect cardiac tamponade (📖 p168) prepare for re-sternotomy.
- If patient is warm and vasodilated draw up 10mcg metaraminol into 10mL saline, give *1mL* through a central line, and flush.
- If patient is still profoundly hypotensive, give 1mL 1:10 000 adrenaline (epinephrine) IV.

Poor gases (📖 p188)
- If sats <85% and falling, get immediate help.
- Increase the fraction of inspired oxygen (FiO_2) to 100% temporarily; check pulse oximeter.

Contd

- Look at expansion, auscultate the chest, check arterial oxygen tension (PaO_2).
- If you suspect tension pneumothorax, treat immediately.
- Suction the endotracheal (ET) tube; check patient is not biting on it.
- Check the drain tubing is patent, and drains are on suction.
- Treat bronchospasm with salbutamol 5mg nebulizer.
- Disconnect from the ventilator and hand-ventilate the patient.
- Get a CXR; look for pneumothorax, haemothorax, atelectasis, ET tube position and lobar collapse, and treat problems.

Poor urine output (📖 p200)

- Check that the Foley catheter is patent.
- If the patient is hypotensive, treat this first (📖 p184).
- Give a fluid challenge of Gelofusine® to raise the CVP to 14mmHg.

If the patient is well perfused and the CVP is >14mmHg, give 20mg furosemide IV and repeat if indicated.

Normal ward management

Preoperative management

Unless your unit has a different policy it is particularly important to clerk cardiothoracic elective admissions in fully, even if they are admitted out of hours. These patients are frequently unwell, with multiple co-morbidity that needs basic assessment and management before surgery.

- Take a full history, paying particular attention to:
  - Angina, breathlessness, recent changes in symptoms.
  - Cardiac patients—angiography, echocardiography, carotid Dopplers.
  - Thoracic patients—CXR, CT, positron emission tomography (PET), histology , lung function tests (LFTs).
- Carry out a full examination, paying particular attention to:
  - Cardiac patients—carotid bruits, heart murmurs, peripheral pulses, varicose veins or scars from varicose vein surgery, Allen's test (patient makes a fist, occlude radial and ulnar pulses, patient's hand should go pink in <5sec when radial pulse released).
- Request FBC, U&Es, LFTs, cross-match 4 units, CXR.

Normal postoperative course in cardiac patients

First 6hr

- Inotropic support usually increases during the first 6hr.
- Pacing may be required (📖 p198).
- Many patients are extubated within 6hr.
- A diuresis of at least 1mL/kg/hr is usual.
- Mediastinal drainage should decrease steadily.
- Insulin requirements increase—aim to keep glucose 5–8mmol/L.
- Prophylactic antibiotics are continued for three doses.
- Aspirin 75mg PO started, preoperative antianginals are discontinued.

Day 1

- Inotropes are weaned.
- Most patients are extubated.
- Chest drains are removed after 3hr of consecutive zero drainage.
- Following drain removal, CXR is taken.
- Patient is transferred from ITU to HDU, and mobilized.
- Routine oral medication is commenced:
  - Aspirin 75mg OD.
  - Low molecular weight (LMW) heparin, e.g. clexane 40mg OD SC.
  - Furosemide 40mg OD.
  - Preoperative statin,
  - Angiotensin converting enzyme (ACE) inhibitor and/or β-blocker if tolerated.
  - Paracetamol 1g QDS,
  - Lactulose 10mL BD, senna two tablets,
- Patients who require formal anticoagulation are started on warfarin.
- Patients should be eating and drinking.

Day 2

- Monitoring lines (arterial, CVP and urinary catheters) are removed.
- The patient is transferred from HDU to the ward.
- Patient-controlled analgesia (PCA) should be discontinued.
- Insulin sliding scales are discontinued and normal antihyperglycaemic regimens commenced if the patient is eating and drinking.

Day 3

- Anticoagulation should be therapeutic for mechanical valves: start IV heparin or therapeutic dose of LMW heparin if this is not the case.
- If there are no contraindications (e.g. heart block, bradycardia, international normalized ratio [INR] >3.0), remove temporary pacing wires.

Day 4

- Patient should complete a satisfactory stairs assessment with a physiotherapist.
- All blood results and imaging should be returning to normal values.
- Adequate pain control should be possible with regular paracetamol.

Day 5–7

- The patient should be ready for discharge home.
- Weight should be back to baseline, and diuretics may be discontinued in patients with good LV (left ventricle).

Routine tests

Protocols vary. The following is a common standard.

Blood tests

FBC, clotting, U&Es on days 1, 2, 3, 5 and 7.

ECG

1–2hr, 12hr and 2 days postop.

Chest X-rays

Daily if chest drains are present on suction, immediately after drain removal, and on days 2, 4 and 7 thereafter.

Transthoracic echocardiography

Day 5 for patients having valve surgery, particularly mitral valve repairs.

Thoracic patients

Drain management is described on 📖 p202.

- Epidurals should be continued for 3–4 days if possible; effective pain control helps optimize lung function; urinary catheter should remain in situ while patient has an epidural.
- Drug chart should contain:
  - LMW heparin, e.g. clexane 40mg SC OD.
  - Saline nebulizers 5mL QDS.
  - COPD/asthma—salbutamol 5mg and Atrovent® 250mg nebulized 2°.
  - Analgesia, e.g. paracetamol 1g QDS (IV more effective than PR/PO) and opiate analgesia, e.g. tramadol 1g QDS PO, if required.
  - Prophylactic antibiotics, e.g. cefuroxime 1.5g IV TDS, three doses.
- While the patient has drains, request and review daily CXR.
- Mediastinoscopy patients can normally go home on day 1 postop.
- Other patients can usually go home once all drains have been removed and CXR is satisfactory.

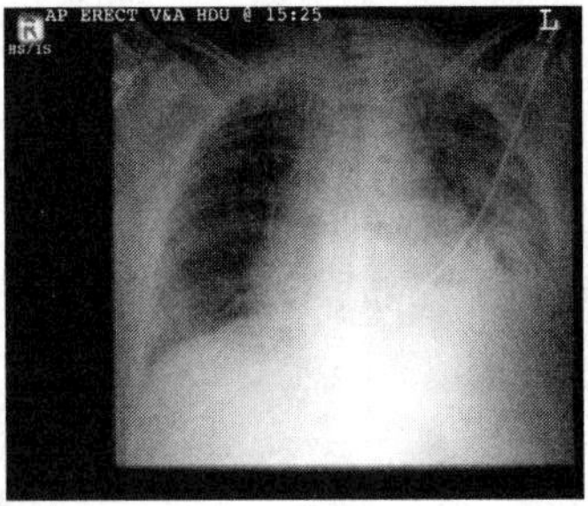

Fig. 5.4 Normal post-CABG CXR.

On this routine post CABG film, the bilateral pleural drains are present, along with sternotomy wires and a RIJv (right internal jugular vein) central line.

There is a moderately sized left pleural effusion and probable pulmonary oedema.

After central line insertion, the things to look for are new pleural effusions and pneumothorax, as well as the position of the tip, ideally in the distal SVC, as in this case.

Drugs

Inotropes increase contractility, pressors vasoconstrict

- α-adrenergic receptor stimulation leads to ↑ SVR and PVR.
- β_1 stimulation leads to ↑ contractility, heart rate and conduction.
- β_2 stimulation causes peripheral dilatation and bronchodilatation.
- DA (dopamine) stimulation causes coronary, renal and mesenteric vasodilatation.

Inotropes

Adrenaline (epinephrine) 0.03–0.5mcg/kg/min or bolus

Action

Direct agonist at α, β_1 and β_2 receptors.

Pharmacodynamics

Instant onset, half-life 2min.

Indications

- Cardiac arrest (asystole, VF, electromechanical dissociation [EMD]).
- Anaphylaxis.
- Low CO states.
- Bronchospasm.

Clinical use

- *Cardiac arrest*—high dose, 0.5–1mg bolus IV (5–10mL 1:10 000).
- *Anaphylaxis*—low to moderate dose, 0.5–2mL 1:10 000 bolus IV.
- *Low CO states*—0.5mL bolus 1:10 000 IV (1mL 1:10 000), then infusion (0.03–0.5mcg/kg/min).
- Administration by central line—extravasation causes skin necrosis.
- Infusions require continual arterial line BP monitoring.
- With high-dose adrenaline, extreme hypertension, cardiovascular accident (CVA) or myocardial infarction (MI) may result. Reserve bolus administration for the periarrest patient.
- Lactic acidosis is common; urine output may fall.
- Serum lactate and glucose levels rise, particularly in diabetic patients.

Dopamine 3–10mcg/kg/min

Action

α, β_1, β_2 and DA_1 agonist, and release of stored neuronal noradrenaline (NA).

Pharmacodynamics

Fast onset, slow offset. Metabolized by monoamine oxidase (MAO).

Indication

- Low CO state.
- Renal insufficiency.

Clinical use

Optimize preload, commence dopamine at 3mcg/kg/min and titrate upwards depending on blood pressure/cardiac output. If no improvement at high doses, reassess with a view to a second inotrope.

- Administration by central line—extravasation causes skin necrosis.
- Improvement in urine output is 2° to ↑ CO.

Dobutamine 3–10mcg/kg/min

Action

Direct β_1 agonist (inotropy), small β_2 effect (↓SVR) with minimal α or DA receptor action. Metabolite of dobutamine is an α antagonist.

Pharmacodynamics

- Half-life is 2min.
- Hepatic metabolism.

Indication

Low CO 2° to ↑ afterload.

Clinical use

As for dopamine. Reduce vasodilator infusions, as dopexamine acts like a combination of an inotrope and a vasodilator.

Pressors

Noradrenaline (norepinephrine) 0.03–1.0mcg/kg/min

Action

Direct α agonist: potent vasoconstriction + β_1 effect = ↑BP.

Pharmacodynamics

Immediate onset; half-life 2min.

Indication

Hypotension because of low SVR in good to high CO states.

Clinical use

Low-dose noradrenaline (0.03–0.06mcg/kg/min) is often started *empirically* in the well filled patient with warm peripheries, where low BP and filling pressures are thought to be a result of vasodilatation.

- Administration by central line: extravasation causes skin necrosis.
- In hearts with borderline CO, noradrenaline should be avoided or used in conjunction with another inotrope, for the reasons below.

Metaraminol (Aramine®) Dilute 10mg in 10mL N saline; give 0.5mL IV

Action

Direct α agonist: potent vasoconstrictor + β1 effect = ↑BP.

Pharmacodynamics

- Metaraminol has a longer duration of action than noradrenaline (norepinephrine).
- Immediate onset; half-life 4–5min.
- Metabolized by MAO.

Indication

Temporizing measure to treat hypotension.

Clinical use

If boluses of metaraminol in the ICU achieve a good but not sustained response, an infusion of noradrenaline (norepinephrine) is indicated.

Vasodilators

GTN (glyceryl trinitrate) 1–10mg/hr

Action

Dilates veins, reducing venous return to the heart, decreasing heart size, stroke volume and CO. This reduces myocardial oxygen demand. Dilates coronary vasculature, reducing vasospasm, redistributing more flow to ischaemic myocardium.

Pharmacodynamics

Half-life 1–3min.

Indications

- Routine prophylaxis/treatment of myocardial ischaemia and coronary spasm.
- Hypertension.

Clinical use

- GTN is routinely started at the lowest end of the range above and titrated against blood pressure to maintain MAP of 70–75mmHg.
- Administration may be by peripheral line, sublingually or topical GTN patches 5–15mg over 24hr.

Antiarrhythmics

Potassium chloride (10–40mmol)

Action:

Hypokalaemia increases the resting membrane potential resulting in ↑ excitability and tachyarrhythmias such as atrial fibrillation.

Pharmacodynamics

Renal excretion.

Indication

Maintenance of serum K^+ 4.5–5.0mmol/L after surgery.

Clinical use

- 10–20mmol in 50mL 5% dextrose can be administered by central line over 20min, or 40mmol in 1L 5% dextrose can be administered peripherally over 8hr.
- Cardiac arrhythmias result if infusion is too fast.
- Potassium should be administered cautiously in patients with renal impairment as hyperkalaemia can quickly result.

Emergency re-sternotomy: call for senior help

Indications

1. **Incipient or actual cardiac arrest** due to cardiac tamponade, torrential haemorrhage: **do on ITU if no time to transfer patient**
2. **Excessive bleeding**: Re-exploration is indicated for excessive bleed that persists after coagulopathy has been corrected.

Theatre

- **Think!** Do you need a perfusionist? Ask someone to phone the surgical consultant responsible for the patient.
- While the anaesthetist sedates the patient, prep and drape.
- Open the wound down to the sternum with a knife.
- Cut the sternal wires with a wire cutter; if there is no wire cutter, use a heavy needle-holder to twist wires until they fracture.
- Pull **all** the wires out—wire fragments will lacerate the heart.
- Gently lever the sternum open with your fingers.
- Place the sternal retractor and carefully expose the heart.
- You should see an immediate improvement in filling and perfusion pressures if there was tamponade.

Magnesium sulfate (2–4g)

Action:

Normal serum Mg^{2+} concentration is 1.0mmol/L. Magnesium promotes cardiac electrical stability by affecting ion transport across membranes.

Pharmacodynamics

Renal excretion.

Indication

Mg^{2+} may be given empirically to treat arrhythmias in cardiac surgical patients, who are normally Mg^{2+} depleted.

Clinical use

2–4g magnesium sulfate in 50mL 5% dextrose may be given via central line over 20min; 1–2g MgCl may be given orally.

Bleeding and tamponade

Excessive bleeding is bleeding that falls outside the 'normal' pattern of bleeding following cardiotomy. **Call for senior help if the patient is haemodynamically compromised.**

'Normal' bleeding

Mediastinal bleeding is normally greatest in the hours immediately after theatre, tailing off to near zero over the course of the following 6–12hr. Although bleeding varies depending on a number of perioperative factors, acceptable rates of bleeding are *roughly*:

- Less than 300mL/hr for 1hr.
- Less than 200mL/hr for 2 consecutive hrs.
- Less than 100mL/hr for 3 consecutive hrs.
- The trend should be decreasing.

Think about

- Is the patient haemodynamically compromised?
- Does the patient need re-opening to sort out a surgical problem?
- Is the bleeding due to coagulopathy?

Ask about

- BP, pulse and CVP.
- The exact amount of bleeding in the past hour.
- The amount of volume replacement needed.
- Fall in Hb (estimated regularly in the blood gases).
- Most recent APTT, activated prothrombin time ratio (APTR) or INR, platelets, fibrinogen, heparin levels.
- Whether the patient has been sat up or rolled—this may cause an old collection of blood to drain suddenly, simulating active bleeding.
- Whether the patient was on aspirin or clopidogrel until surgery.

Look for

- **Cardiac tamponade is a life-threatening emergency (📖 p168) and is an indication for URGENT re-sternotomy (📖 p182). Call for senior help.**
- Blood rising rapidly up the drainage tubing when you lift it up.
- Bright red blood in the drainage tubing, suggesting an arterial bleed.
- Bleeding cannula sites, suggesting coagulopathy.

Investigations

- APTT, APTR, platelets, fibrinogen levels, heparin levels.
- CXR (blood may be collecting in the pleura).

Management

- **If bleeding approaches 500mL in 30min, or the patient is haemodynamically unstable, call for senior help and prepare for emergency re sternotomy (📖 p182).**
- Give blood, or Gelofusine® if no blood available, to maintain MAP of 70–75mmHg, and CVP of 8–10mmHg.
- Put the bed flat or head down if you have trouble achieving these parameters.
- If you do not have recent clotting results:
  - Order 4–6 units blood and 2 units FFP.
  - Ask for platelets if the patient was on clopidogrel or aspirin until surgery.
  - Give 25mg protamine empirically—if this was well tolerated in theatre it should be well tolerated in ICU.
  - If the patient was on aspirin or clopidogrel before surgery consider *either* starting aprotinin infusion at ½ million units (50mL) per hr for 6hr, *or* giving tranexamic acid 2g—but discuss this with your senior cover.
- If you do have clotting results:
  - Order 4–6 units blood and give to maintain Hb >8.0g/dL.
  - Give platelets to maintain platelet count $>100^9$/L (1U increases platelets by about 10^9/L in a 70kg adult).
  - Give protamine to correct raised APTT or APTR.
  - Give FFP to correct raised APTT or APTR (roughly 5–10mL/kg will be issued).
  - Give cryoprecipitate to achieve fibrinogen 1–2mg/L (10 bags will raise fibrinogen by about 0.6mg/L).
- Avoid giving large volumes of cold fluid: use infusion warmers.
- Warm the patient to 37°C—hypothermia suppresses coagulation mechanism and platelet function.
- Control hypertension with adequate sedation and ↑GTN, and control shivering with 25mg pethidine IM/IV.
- Avoid the use of colloid volume expanders unless blood products are unavailable and the patient is hypovolaemic.
- Withhold postoperative aspirin and any anticoagulants.
- Ensure patency of chest drains by milking them regularly.

Hypotension

Normally we aim for a systolic BP of 110–130mmHg, or MAP of 70–75 mmHg. Some patients need higher and some lower pressures than this; if the patient is passing >1mL/kg/hr urine and is not acidotic, their blood pressure is probably adequate.

Think about

- Is the patient haemodynamically compromised?
- Is there an acute cause?

Ask about

- *Exact* BP, pulse rate and rhythm, and CVP.
- Dizziness and chest pain if the patient is awake.
- Rate of bleeding if the patient has chest drains.
- Amount of volume replacement required.
- Amount of inotrope infusion.
- Recent changes such as removal of pacing wires, new drug regimens.
- Pyrexia, abdominal symptoms, blood sugar.

Look for

- **Evidence of poor tissue perfusion**—cool clammy peripheries, ↓urine output, ↑Cr, confusion, myocardial ischaemia, metabolic acidosis.

Causes

- Cardiac tamponade:
  - ↑CVP or JVP, ↓BP, ↑pulse (if not β-blocked).
  - Excessive widening of the mediastinum on CXR.
  - Tachycardia and dysrhythmias, including VF and EMD.
  - ECHO may show clot in pericardium + right ventricular (RV) diastolic collapse.
- Impaired left ventricular (LV) function:
  - ↑CVP or JVP, ↓BP, ↑pulse (if not β-blocked).
  - ↓BP with fluid challenge.
  - History of poor LV function preop.
- Hypovolaemia:
  - Causes—surgical bleeding, polyuria, GI bleed.
  - ↓CVP (<8mmHg) or JVP, ↑HR.
  - Reduced skin turgor, dry mucous membranes, patient thirsty.
  - Overall negative fluid balance.
- Peripheral vasodilatation:
  - Causes—GTN, propofol, sepsis, ACE inhibitors, epidurals.
  - Patient peripheries feel warm; palpable peripheral pulses.
- Other causes:
  - Arrhythmias, changes in inotropes and antihypertensives.
  - Systemic problems (GI bleed, tension pneumothorax, hypoglycaemia, sepsis).
  - Myocardial ischaemia (angina, ST segment changes).

Causes of postoperative hypotension

Ten commonest causes

- Patient is vasodilated—reduce GTN, think about noradrenaline (norepinephrine).
- Patient is hypovolaemic—give fluid and assess bleeding (📖 p180).
- Temporarily impaired LV function—start inotropes (📖 p176).
- Arrhythmia—treat aggressively (📖 p198).
- Sedation—give careful fluid bolus and consider metaraminol.
- Cardiac tamponade—call for immediate senior help (📖 p168).
- Postural—patient has been sat up or out: give fluids.
- NOT hypotension—normal BP for patient! Check preop BP.
- NOT hypotension—artefact: check non-invasive BP manually.

Other causes

- Pump failure:
  - Poor LV function preop.; RV dysfunction.
  - Hypoxia, acidosis, hypercarbia, hypoglycaemia, hyperkalaemia.
  - Arrhythmias, myocardial ischaemia.
  - Drugs—amiodarone, β-blockers, propofol, fentanyl.
- Hypovolaemia:
  - Actual—haemorrhage, polyuria, inadequate volume replacement.
  - Relative—sepsis, vasodilatation (propofol, GTN), epidural anaesthesia, anaphylactoid reactions).
- Mechanical causes:
  - Intracardiac: valve thrombosis, acute regurgitation, pulmonary embolism.
  - Extracardiac—cardiac tamponade, tension pneumothorax.

Investigations

- Usually cause is apparent from focused history and examination.
- ECG, CXR, arterial blood gases for PaO_2, $PaCO_2$, Hb, K^+, glucose.

Management

- Treat obvious specific causes: **immediately life-threatening causes are**:
  - **Cardiac tamponade**: definitive treatment emergency re-sternotomy—fluids, inotropes and pressors are temporary measures.
  - **Arrhythmias**: VF, VT, asystole, loss of pacing, heart block (📖 p198).
  - **Massive haemorrhage**.
  - **Tension pneumothorax**: 14G cannula, 2nd intercostal space in midclavicular line; definitive management is a chest drain.
- Treat hypovolaemia:
  - Give colloid to achieve CVP of 12–16mmHg or systolic BP >100mmHg.
  - Lie the patient down; if necessary put the bed-head down.
  - Treat bleeding (📖 p180).

- Treat peripheral vasodilatation:
  - Reduce GTN, remove warming blankets.
  - Dilute 10mg metaraminol in 10mL N saline, give 0.5mL IV and flush.
  - Consider noradrenaline (norepinephrine) infusion (📖 p176).
- Treat poor LV function:
  - Correct hypoxia (📖 p187), hyperkalaemia, and acidosis (📖 p190).
  - Treat hypoglycaemia.
  - Stop recent infusions that may cause ↓LV function (amiodarone, propofol).
  - Start small dose of dopamine or adrenaline (epinephrine) (📖 p176).
  - Treat myocardial ischaemia by starting GTN—discuss with senior as patient may need re-sternotomy or intra-aortic balloon pump.

The ventilated patient with poor gases

Most patients, however, recover respiratory function and are weaned from ventilatory support within 24hr; 5% require additional support.

Think about

- Is the patient severely compromised?
- Requesting a CXR as you go to see the patient.

Ask about

- PaO_2, $PaCO_2$, oxygen saturations, FiO_2. If the patient is not already on 100%, ask the nursing staff to do this.
- Mode of ventilation.
- BP, HR.

Look for

- ET tube—displaced, patient biting it.
- Asymmetrical chest expansion—suggests malpositioned ET tube, pnemothorax, haemothorax.
- For bilateral breath sounds—if unilateral:
  - The ET tube may be displaced down one bronchus,
  - There may be a large haemothorax or pneumothorax.
- Bronchospasm.
- Incorrect ventilator settings (see box),
- Artefact—hypotension, vasoconstriction, shivering, misplacement can all cause pulse oximetry readings to be too low.

Investigations

- PaO_2, $PaCO_2$, oxygen saturations.
- CXR.

Management

- **If oxygen saturation is falling with no obvious cause, call for immediate anaesthetic help.**
- *Treat bronchospasm with* nebulized salbutamol 5mg.
- *Increase the* FiO_2—100% oxygen can be given for short periods without causing oxygen toxicity, and usually reverses hypoxia.
- Is the patient biting on the ET tube? If they are uncooperative, they are not ready for weaning and should be re-sedated—*sedation or paralysis* improves gas exchange by improving efficiency of ventilation and reducing the energy demands of spontaneous ventilation.
- Assess position of the ET tube on CXR—it should be ≥2cm above the carina; the anaesthetist should pull it back if this is not the case.
- Treat *pneumothoraces* or *haemothoraces* with a chest drain.
- Treat *atelectasis*—should be managed with intermittent ET tube suction and ↑ positive end-expiratory pressure (PEEP).
- Check the *ventilator settings*—enlist the help of an anaesthetist.
- If worsening O_2 sats, *suction the ET tube* and *hand-ventilate*—should be done by the most experienced, usually the nursing staff looking after the patient.

The extubated patient with poor gases

Think about

- Does the patient need intubating urgently?
- If not, for how long is the current level of respiratory effort sustainable?
- Is there an easily reversible cause?
- Request a CXR as you go to see the patient.

Ask about

- Oxygen saturations, FiO_2—if the patient is not already on 6L by face mask, ask the nursing staff to do this.
- BP, RR.
- Level of consciousness.
- PaO_2, $PaCO_2$ if available.
- Chest pain, cough, sputum.

Look for

- Stridor.
- Cyanosis, pallor; cold, clammy peripheries.
- Hypotension, tachycardia, raised JVP (think tension pneumothorax).
- Tachypnoea.
- Surgical emphysema (swelling around wound, drain sites, sometimes neck and facial swelling with 'bubble wrap' crackling texture, representing air in the subcutaneous tissues suggesting major air leak, and often associated with a pneumothorax).
- Asymmetrical chest expansion (pneumothorax, haemopneumothorax).
- Auscultate for absent breath sounds (pneumothorax, haemothorax, mucus plugging), wheeze (asthma/COPD), crepitations, bronchial breath sounds (chest infection).
- If the patient has chest drains, check them carefully (📖 p202).

Investigations

- PaO_2, $PaCO_2$, pH, base excess, oxygen saturations.
- CXR.
- Ultrasound—differentiate between fluid collection and consolidation.

Management

- **The exhausted or tiring acidotic patient may need intubating.**
- **The patient with stridor may need intubating—call an anaesthetist.**
- **Lobectomy and pneumonectomy patients have minimal respiratory reserve—if they do not improve quickly call senior cover.**
- Sit the patient up and give 6–8L oxygen via a face mask.
- Treat large pneumothorax or haemothorax with a chest drain (📖 p202).
- Treat chest infection with antibiotics (e.g. ciprofloxacin 500mg PO BD), nebulized saline (5mL QDS) and regular chest physiotherapy.
- Treat mucus plugging and lobar collapse with broncheoalveolar lavage (BAL) or continuous positive airway pressure (CPAP), nebulized saline (5mL QDS), and chest physiotherapy.

- Treat COPD with nebulized saline (5mL QDS), salbutamol (5mg every 2hr max) and Atrovent® (250mcg QDS), chest physiotherapy and CPAP.
- Treat pulmonary oedema with 40mg furosemide IV; start fluid balance.

The acidotic patient

Acidosis is a pH <7.45. *Base deficit* or *negative base excess* (millimoles per litre of base required to titrate the blood pH back to 7.45) is often quoted instead of pH. Normal base deficit is from −2 to +2; > −5 is very significant, The trend is important. Acidosis reduces myocardial function and often suggests a significant underlying problem (see box).

Think about

- Is this a metabolic or a respiratory or metabolic acidosis? (See box).
- If it is a metabolic acidosis, is it a sign of low CO?
- Is the acidosis severe enough to compromise LV function?

Ask about

- Base excess, $PaCO_2$, blood glucose, K^+, lactate.
- Hypotension, urine output.
- Infusions such as adrenaline (epinephrine), SNP.
- Peripheral pulses and perfusion, abdominal distension.

Look for

- Signs of peripheral limb ischaemia—pallor, absent peripheral pulses.
- Mesenteric ischaemia is difficult to diagnose (see below).

Investigations

- Base excess, $PaCO_2$, serum HCO_3^-, blood glucose, lactate, K^+.
- Urinary ketones.

Management

The picture is often mixed. A significant lactic acidosis is uncommon, but when it occurs it often indicates a major problem. Identify and treat the other common causes of a metabolic acidosis quickly, while identifying and investigating a possible lactic acidosis. *Give sodium bicarbonate* 25–50mL 8.4% IV where the underlying cause of a severe metabolic acidosis cannot be treated immediately.

Lactic acidosis (lactate >2.5mmol/L)

This suggests profound tissue hypoperfusion. Causes are listed in the box.

- Treat hypotension, hypoxaemia and hypovolaemia (📖 p184).
- Look hard for causes:
  - Examine the distal pulses and capillary refill.
  - *Treat peripheral hypoperfusion* by using a warming blanket if necessary, to achieve core temperature of 36.5–37.5°C.
  - Adrenaline (epinephrine) infusions often cause a lactic acidosis—discuss alternative inotrope regimens with a senior.
  - The only way to exclude infarcted bowel is via a laparotomy (bowel sounds, abdominal X-ray and CT all have low sensitivity) but laparotomy after cardiac surgery is associated with high morbidity and mortality rates.

1. Distinguish between metabolic and respiratory acidosis

- Look at the pH—it must be <7.45 for an acidosis.
- Look at the $PaCO_2$—is it >5.5? If so, there is a **respiratory acidosis.**
- Look at the base deficit (or anion gap)—if BE > −2.0 there is a **metabolic acidosis.**
- Look at the blood glucose—if it is >10mmol/L there is probably a ketoacidosis.
- Look at the lactate—if it is >2.0mg/dL there is a lactic acidosis.

2. Establish the causes of the acid–base disturbance

Metabolic acidosis due to ↑ metabolic acids (↑anion gap)

- Lactic acid—global and/or regional hypoperfusion, especially mesenteric ischaemia (this is very difficult to detect in the sedated patient; lactic acidosis may be the only sign), profound hypoxia, sepsis, adrenaline infusions, hepatic failure as the liver normally metabolizes lactate).
- Uric acid, loss of bicarbonate (renal failure).
- Ketones (diabetic ketoacidosis, alcoholic and starvation ketoacidosis).
- Drugs/toxins (salicylates, SNP overdose).
- Hyperchloraemia (N saline infusion).

Due to loss of bicarbonate or hyperchloraemia (normal anion gap)

- Renal tubular acidosis (loss of bicarbonate).
- Diarrhoea, high-output ileostomy (loss of bicarbonate).
- Pancreatic fistulae (loss of bicarbonate).
- Hyperchloraemic acidosis (excessive saline administration).

Respiratory acidosis

- Any cause of respiratory failure, or hypoventilation.
- ↑ production of CO_2, e.g. sepsis, malignant hyperpyrexia.
- Rebreathing CO_2 (circuit misconnections, soda lime exhaustion).

Ketoacidosis (urinary glucose + ketones; BG >14)

- Common after cardiac surgery.
- Increase sliding scale to ↓ blood glucose to <8mmol/L; it may be necessary to increase this several times to achieve tight control.
- Discuss changing adrenaline (epinephrine) infusions with a senior.

Hyperchloraemic acidosis (serum Cl >120mEq/L)

Common where N saline is used as maintenance: change to dextrose.

Renal failure (↑creatinine, urine output usually <1mL/kg/hr)

- See 📖 p200 for diagnosis and management of renal failure.
- A deteriorating base deficit, refractory to medical management, in the patient with renal failure is an indication for urgent *haemofiltration.*

Respiratory acidosis

- Treat respiratory acidosis by increasing respiratory rate and tidal volumes of the ventilator settings: aim for a minute volume of 100mL/kg/min.
- The weaning process should be reversed in the patient who develops a respiratory acidosis whilst being weaned from ventilation; extubated patients should be started on CPAP to reduce the work of breathing.

Chest pain

Chest pain is very common after cardiothoracic surgery, but normally reflects the effects of a median sternotomy, rib retraction and drains. Taking a careful pain history should help differentiate between the causes of chest discomfort listed in the box. **Wound pain is usually sharp or sore, and worse with deep breathing or coughing.**

Think about
- Is this normal wound pain, or does it reflect serious problems?

Ask about
- Whether the patient is haemodynamically unstable.
- Whether pain is worse with breathing deeply or coughing.
- Whether pain is sharp/sore or dull/heavy.
- Whether pain is like angina before the operation.
- What brought the pain on and for how long the pain has lasted.
- Whether there are associated symptoms, e.g. dyspnoea, nausea.

Look for
- Hypotension, tachycardia, tachypnoea.
- Evidence of infection—pyrexia, cellulitis, pus.
- Level of epidural cover in thoracic patients—if your touch feels the same bilaterally in the incision dermatomes, the block is ineffective.
- Sternal 'click' (palpable movement of the sternal edges on coughing in a patient with a median sternotomy incision suggests unstable sternum).
- Recent reduction in analgesia, or failure to take regular analgesia.

Investigations
- Troponin for ?MI (TropT >3.4mcg/L more than 48hr post-CABG has a 90% sensitivity and almost 95% specificity for MI).
- White cell count (WCC) and C-reactive protein (CRP) for suspected infection, wound swabs.
- ECG.
- Transthoracic ECHO if you suspect cardiac tamponade.
- CXR.

Management
'Normal' wound pain
- Reassure the patient that their operation has not 'gone wrong'.
- Remember regular analgesia is usually more effective than PRN.
- Avoid non-steroidal anti-inflammatory drugs (NSAIDs) in patients with asthma, renal impairment, peptic ulcer disease and the elderly; if you have to prescribe them, limit to PRN for 48hr, and prescribe omeprazole 20mg OD.

Causes of postoperative chest pain

Dull central ache

- Myocardial ischaemia (usually brought on by exertion), ECG changes usually suggest the source of the problem:
  - V1–V4: LAD territory—problem with LIMA.
  - I, II, aVF: inferior wall—problem with vein graft to posterior descending artery (PDA) or right coronary artery (RCA).
  - V3–V6: possibly a problem with vein graft to obtuse marginal (OM)/ intermediate.
- Cardiac tamponade (📖 p168).
- Pericarditis (classically soreness rather than ache).
- Peptic ulcer disease, oesophagitis, rarely pancreatitis.

Pain on movement

- Musculoskeletal pain, wound infection, unstable sternum.
- Chest drains.

Pleuritic pain

- Chest infection.
- Pneumothorax (📖 p168).
- Haemothorax, pleural effusion, empyema (📖 p168).
- Chest drain in situ.
- Pulmonary embolism.

- Remember the analgesic ladder, escalate appropriately:
  - Paracetamol 1g QDS PO, PR or (most effective) IV.
  - Co-dydramol® two tablets QDS PO.
  - Paracetamol 1g QDS PO/R and tramadol 100mg PO QDS.
  - Paracetamol 1g QDS PO/R and tramadol 100mg PO QDS and ibuprofen 2–400mg PO PRN for breakthrough pain (max QDS).
  - Paracetamol 1g QDS PO/R and morphine PCA or infusion.
- Ask an anaesthetist to review the epidural if the block is inadequate.

Wound problems

- Unstable sternum may reflect underlying wound infection:
  - Swab the wound and start empirical antibiotics (e.g. ciprofloxacin 500mg BD).
  - Give analgesia as above—a 'cough-lock' sometimes helps.
  - Discuss with senior cover—the definitive management is re-sternotomy.
- Treat wound infection very aggressively—mediastinitis and bronchopleural fistulae are potential complications with high mortality:
  - Infected wounds should be swabbed and empirical antibiotics started (e.g. cefuroxime 1.5g TDS IV and metronidazole 500mg TDS).
  - Consider a vacuum pump dressing or surgical debridement if there is frank pus—discuss with senior cover.

Myocardial ischaemia

- Uncommon but serious complication following cardiac or thoracic surgery.
- Sit the patient up, give 6–8L O_2 by face mask.
- Give 75mg aspirin and start IV GTN infusion.
- Give 40mg clexane SC daily.
- Discuss with senior cover immediately and cardiology registrar—*intra-aortic balloon pump*, coronary angiography, re-sternotomy may be indicated in patients after CABG.
  - An *intra-aortic balloon pump* is a sausage-shaped balloon inserted into the aorta via the femoral artery. It inflates during diastole and deflates during systole. This reduces the work of the ventricle and improves coronary perfusion, reducing myocardial ischaemia. Limb ischaemia is one complication.

Arrhythmias and pacing

VF, ventricular tachycardia (VT), peak endocardial acceleration (PEA), asystole in cardiac surgery patients

Use the ALS algorithm *and* talk to senior cover. The following adjuncts must be considered as they are potentially life-saving measures:
- In bradycardia, asystole and PEA, connect temporary pacing wires to a pacing box and pace (see box).
- *Emergency re-sternotomy* to correct underlying problem, e.g. graft occlusion, tamponade, allow internal cardiac massage, or addition of pacing wires.

Common postoperative arrhythmias are:
- Atrial fibrillation (AF) and atrial flutter.
- Atrial ectopics.
- Ventricular ectopics, ventricular tachycardia (VT).
- Sinus tachycardia.
- Junctional bradycardias and tachycardias.
- Bradycardias.
- Heart block.

More than one-third of patients after cardiothoracic surgery experience arrhythmias. They are rarely benign: complications include major haemodynamic compromise as well as stroke and other embolic complications.

Think about
- Is the patient haemodynamically compromised? **Immediate definitive management is needed**.
- Is this a sign of a serious underlying surgical problem?

Ask about
- If patient is symptomatic, including unresponsive, chest pain—**needs immediate definitive management**.
- BP, pulse rate.
- K^+.
- Oxygen saturations, PaO_2.

Look for
- Preoperative anti-arrhythmics (particularly β-blockers) not recommenced.
- ECG changes suggesting myocardial ischaemia.
- Temporary pacing wires (see box).

Investigations
- K^+, Mg^{2+}.
- pH, $PaCO_2$, PaO_2.
- 12-lead ECG.

Pacing after cardiac surgery

- Temporary pacing wires are commonly attached to the epicardium and brought out to the skin after cardiac surgery, especially AVR.
- Wires may be attached to the right ventricle or right atrium.
- You can ∴ pace the ventricles or the atria.
- To pace you must know whether the wires are atrial or ventricular; connect a pair of wires to a pacing box, usually via a pacing lead.
- The safest mode of pacing is demand (DDD): the box will not pace the heart unless it senses no activity, at a rate of 60–90 beats per minute (bpm), 5–10mV.
- If patient loses pacing and cardiac output, **get immediate help, check all connections and start basic life support.**

Management

- Ask nurses to place patient on monitor.
- If haemodynamically unstable, go straight to **definitive management**.
- Aim for serum K^+ 4.5–5.0mEq/L:
  - Give 10–40mmol KCl in 100mL 5% dextrose via CVP line over 20min (fastest); or
  - 40mmol KCl in 1L 5% dextrose or N saline via peripheral line over 8hr; or
  - 3 tablets Sando-K® TDS for 48hr.
- Hyperkalaemia is not usually a problem—if serum K^+ >6.0mEq/L, give 50mL 50% dextrose with 15 units Actrapid® over 20min, check BMs and repeat if necessary.
- Aim for serum Mg^{2+} of 1.0mEq/L:
  - Give 2.5–5g $MgSO_4$ via central line over 20min.
- Correct hypoxia and hypercarbia (📖 p188), and acidosis (📖 p190).

Definitive management

Atrial fibrillation and flutter

- Amiodarone for cardioversion (avoid when poor LV function):
  - Loading via central line—300mg IV over 1hr, then 900mg over 23hr.
  - Loading orally—400mg TDS for 24hr.
  - Maintenance—200mg TDS PO for 1 week, 200mg BD PO for 1 week, 200mg OD for 6 weeks.
- Digoxin for rate control (better than amiodarone in poor LV function):
  - Loading via central line—125mg over 20min, repeated up to a maximum of 1250mg, or until rate control achieved.
  - Maintenance—62.5–250mg PO OD titrated to digoxin levels.
- DC cardioversion for persistent or compromising AF—patient should be sedated with anaesthetic assistance. Give **synchronized** DC shocks of 50J, then 100J, then 200J, then 360J until sinus rhythm restored. If unsure ask senior cover or cardiology for assistance.

Bradycardia

- Pacing if epicardial wires are present (see box).
- Atropine 300–900mcg IV.
- Adrenaline 0.5mL 1:10 000 IV; consider isoprenaline infusion.

The oliguric patient

Glomerular filtration rate and hence urine output is a sensitive measure of renal perfusion and hence cardiac function. Oliguria in cardiac patients may be a sign of serious problems, so treat early and aggressively.

Definition of oliguria after cardiac surgery

- Urine output <1mL/kg/hr.

Think about
- Is this primarily a renal problem or a cardiac problem?
- Is the patient adequately hydrated, or fluid overloaded?

Ask about
- Exact urine output each hour for last 3hr.
- Total fluid balance.
- BP and CVP.
- K^+, pH, PaO_2, serum creatinine.
- Is the catheter working—has the nurse tried a bladder washout?
- Preoperative creatinine.

Look for
- Signs of dehydration:
  - Dry mucous membranes, ↓ skin turgor.
  - ↓CVP or JVP, rises then falls (or unchanged) with fluid challenge.
  - No peripheral oedema.
  - No pulmonary oedema, sharp costophrenic angles on CXR.
- Signs of fluid overload:
  - Hydrated mucous membranes, peripheral oedema.
  - ↑CVP or JVP, rises and remains high with fluid challenge.
  - Pulmonary oedema and/or effusions on CXR.
- Distended bladder.
- Nephrotoxic drugs and consider stopping them:
  - NSAIDs.
  - Antibiotics including vancomycin, gentamicin.

Investigations
- K^+, creatinine and urea.
- pH, base excess.
- CXR.
- Bladder ultrasonography if concern that there is a distended bladder.

Management

- Aim for CVP 12–14mmHg and systolics >120mmHg:
    - If CVP is low, give colloid, e.g. 250mL Gelofusine®, and repeat if necessary.
    - If CVP >14mmHg and BP >110mmHg, give 20mg furosemide IV.
    - If CVP is high and BP low, discuss with senior cover—you may need to start inotropes, e.g. adrenaline (epinephrine) 0.03mcg/kg/min or dopamine 5.0mcg/kg/min, and exclude cardiac tamponade.
- Treat any arrhythmias (📖 p198).
- Treat hypoxia (📖 p187).

Treat the important problems associated with severe oliguria

These are all indications for haemodialysis if they do not respond to basic measures.

- Pulmonary and potentially cerebral oedema:
    - Sit the patient up if possible.
    - Give 6–8L O_2 by tightly fitting face mask.
    - Furosemide 20–40mg IV.
- Hyperkalaemia:
    - 50mL 50% dextrose with 15 units Actrapid® over 20min.
    - Repeat if necessary, checking BMs.
    - Calcium resonium.
    - Sodium bicarbonate.
- Acidosis:
    - Hydrate the patient if no evidence of volume overload.
    - Furosemide 20–40mg IV if patient adequately hydrated.
    - $NaHCO_3$ 50–100mL IV if patient ventilated/$PaCO_2$ <5.0kPa
- Drug toxicity—reduce doses and monitor levels of drugs that depend on renal excretion:
    - Digoxin.
    - Heparin.
    - Vancomycin.
    - Opiates.

Chest drains

Management of chest drains

Chest drainage should always be into a container with an underwater seal.

Clamping chest drains

Some nurses have been trained to do this when transferring patients. This stems from the days of treatment for tuberculosis with caustic solutions, and was aimed to prevent drain effluent draining back into the chest. In modern practice the **ONLY** indications for clamping drains are: (1) in the trauma setting if the patient is exsanguinating through it (>1500mL blood after insertion) and (2) under specialist supervision prior to drain removal in a patient with a chronic air leak.

- Clamping a thoracic drain in a patient with an air leak may rapidly result in a **tension pneumothorax**.
- Clamping a mediastinal drain in a patient who is bleeding may rapidly result in **cardiac tamponade**.
- The safest mode is an **unclamped** drain connected to an underwater seal that is kept **below** the level of the patient at **all** times.
- If you connect the drain to wall suction, but do not put the wall suction on. this is effectively clamping the drain. If you and the nurses do not know what you are doing, ASK FOR HELP.
- If you press the one-way valve on the top of the underwater seal in too tightly, this is effectively clamping the drain. If in doubt, pull it out!

Management of chest drains inserted for pneumothorax

- Put the drain on low-pressure high-volume wall suction (–3 to –5kPa) initially (NOT the high-pressure wall suction used for tracheal toilet).
- Request CXR daily.
- Bubbling in the underwater seal, either continuously or only when the patient coughs, indicates an air leak, and that the lung parenchyma has not healed. You can only **remove the drain when there is no air leak**, otherwise a pneumothorax will rapidly re-form.
- When the air leak stops, take the drain off suction for 12hr and repeat CXR. If the lung is fully up, the drain can be removed.
- Always perform a CXR after drain removal to check for a pneumo thorax.

Management of chest drains inserted to drain collections

Management of chest trauma is described on 📖 p166.

- There is no evidence that placing these drains on suction improves outcome.
- Make sure that the nursing staff measure the drainage—hourly in the postoperative patient, every 24hr in longer-term drains.

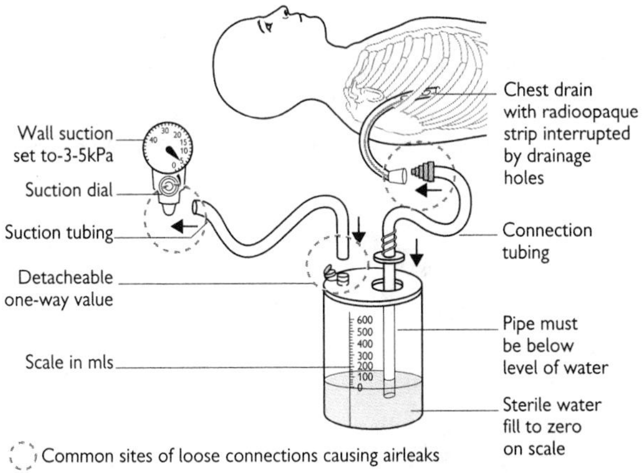

Fig. 5.5 Diagram showing chest drain, underwater seal, and connection and drainage tubing.

A haemodynamically unstable postoperative patient, or one who is draining more than 300mL blood per hr, should be discussed urgently with the thoracic surgeons.

- Postoperative thoracic drains are normally removed when they drain nothing for two consecutive hours, unless there is an air leak.
- Drains for pleural effusions can be removed when they drain less than 250mL in 24hr.
- Drains for empyemas can be removed when they stop draining completely.
- Always request and review a CXR after drain removal to check for pneumothorax.

Problems with chest drains

Air leak at site of insertion ± surgical emphysema

- In inspiration, air is sucked into the pleural cavity.
- In expiration, air is blown out around the drain and/or, if there is surgical emphysema, into the subcutaneous tissues.
- There are four main causes:
  - Drain site loose—put a horizontal mattress stitch in the skin around the drain and tie quite tightly.
  - Drain holes in contact with air—remove the drain (the drain is not sterile so you cannot simply push it back in). If there is a large residual pneumothorax, insert a new drain.
  - Massive air leak, too large for drain—patient needs multiple drains or definitive surgical repair.
  - Drain is blocked—check for and correct kinking, clamping, occluded one-way valve, suction connected but not turned on.

No respiratory swing

- Usually the fluid in the drain moves up and down with respiration, reflecting changes in intrathoracic pressure; no swing suggests:
  - Pleural space is obliterated and a drain is not necessary.
  - Drain is not in the pleural cavity—check with CXR.
  - Drain is clamped, kinked or blocked—check and correct.

Chapter 6

Neurosurgery

James Laban

Introduction

Swift optimal management of neurosurgical emergencies can drastically improve prognosis—truly, you can save lives. The principles of management, however, are fairly straightforward.

- Always think 'ABC', ensuring adequate brain and spine oxygenation.
- Ensure all patients have well documented, regular neurological observations.
- Never disregard a change in a patient's neurological status.
- Head and spine injuries often coexist—if your patient has one, consider the other.
- Remember that CT scanners have been nicknamed 'doughnuts of death' for a reason—if necessary, protect the airway beforehand.
- Finally, and most importantly, ensure your registrar or consultant is aware of all changes—neurosurgeons want to know everything about their patients.

In most centres, unlike other specialties, the registrar takes the referrals. This chapter includes a section on all the basic information needed for a satisfactory referral. In the simplest terms, three things are of interest:

- Neurology.
- Mass effect.
- Premorbid status.

The more junior medical staff tend not to be involved in the emergency patient who is rushed to theatre from the emergency department; only postoperatively (and sometimes following a lengthy intensive care stay) will you manage those patients. You will admit the more stable patients, usually with a confirmed diagnosis; arrange full preoperative work-up, care for the patients postoperatively and organize rehabilitation and discharge.

Considered here for each pathology is the care of those patients who are stable enough for the ward. Should these ward patients with intracranial pathologies deteriorate neurologically, you should refer to the sections on ↓ Glasgow Coma Score (GCS) and intracranial pressure (ICP) management.

Anatomy

Understanding anatomy is the key to understanding the symptoms and deficits that various pathologies can cause. Some 90% of the population is right-handed, of whom 95% are estimated to be left hemisphere dominant for expressive and receptive linguistic functions and fine motor control. About half of left-handed people are also left hemisphere dominant. This cerebral dominance is of particular relevance when considering outcome.

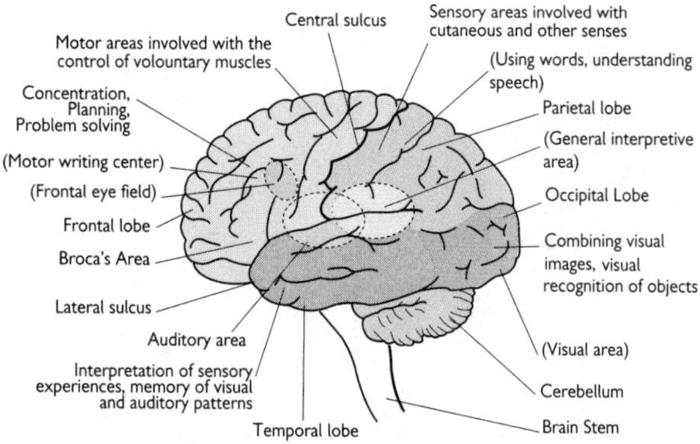

Fig. 6.1 Lateral view of the brain (functional area description in brackets).

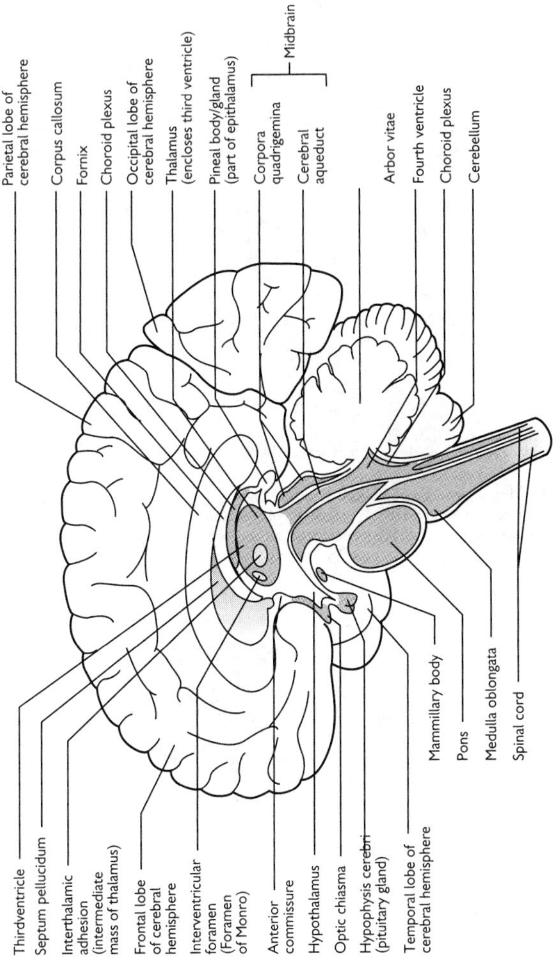
Parietal lobe of cerebral hemisphere
Corpus callosum
Fornix
Choroid plexus
Occipital lobe of cerebral hemisphere
Thalamus (encloses third ventricle)
Pineal body/gland (part of epithalamus)
Corpora quadrigemina
Cerebral aqueduct
Midbrain
Arbor vitae
Fourth ventricle
Choroid plexus
Cerebellum
Thirdventricle
Septum pellucidum
Interthalamic adhesion (intermediate mass of thalamus)
Frontal lobe of cerebral hemisphere
Interventricular foramen (Foramen of Monro)
Anterior commissure
Hypothalamus
Optic chiasma
Hypophysis cerebri (pituitary gland)
Temporal lobe of cerebral hemisphere
Mammillary body
Pons
Medulla oblongata
Spinal cord

Fig. 6.2 Sagittal view of the brain.

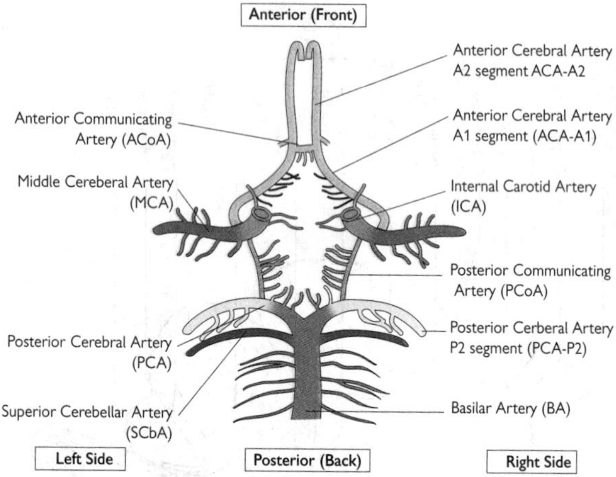

Fig. 6.3 Intracranial arterial blood supply. ACA: leg, motor and sensory; MCA: arm and face, motor and sensory; PCA: visual area and 5Ds (dysarthria, dysphagia, diplopia, dizziness, dysmetria); BA: cerebellum and brainstem.

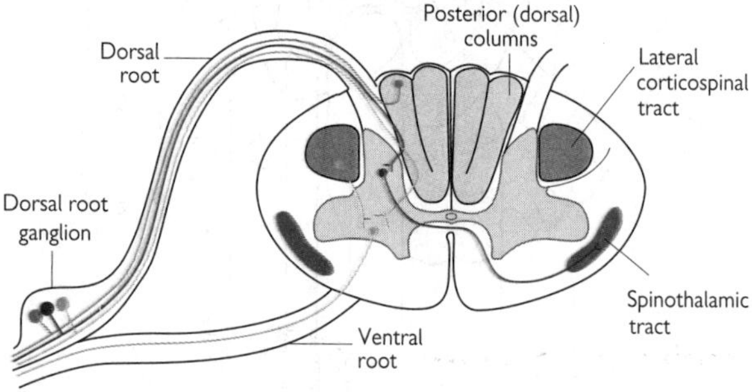

Fig. 6.4 Axial spinal cord.

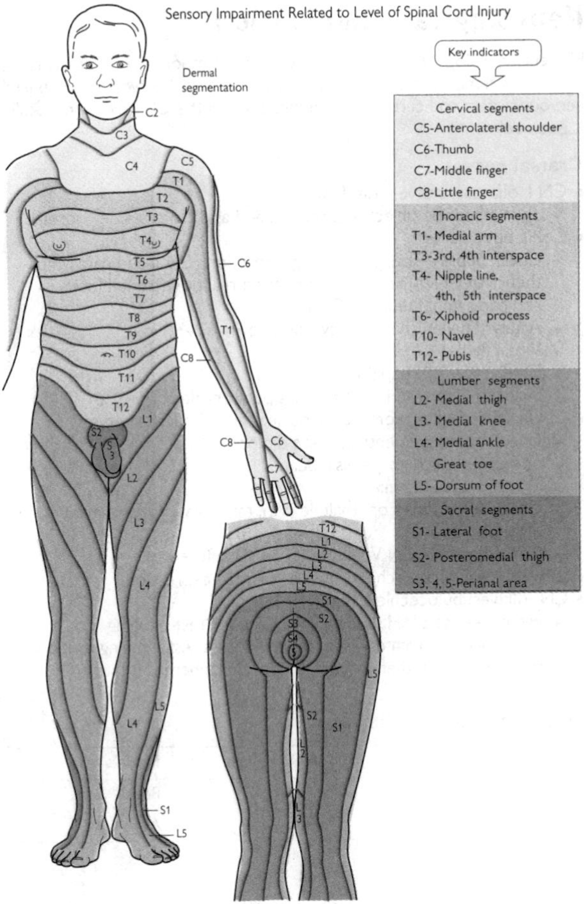
Sensory Impairment Related to Level of Spinal Cord Injury
Dermal segmentation
Key indicators
Cervical segments
C5-Anterolateral shoulder
C6-Thumb
C7-Middle finger
C8-Little finger
Thoracic segments
T1- Medial arm
T3-3rd, 4th interspace
T4- Nipple line,
4th, 5th interspace
T6- Xiphoid process
T10- Navel
T12- Pubis
Lumber segments
L2- Medial thigh
L3- Medial knee
L4- Medial ankle
Great toe
L5- Dorsum of foot
Sacral segments
S1- Lateral foot
S2- Posteromedial thigh
S3, 4, 5-Perianal area
C2
C3
C4
C5
T1
T2
T3
T4
T5
T6
T7
T8
T9
T10
T11
T12
L1
L2
L3
L4
L5
S1
S2
C6
C7
C8

Fig. 6.5 Dermatomes.

Neurological examination

Efficient neurological examination is of utmost importance in determining neurosurgical management. A short summary of cranial nerves, the peripheral nervous system and cerebellar examination, and the Glasgow Coma Scale, is given below.

Cranial nerves

- CN I: olfactory nerve—rarely tested.
  - Take a bedside object, e.g. orange, and ask 'Does it smell normal?'
- CN II: optic nerve:
  - Check pupils—size, pupillary light reaction (CN II and parasympathetics of CN III) and accommodation reaction (frontal lobes and parasympathetics of CN III).
  - Acuity (Snellen chart or newspaper print size).
  - Visual fields.
  - Fundi, especially papilloedema.
  - Swinging light test, for an afferent pupillary defect.
- CN III, IV and VI: oculomotor, trochlear and abducens nerves:
  - Check eye movements. Is there diplopia? Where is it worst? Cover one eye—which image disappears?
- CN V: trigeminal nerve:
  - Check sensation in ophthalmic (Va), maxillary (Vb) and mandibular divisions (Vc).
  - Corneal reflex (CN V, afferent; CN VII, efferent).
- CN VII: facial nerve—check muscles of facial expression.
- CN VIII: vestibulocochlear nerve:
  - Hearing—use 516Hz tuning fork. Weber's test—tuning fork on vertex; in which ear is it louder? Rinne's test—tuning fork on mastoid (bone), then in front of ear (air); where is it louder?

Table 6.1 Testing for deafness

Type of deafness	Weber's test	Rinne's test
Conductive deafness	Deaf ear	Bone > Air
Sensorineural deafness	Good ear	Air > Bone

  - Gait.
  - Caloric testing: warm water—nystagmus towards stimulus; cold water—away from stimulus.
- CN IX, X: glossopharyngeal and vagus nerves:
  - Uvula moves away from side of lesion.
  - Check swallow, cough and voice.
  - Gag reflex (CN IX and CN X).
- CN XI: accessory nerve:
  - Check sternocleidomastoid and trapezius.
- CNXII: hypoglossal nerve:
  - Tongue deviates towards side of lesion.

Peripheral nervous system

- Tone:
  - Normal, flaccid or spastic?
- Power.

Table 6.2 Testing for muscle power

Medical Research Council (MRC) grade	Muscle movement
5	Normal power
4	Against resistance
3	Against gravity
2	Gravity eliminated
1	Flicker
0	None

MRC.

Table 6.3 Testing for muscle power

Nerve root	Action
C5	Shoulder abduction
C6	Wrist extension
C7	Elbow extension
C8	Finger flexion
T1	Finger abduction
L2	Hip flexion
L3	Knee extension
L4	Ankle dorsiflexion
L5	Big toe extension
S1	Ankle plantarflexion
S2	Hip extension

Table 6.4 Reflexes

Reflex	Nerve roots or tracts
Biceps	C5, C6
Supinator	C6, C7
Triceps	C7, C8
Knee jerk	L3, L4
Ankle jerk	S1, S2
Babinski	Corticospinal tracts

- Sensation:
  - Spinothalamic—pinprick, temperature and light touch.
  - Dorsal columns—vibration, joint position, light touch, Romberg's sign. If patient falls with eyes open, this suggests a central cause. If falls with eyes closed, there is a problem with the dorsal columns.

Cerebellar examination

- Coordination: finger–nose (past pointing) and heel–shin tests.
- Repeated movements—pat one hand on the back of the other (dysdiadochokinesis).
- Eye movements—nystagmus.
- Gait—ataxia.
- Speech—slurred.
- Tone—hypotonia.

Glasgow Coma Scale

This is the most crucial part of the examination on neurosurgical wards.

Published in 1974 by Graham Teasdale and Bryan J. Jennett of the University of Glasgow, the Glasgow Coma Scale (GCS) is composed of three parameters:

- Best eye response.
- Best verbal response.
- Best motor response.

The worst score is 3 and the best is 15. However, it is important always to describe the GCS in terms of its three components.

If a potential neurosurgical patient is on a non-neurosurgical ward, ensure the nursing staff are experienced in assessing the GCS.

Best eye response

1 No eye opening.
2 Eye opening to pain.
3 Eye opening to verbal command.
4 Eye opening spontaneous.

Best verbal response

1 No verbal response.
2 Incomprehensible sounds.
3 Inappropriate words.
4 Confused.
5 Orientated.

Best motor response

1 No motor response.
2 Extension to pain (decerebrate response).
3 Flexion to pain (decorticate response).
4 Withdrawal from pain.
5 Localizing pain.
6 Obeys command.

Neuroradiology

Normal head CT scan

In most hospitals in the UK, the on-call radiology service is usually involved in the approval for and interpretation of out-of-hours CT head scans. Even so, it is useful for all doctors involved with these cases to be familiar with some basic concepts of interpreting CT brains. Even without a detailed understanding of neuroanatomy it should be relatively easy to identify gross abnormalities.

Tips

- Blood is bright (high density).
- Infarcts are dark (low density).
- Cerebrospinal fluid (CSF) is dark (low density).
- CSF spaces should be reviewed to check for presence of blood.
- A CT head is performed with patient supine, so blood tends to layer in dependant regions of the CSF spaces.
- Altering the windowing of the scan on your local Picture Archiving and Communication System (PACS) will aid identification of abnormalities—look for fractures using bone windows (W500/L4000). Blood is made more conspicuous by widening the window width (~W250/L35).
- Check to see whether the scan is with or without contrast (usually annotated—otherwise, the cerebral vessels will be bright on an enhanced scan).

Normal axial CT brain

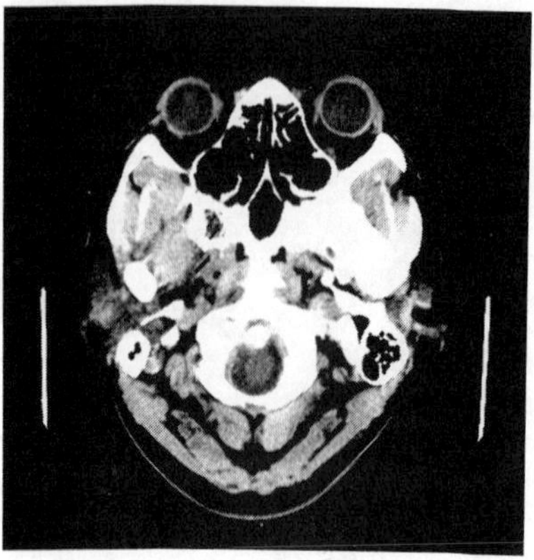

Fig. 6.6 Normal axial CT brain at foramen magnum.

Base of the scan showing the foramen magnum. Note the brainstem in the centre with rim of low density surrounding it—this is CSF. Absence of this low-density rim suggests descent of the cerebellar tonsils—coning!

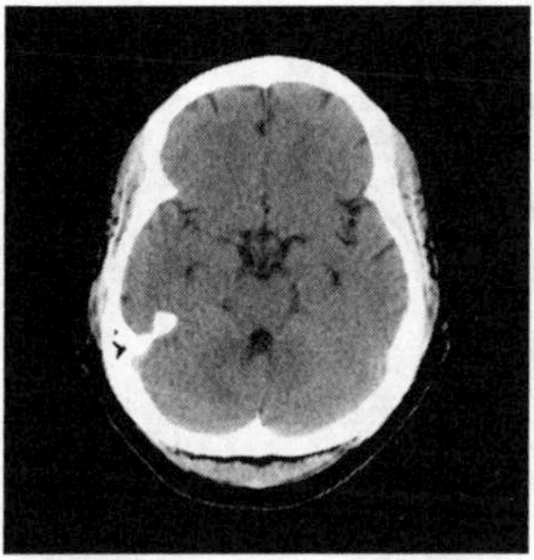

Fig. 6.7 Normal axial CT brain at midbrain.

This is a slice taken at the level of the midbrain; posteriorly the cerebellum can be seen. Check the fourth ventricle, the Sylvian fissures and basal cisterns (prepontine and ambient)—these should contain only CSF; if any was blood present in these CSF spaces, it would be bright (white/high density). The temporal horns of the lateral ventricles are also shown; they should be slit-like and of equal size. In subtle subarachnoid haemorrhage (SAH), dilatation of the temporal horns, either unilateral or bilateral, due to the development of non-communicating hydrocephalus may be the only sign of the presence of blood.

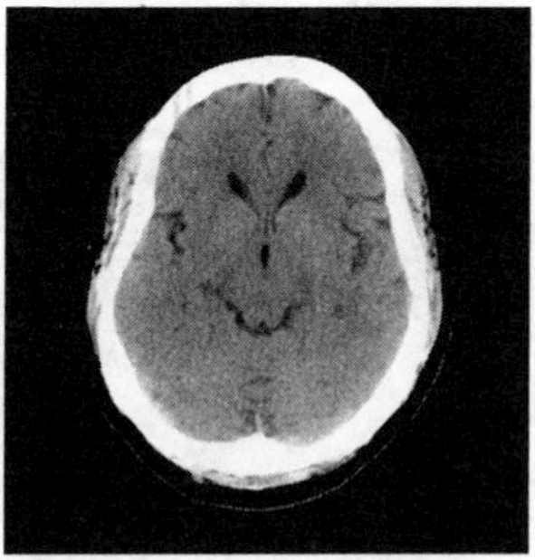

Fig. 6.8 Normal axial CT brain at basal ganglia.

This slice is taken at the level of the basal ganglia. The quadrigeminal cistern should be checked—look for the 'bum on seat', made up of the humps of the tectal plate and the CSF space. If there is a marked ↑ in intracranial pressure (ICP), this is effaced early on. Note also the normal slit-like third ventricle and the frontal horns of the lateral ventricles.

Signs of raised intracranial pressure

- Effacement of the sulci overlying the cerebral hemispheres.
- Effacement of basal cisterns (including loss of 'bum on seat').
- No space in the foramen magnum, due to descent of cerebellar tonsils—the patient is coning!

Extradural blood: axial unenhanced CT brain

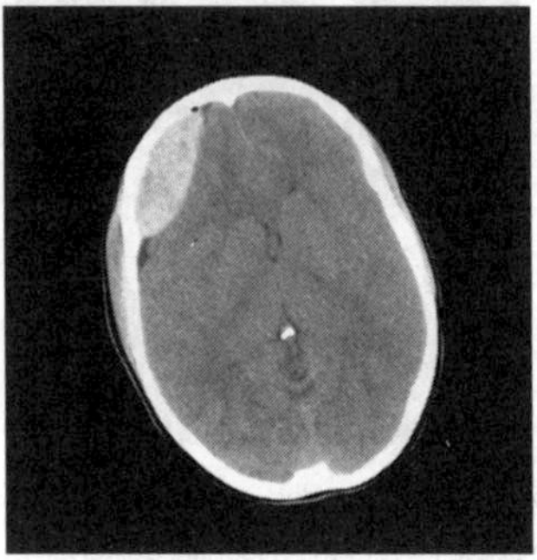

Fig. 6.9 (A) Classical right frontal extradural haematoma.

Note that the haematoma is biconvex (lentiform) in shape and of high density. There is a tiny pocket of gas in its most superior part, which raises the possibility of underlying bony disruption. Note that the anterior midline structures of this rotated scan are deviated to the left due to mass effect from the haematoma. In addition, none of the normal sulci overlying the cerebral hemispheres are visible due to compression as a result of ↑ ICP. The right frontal horn of the lateral ventricle has been effaced.

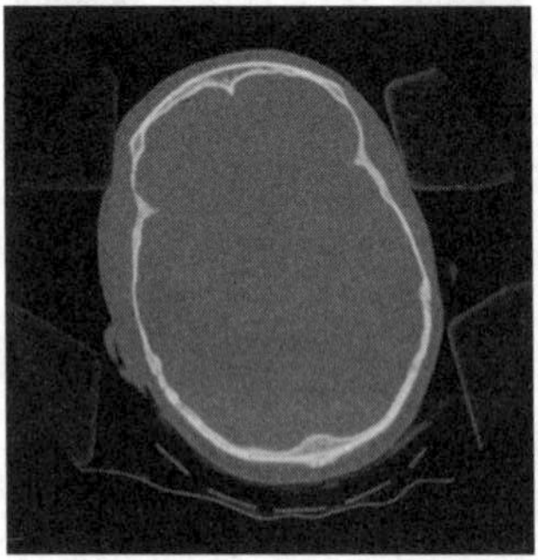

Fig. 6.9 (B) Shows the same slice as in Fig. 6.9A with bone windows.

A non-depressed right frontal bone fracture is marked. There is soft tissue swelling over the right frontoparietal region and the patient's head is in sand-blocks. The patient had been involved in a road traffic accident (RTA) and was intubated on arrival in A&E. Urgent neurosurgical intervention was undertaken.

Subdural blood: axial unenhanced CT brain

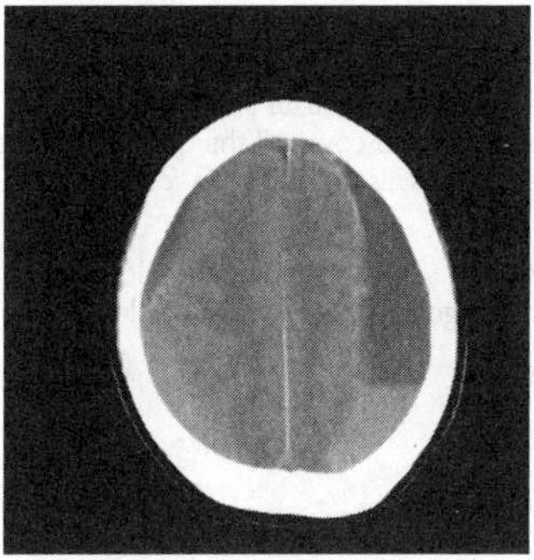

Fig. 6.10 Acute on chronic subdural blood—axial unenhanced CT brain.

This 82-yr-old man was admitted from a nursing home with worsening of chronic confusion and a recent fall. There are bilateral subdural haematomas on the left extending over the entire cerebral convexity, and on the right overlying the frontoparietal convexity. The shape is typically crescentic. On the left, fresh blood can be seen layered in a dependant location (presumably due to trauma in the recent fall), the low-density anterior to this represents old haematoma. Notice that the left cerebral parenchyma is very compressed.

Subarachnoid blood: axial unenhanced CT brain

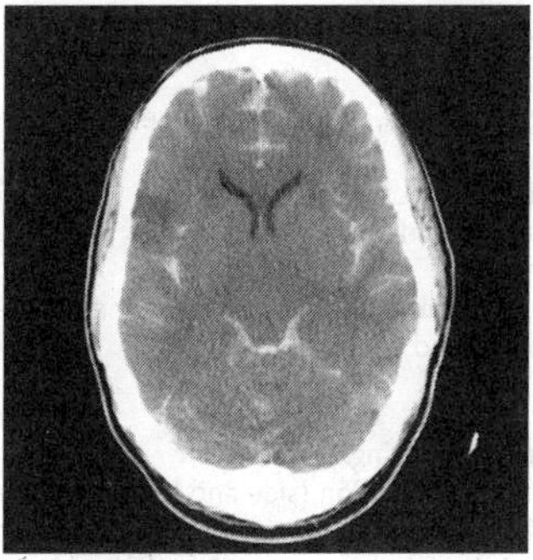

Fig. 6.11 Subarachnoid blood–axial unenhanced CT brain.

High density is seen within all sulci and within the quadrigeminal cistern, which is effaced. This is a gross example of diffuse SAH, in this case due to rupture of an aneurysm.

Neurosurgical referrals

The neurosurgical registrar will usually take all referrals, but there may be circumstances in which you are asked to answer the bleep (e.g. the registrar is scrubbed up and about to evacuate an extradural).

This section endeavours to cover all the questions you should ask before informing your senior. It is also a proforma for any doctor referring to the neurosurgeon on-call.

Note: In the event that you are holding the bleep, all referrals should be discussed with your registrar as soon as possible.

Patient details

- Name.
- Age.
- Sex.
- Ward.
- Referring hospital.
- Referring consultant.
- Referring specialty.
- Referring doctor.
- Contact number—bleep or extension.

Ask about

- History of presenting complaint, including mechanism of injury if trauma.
- Current symptoms.
- Sphincter disturbance in spinal patients.
- Previous medical history.
- Medication—specifically *anticoagulants* inc. aspirin and clopidogrel.

Look for

- GCS initially and now.
- Pupil size and reactivity.
- Focal neurological deficits, especially reflexes and sphincters in spinal patients.
- CSF otorrhoea and rhinorrhoea if relevant.
- Blood pressure (BP) and pulse.
- Oxygen saturation.
- Other injuries, especially spinal, if trauma (remember ATLS).
- Is patient intubated and ventilated?

Investigations

- FBC, U&Es, glucose, clotting.
- CT head—anatomical location (side and lobe) of the lesion, contrast enhancement and oedema if relevant, amount of midline shift (in centimetres), ventricular size, effacement of sulci and basal cisterns, skull fractures if relevant (seen on scout view), intracranial air, opacification of sinuses.
- Other, including other imaging (e.g. C-spine).

NICE head injury guidelines

National Institute for Health and Clinical Excellence: www.nice.org.uk

Patients who have sustained a head injury and present with any one of the following risk factors should have a CT scan of the head requested immediately.

Risk factors

- GCS <13 at any point since the injury.
- GCS of 13 or 14 at 2hr post-injury.
- Suspected open or depressed skull fracture.
- Any sign of basal skull fracture—haemotympanum, 'panda' eyes, CSF otorrhoea, Battle's sign.
- Post-traumatic seizure.
- Focal neurological deficit.
- > one episode of vomiting—clinical judgement should be used regarding the cause of vomiting in those aged ≤12yrs and whether imaging is necessary.
- Amnesia >30min of events before impact—assessment of amnesia will not be possible in pre-verbal children and is unlikely to be possible in any child <5yrs.

CT should also be immediately requested in patients with any of the following risk factors, provided they have experienced some loss of consciousness or amnesia since the injury.

Risk factors

- Age ≥65yrs.
- Coagulopathy—history of bleeding, clotting disorder, current treatment with warfarin.
- Dangerous mechanism of injury (e.g. pedestrian struck by motor vehicle or fall from height >1m or five stairs). A lower threshold for height of falls should be used when dealing with infants and young children aged <5yrs.

General points

- Current NICE guidelines indicate that the 1° investigation of choice for the detection of acute, clinically significant, brain injuries is CT imaging of the head. Skull X-rays may be used in the detection of non-accidental injury (NAI) in children, or in conjunction with high-quality inpatient observation where CT s unavailable.
- If the head injury is minor, patients should be discharged with a responsible adult who can call for assistance when required. If this is not possible, the patient should be admitted overnight.

Which head injuries to refer to neurosurgery?—NICE guidelines

- All patients with new, surgically significant, findings on imaging.
- Persisting coma (GCS ≤8) after initial resuscitation—most will have a toxic metabolite aetiology.
- Unexplained confusion >4hr.
- Deterioration in GCS after admission.
- Progressive focal neurological signs.
- Seizure without full recovery.
- Penetrating injury.
- CSF leak.

Which head injuries to admit to hospital?

- All patients with new, clinically significant, findings on imaging.
- Patients who have not returned to GCS 15, regardless of imaging results.
- Patients who fulfil the criteria for CT but are unable to undergo CT.
- Continuing worrying clinical signs, e.g. persistent vomiting or severe headaches.
- Other clinical concerns, e.g. other injuries, CSF leak, meningism, shock, intoxication.

☠ Decreased GCS

Timely, effective intervention in a patient with a ↓ GCS may be life saving.

Think about

If you get a call about a patient with a deterioration of GCS, including ↑ confusion or agitation, you must see them urgently. Even a drop of one point can be highly significant and timely intervention can prevent significant morbidity, e.g. vasospasm following SAH causing dominant hemisphere infarct. Never ignore any drop in GCS!

At GCS ≤8 the patient will have an impaired ability to protect the airway and an anaesthetist should be called.

In normotensive patients with a normal PaO_2, the following causes of a ↓ GCS should be considered:

- Hypo/hyperglycaemia.
- Alcohol.
- Drugs, e.g. benzodiazepines, opiates, anaesthetic agents.
- Electrolyte disturbances, e.g. hypo/hypernatraemia.
- Seizures.
- Meningitis.
- Encephalitis.
- Encephalopathy, e.g. hypoxic, hepatic, uraemic.
- Intracranial lesion, e.g. haematoma, diffuse axonal injury (DAI), hydrocephalus, abscess, tumour.

Ask about

- Current inpatient management.
- Previous medical history inc. seizures, diabetes.
- Medication inc. analgesia and sedatives.

Look for

- What is the GCS?
- Any focal neurological deterioration, esp. pupillary reaction.
- Cardiorespiratory compromise.
- Signs of seizure activity.
- Fever.
- Meningism—neck stiffness, photophobia, Kernig or Brudzinski sign.

Investigations

- FBC, U&Es, glucose, clotting, group and save.
- ABG (oxygenation, acidosis).
- CT.
- Consider lumbar puncture.
- Consider EEG.

Management

- ABC.
- ATLS—assume cervical spine injury (trauma).
- Maintain oxygenation and normal BP—to ensure adequate cerebral perfusion.
- Nil by mouth—possible surgery or impaired ability to protect airway.
- Inform neurosurgical specialist registrar (SpR).
- Call anaesthetic SpR if GCS ≤8 or not protecting airway.
- Determine, and if possible reverse, cause of ↓ GCS.

General points

- Well documented, regular neurological observations.
- Ensure adequate hydration.
- Consider nasogastric (NG) or orogastric (OG) feed.
- Consider laxatives.
- Consider antithrombotic prophylaxis.
- Consider gastrointestinal ulcer protection.

ICP and ICP management

Acute neurosurgical management is based on maintaining optimal brain tissue oxygenation and preventing brain herniation whereby the brain is squeezed past structures within the skull, severely compressing it. If brainstem compression is involved, this may lead to ↓ respiratory drive and is potentially fatal. This herniation is often referred to as 'coning'.

Monro–Kellie doctrine

In 1783 Alexander Monro deduced that the cranium was a 'rigid box' filled with a 'nearly incompressible brain' and that its total volume tended to remain constant. The doctrine states that any increase in the volume of the cranial contents (e.g. brain, blood, CSF) will ↑ ICP. Further, if one of these three elements increases in volume, it must occur at the expense of volume of the other elements. In 1824 George Kellie confirmed many of Monro's early observations.

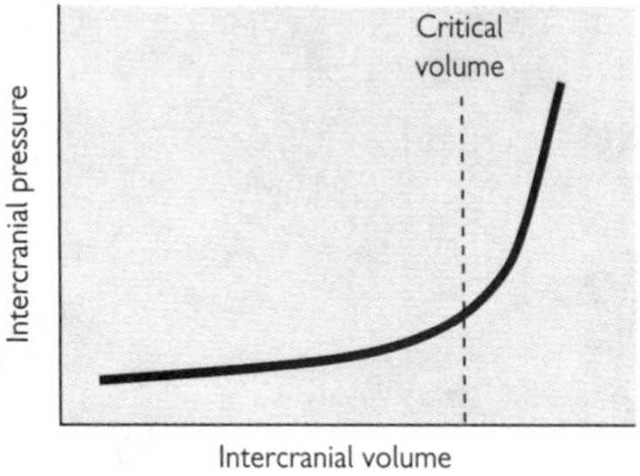

Fig. 6.12 Monro–Kellie doctrine.

Initially some compensation is possible as CSF and blood move extracranially (into the thecal sac around the spine). However, there is a critical point beyond which minimal changes in volume (such as intubation, coughing or even lying flat) will cause dramatic rises in ICP and may cause coning (herniation of the brain into the foramen magnum), and thus lead to death.

Brain tissue oxygenation

In simplest terms, this depends on cerebral perfusion pressure and oxygen content in the blood (Hb and oxygen saturation). Once Hb and oxygen saturation have been optimized, cerebral perfusion pressure becomes singularly important:

$$CPP = MAP - ICP$$

where CPP is cerebral perfusion pressure, MAP is mean arterial pressure and ICP is intracranial pressure.

ICP is normally 0–10mmHg, but can rise much higher in pathological states. When ICP >20mmHg, treatment should be considered.

CPP should be maintained >70–80mmHg; consequently MAP and ICP management is critically important.

ICP management

Timely, effective ICP management may be life saving.

Raised ICP is the final common pathway to brain damage and death from various acute intracranial conditions. Various steps can be taken to try to manage ICP and thereby optimize CPP. Current management algorithms are based on maximizing cerebral perfusion and minimizing cerebral metabolism.

Monitoring

All patients with or at risk of intracranial hypertension must have:

- Invasive arterial line.
- CVP line.
- ICP monitor if unable to assess neurologically, i.e. anaesthetized.
- Urinary catheter.

Primary targets

- 10–15° head up–once C-spine is cleared.
- No venous obstruction—check endotracheal tube ties, avoid excessively constrictive hard collar.
- CPP >70mmHg.
- ICP <25mmHg.
- SpO_2 >97%, PaO_2 >11kPa, $PaCO_2$ 4.0–4.5kPa (or 4.5–5.0 if SAH).
- Temperature—35–37°C.
- Blood sugar 4–7mmol/L.
- CT brain and evacuate significant space-occupying lesions.

Initial anaesthetic agents

- Propofol 2–5mg/kg/hr—check plasma lipids daily if patient cooled.
- Fentanyl 1–2mcg/kg/hr.
- Atracurium 0.5mg/kg/hr.
- Norepinephrine (noradrenaline).

Secondary intervention
If ICP >25mmHg, CPP <60mmHg:
- Check 1° targets.
- Check probe.
- Repeat CT and evacuate significant space-occupying lesions—some centres drain CSF via extraventricular drain if possible.

If repeat CT does not indicate surgical intervention:
- Cool patient—temperature 34–35°C.
- EEG—is the patient in status epilepticus?
- 5% NaCl IV at 2mL/kg—repeat if Na <155mmol/L, Posm <320mOsm/L).
- 20% mannitol IV at 2mL/kg—repeat if Posm <320mOsm/L).
- Consider midazolam (0.1–0.2mg/kg/hr) or thiopental (3–8mg/kg/hr) to maintain burst suppression, i.e. minimize cerebral metabolism.

If these measures fail to control ICP, the patient should be considered for decompressive craniectomy.

Severe traumatic head injury

- Alert neurosurgeon immediately.
- Potentially fatal—requires immediate diagnosis; surgical intervention may be necessary.

Think about

Severe traumatic brain injury is the commonest cause of death in those aged 15–45yrs. The most common causes include RTA, assault, falls from a height and sporting accidents. As always, mechanism can acts as a guide to the extent of injury sustained. Alcohol is often involved.

Head and spinal trauma often coexist. Always assume spinal injury until proven otherwise. It is simple to request a CT head and C-spine. Thoracic and lumbar spine can be cleared with plain X-rays if necessary.

The patient may also have sustained other injuries. These may have been missed in the initial ATLS 2° survey and, indeed, may not become apparent for several days. Keep this in mind.

Urgent surgical intervention may be indicated and optimal treatment can significantly improve outcome. Some of the distinct injuries seen in cranial trauma are included here—they often coexist.

Extradural haematoma (EDH)

Typically caused by a blow to the head and usually associated with an overlying skull fracture. Disruption of the vessels interposed between the cranium and dura causes a pathological collection of blood that may lead to a shift of cranial contents and herniation.

Classically, EDH is associated with a lucid interval between initial loss of consciousness and subsequent deterioration; this occurs in only 30% and level of consciousness may be variable.

CT shows a lentiform-shaped high-density collection (see Fig. 6.9) at the peripheral margins of the hemisphere that does not cross cranial suture lines.

Acute subdural haematoma (ASDH)

Tearing of bridging veins between the cortex and the venous sinuses, or laceration of the brain surface, causes a pathological collection of blood between the dura and the arachnoid. ASDH typically is the result of acceleration–deceleration injuries.

CT shows a hyperdense crescent-shaped collection (see Fig. 6.10).

Chronic subdural haematoma (CSDH)

The pathophysiology of CSDH is essentially the same as for ASDH. However, commonly associated with cerebral atrophy, the causative trauma may be minor, and often forgotten. The patient, usually elderly, alcoholic or coagulopathic, typically presents with ↑ confusion and/or motor weakness.

CSDH may be hyperdense (<7 days old), isodense (7–21 days old), or hypodense (>21 days old) (see Fig. 6.10).

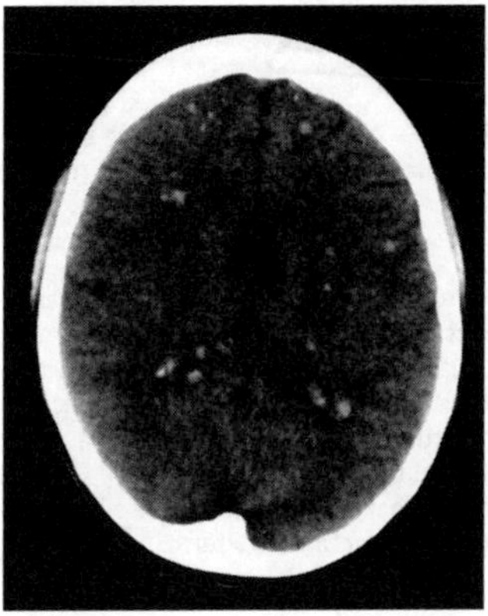

Fig. 6.13 Diffuse axonal injury.

Intracerebral haematoma (ICH) and contusions

ICH usually affect the white matter or basal ganglia (please refer to later section for other causes of ICH). The term contusion refers to more superficial areas of haemorrhage usually affecting the frontal and temporal lobes, sustained as the brain hits the bony protuberances of the skull at the site of impact (coup injury) and then the opposite side during deceleration (contrecoup injury). Contusions may be thought of as bruises of the brain. As ICH and contusions evolve, there is ↑ oedema and infarction, and this may cause neurological deterioration days after injury.

ICH appear hyperdense, whereas contusions may be of variable density.

Diffuse axonal injury

Widespread disruption of axonal sheaths follows the high-energy impact.

CT may show a tight, swollen brain, with petechial haemorrhages and loss of grey–white differentiation (Fig. 6.13). However, CT findings may be normal.

Concussion is thought to be caused by mild DAI and, although the impairment of consciousness is transient, it is sometimes associated with significant long-term sequelae requiring neuropsychological expertise.

Subarachnoid haemorrhage

This is discussed in a separate section (see 📖 p236).

Cranial CSF leak

- Alert neurosurgeon.
- Potentially fatal, requires urgent diagnosis and management.

Think about

- CSF leaks may present as otorrhoea or rhinorrhoea—occasionally patients notice a salty taste as CSF runs down from the nasopharynx.
- CSF leaks are usually caused by trauma or surgery; rarely spontaneous.
- Meningitis is a serious and potentially fatal complication.
- CT may show fracture site, bony defect and pneumocephalus. It may not, however, reveal the site of leak,
- The majority of CSF leaks resolve with conservative treatment.
- Surgical options are extracranial (external, endoscopic) or intracranial.

Ask about

- Trauma—basal skull fracture.
- Previous neurosurgery—typically transphenoidal surgery.
- Cerebral tumour, particularly symptoms of sellar tumours.
- Low-pressure headache.

Look for

- Any neurological deterioration.
- Otorrhoea/rhinorrhoea.
- 'Tramlining'—blood mixed with CSF clots only peripherally as it trickles down the face.
- 'Ring test'—blood clots centrally on blotting paper whilst CSF diffuses outwards.
- Meningism.

Investigations

- FBC, U&Es, glucose, clotting, group and save.
- To confirm CSF leak, test fluid for glucose, β_2-transferrin, tau protein.
- CT head.

Management

- Trial of conservative treatment (1–2 weeks).
- Consider lumbar drain—discuss with registrar.
- Surgical repair (intracranial/extracranial).

General points

- Nurse head-up.
- Avoid coughing, sneezing, nose blowing, heavy lifting.
- Do not use continuous positive airway pressure (CPAP) or bi-level positive airway pressure (BIPAP)—will cause pneumocephalus.
- Consider antithrombotic prophylaxis.

Differential diagnosis

- Blood/mucus from nose or ear.

Skull fractures

Skull fractures often need no specific treatment but may be important because of associated problems. They may be linear, depressed or affecting the skull base. Linear and depressed fractures may be open or closed (see Fig. 6.9B).

Skull fractures are associated with an ↑ risk of intracranial haematoma; however, the importance of this has greatly diminished with the introduction of CT as a first-line investigation.

Basal skull fractures are associated with CSF leaks: look out for otorrhoea, rhinorrhoea, racoon eyes or Battle's sign. 30% of CT scans are negative.

Depressed fractures may require surgical repair if open, causing neurological deficit or for cosmesis, and are associated with an ↑ risk of long-term epilepsy.

Prophylactic antibiotics are not usually indicated as they have not been shown to prevent meningitis.

Differential diagnosis

- Vascular markings—margins are usually poorly defined, running up and posterior from skull base.
- Suture line—curve, consistent width throughout course, at specific anatomical sites.
- Old fracture line—painless on palpation.

Scalp lacerations

Should be cleaned thoroughly and closed primarily, in two layers, unless 2° to a bite. Tissue glue may be used for small lacerations. Rule out underlying fractures or foreign bodies, and consider anti-tetanus prophylaxis and antibiotics.

Subarachnoid haemorrhage

- Alert neurosurgeon immediately.
- Potentially fatal—requires immediate diagnosis and treatment.

Think about

There is pathological collection of blood in the subarachnoid space, most commonly seen following trauma.

Traumatic SAH is seen in 44% of all significant head injuries. It occurs as a result of tears in the small subarachnoid vessels. Initial CT scan will detect blood in the basal cisterns or within the interhemispheric fissures and sulci. The amount of blood within the haemorrhage correlates directly with the outcome. There may be vasospasm, which can be treated with calcium channel blockers. If there is no other brain injury, the prognosis is good.

Spontaneous SAH may be due to rupture of an intracranial aneurysm (70%), arteriovenous malformation (15%), unknown (15%) or rare causes.

Typically CT shows hyperdensity in the subarachnoid space (90%) (see Fig. 6.11), although the scan may be normal (10%) and lumbar puncture for CSF bilirubin (xanthochromia) and cell count are needed to confirm diagnosis (most sensitive 12hr after onset of symptoms).

Localization and confirmation of the presence of an aneurysm by CT angiography, MRI and angiography is then needed.

Patients with poor-grade subarachnoid will be transferred directly to intensive care. You may not be involved in their care until they are discharged to the ward several days or even weeks later.

One-third of patients with aneurysmal haemorrhages will die from the initial bleed and a further third will rebleed within the first 6 weeks. Hydrocephalus and vasospasm (days 3–12) are also frequent, and potentially very serious, complications.

Some patients with World Federation of Neurosurgeons (WFNS) SAH grade I (Table 6.5) look remarkably well on admission. It is worthwhile at this stage, with the patient's permission, explaining to relatives the seriousness of the condition and that complications may occur despite optimal management.

Aneurysm treatment is by endovascular embolization, or craniotomy and clipping of the aneurysm. Endovascular treatment is certainly on the increase, but there remains a place for surgical intervention.

Timing of aneurysmal surgery is controversial ('early', before day 3, versus 'late', after day 12); however, if an aneurysm can be secured early it facilitates treatment of vasospasm and virtually eliminates the risk of rebleeding.

Table 6.5 WFNS grading system

WFNS grade	GCS	Motor deficit
I	15	Present or absent
II	13–14	Absent
III	13–14	Present
IV	7–12	Present or absent
V	3–6	Present or absent

Ask about

- Sudden-onset headache 'thunderclap' with no precedent trauma.
- Maximal in first seconds to minutes.
- Different from previous headaches.
- Previous medical history inc. hypertension, smoking, other related conditions, e.g. polycystic kidneys, connective tissue disorders, familial history.

Look for

- Any neurological deterioration—typically because of hyponatraemia, rebleed, hydrocephalus or vasospasm.
- Cardiovascular or respiratory compromise—maintain cerebral perfusion!
- Fluid status.

Investigations

- FBC, U&Es, glucose, clotting, group and save.
- CT head and lumbar puncture to confirm diagnosis have usually already been done by the referring team.
- CT/MRI/angiography, as discussed with radiology.
- Check sodium and re-CT head if neurological deterioration.
- Transcranial Doppler if available—to detect vasospasm.

Management

- See ↓ GCS (📖 p224) and ICP management (📖 p226) if appropriate.
- Oral nimodipine 60mg 4 hourly for 21 days.
- Consider commencing a statin.
- Normalize any electrolyte abnormalities—see section on sodium balance (📖 p260).
- Definitive treatment with endovascular coiling or surgical clipping.
- Triple H therapy (Table 6.6)—hypervolaemia, haemodilution and hypertension—to treat vasospasm once aneurysm is protected. This is controversial and practice varies between neurosurgeons.

Table 6.6 Triple H therapy for SAH

Hypertension	MAP 100–110 mmHg
Hypervolaemia	CVP 8–15 mmHg
Haemodilution	Haematocrit 0.3–0.34

General points

- Multidisciplinary team approach to rehabilitation.
- Ensure adequate hydration—3L/day.
- Bed-rest.
- Elevate head of bed to 30° angle—some units advocate flat bed-rest, but this may compromise ventilation.
- Analgesia and antiemetics.
- Consider laxatives.
- Consider gastrointestinal ulcer protection.
- Consider antithrombotic prophylaxis.
- Consider neuropsychological referral once stable.
- Patient must be told to inform the DVLA before driving.

Differential diagnosis

- SAH 2° to trauma.

Intracerebral haemorrhage

- Alert neurosurgeon immediately.
- Potentially fatal—requires immediate diagnosis.

Think about

ICH is a common cause of ↓ consciousness in patients with hypertension. Other causes include trauma (as discussed previously), arteriovenous malformation, aneursymal rupture, coagulopathy and intracranial neoplasms. Blood is present pathologically within the brain parenchyma and may extend into the ventricular system.

CT shows acute intracerebral haemorrhage as a hyperdense lesion within the brain parenchyma (Fig. 6.14).

Treatment is usual conservative (STICH trial), in which case the patient should be referred to a specialist stroke unit; however, craniotomy and evacuation of haematoma may be performed. Indications for surgery are controversial and ∴ the decision should be made on an individual basis, taking into account the size and location of haematoma, patient's neurological condition, age and well-being, and family and patient's wishes.

Differential diagnosis

- Intracranial tumour.
- Intracranial abscess.

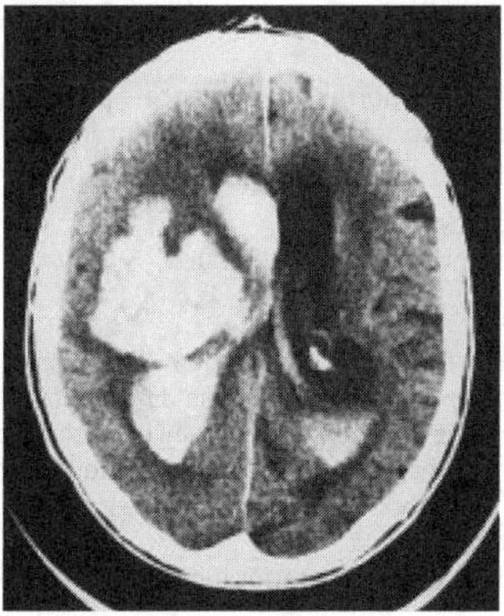

Fig. 6.14 Intracerebral haemorrhage.

Intracranial tumours

- Alert neurosurgeon immediately.
- Potentially fatal—must be taken seriously.

Think about

Cerebral tumours are classified as 1° or 2°. 1° brain tumours arise from central nervous system (CNS) tissue whereas 2° tumours have metastasized from outside the CNS. The commonest 1° brain tumours are meningiomas and gliomas.

Patients usually present with progressive neurological deficit, headache (and other associated signs of raised ICP) or seizures, and often, for 1° brain tumours, no associated previous history. Malignant tumours tend to have a shorter history than benign tumours (weeks/months vs. months/years), and, by comparison, abscesses tend to have the shortest history (days/weeks).

CT may show an irregular enhancing lesion, cystic or solid, with mass effect and surrounding oedema.

Diagnosis is confirmed by histology obtained intraoperatively. This may be biopsy, debulking or excision of tumour. Intraoperatively, the surgical team may send a frozen section, which gives a preliminary indication of the diagnosis. Formal histology results can take days.

Definitive treatment may be conservative, with chemotherapy and radiotherapy, or purely surgical. A multidisciplinary team approach is ∴ a necessity.

Ask about

- Length of symptoms, e.g. headaches (especially in morning), vomiting, focal weakness, seizures.
- Visual impairment and hormonal imbalance—pituitary tumours.
- Previous medical history inc. malignancy, prior irradiation, HIV.

Look for

- Any neurological deterioration.
- Hormonal imbalance—pituitary tumours.

Investigations

- FBC, U&Es, glucose, clotting, cross-match if necessary.
- Endocrine work-up and formal visual fields if pituitary tumour.
- CT and MRI brain ± contrast have usually been done by the referring team; however, further radiology may be needed for image guidance localization of the tumour intraoperatively, e.g. stealth, frame-based stereotactic surgery.
- Re-CT head if neurological deterioration.

Management

- See ↓ GCS (📖 p224), ICP management (📖 p226) and postoperative management (📖 p252) sections as appropriate.
- Ensure full preoperative work-up.
- Inform radiology if intraoperative imaging is necessary, e.g. frame-based stereotactic surgery.
- Place and mark fiducials (little stickers like corn pads; they may fall off) to localize tumour if image guidance is to be used.
- Commence dexamethasone 4mg QDS if indicated (decreases oedema), then wean as appropriate.
- Anticonvulsants—if history of seizures or prophylactically following discussion with neurosurgeon.
- Postoperatively, chase histology and refer to oncologists if necessary.
- Following pituitary surgery, keep a close eye on fluid status as diabetes insipidus may occur—see section on sodium balance (📖 p260).

General points

- Multidisciplinary team approach.
- Gastrointestinal ulcer protection if on steroids (beware: bowel perforation!).
- Consider antithrombotic prophylaxis.

Differential diagnosis

- Intracranial haemorrhage, infarct, or even aneurysm.
- Intracranial abscess.

Hydrocephalus

- Alert neurosurgeon immediately.
- Potentially fatal—requires immediate diagnosis and may require immediate surgical intervention.

Think about

Hydrocephalus is an excessive accumulation of CSF within the ventricles of the brain and is caused by a disturbance in its formation, flow or absorption. Presentation is usually with symptoms of raised ICP, e.g. headache, vomiting and confusion.

Note: Papilloedema may take weeks or months to develop and is a late sign.

In *communicating hydrocephalus* there is free flow of CSF from the ventricular system to subarachnoid space, usually caused by a failure in absorption, i.e. CSF circulation is blocked at the level of the arachnoid granulations. It is safe to perform a lumbar puncture and treatment is by shunt placement.

In *non-communicating hydrocephalus* there is an obstruction within the ventricular system (proximal to the arachnoid granulations) and ∴ CSF cannot reach the subarachnoid space. It is not safe to perform a lumbar puncture and treatment options include conservative treatment, external ventricular drain (EVD), reservoir, shunt or third ventriculostomy.

CT may show ventricular dilatation (in normal subjects the temporal horns are barely visible and the third ventricle is slit-like) and periventricular lucency (hypodensity in the white matter around the ventricles 2° to extravasation of CSF) (see Fig. 6.15). However, in benign intracranial hypertension, despite raised CSF pressures, the ventricular size is normal. In non-communicating hydrocephalus only that part of the ventricular system proximal to the obstruction will be dilated.

Medical management of hydrocephalus, e.g. acetzolamide, furosemide, is rarely seen on neurosurgical wards.

Ask about

- Duration of symptoms—headache, vomiting, visual disturbances, ataxia, incontinence.
- Previous medical history inc. intracranial congenital abnormalities, tumour, infection and haemorrhage.

Look for

- Any neurological deterioration inc. fundal changes (subhyaloid/retinal haemorrhage, papilloedema).
- Tense fontanelle in children.
- Hakim triad—gait apraxia, incontinence, dementia (seen in normal-pressure hydrocephalus).

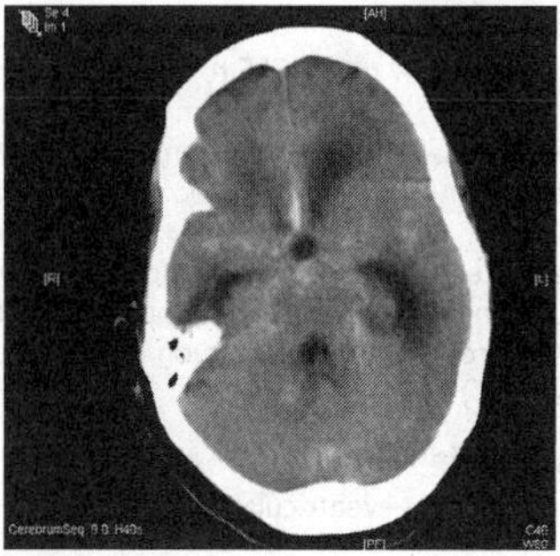

Fig. 6.15 Hydrocephalus—prominent temporal horns and third ventricle with effacement of the sulci and basal cisterns.

Investigations

- FBC, U&Es, glucose, clotting, group and save.
- CT head—usually done by referring team.
- Consider MRI to elucidate underlying cause, e.g. tumour, aqueduct stenosis.

Management

- See ↓ GCS (📖 p224), ICP management (📖 p226) and postoperative management (📖 p252) sections as appropriate.
- Insertion of EVD, reservoir, shunt or third ventriculostomy.
- Repeat CT if deterioration (shunt failure).
- Consider tapping shunt, reservoir or EVD for CSF if deterioration (ventriculitis/under-shunting/over-shunting).

Stepwise approach to tapping a shunt

- First, you must know what type of shunt you are dealing with. Different shunts have different components specifically designed to be tapped. If there is any uncertainty get an X-ray.
- Immaculate sterile technique.
- Insert 25G (orange) butterfly needle or smaller into the tapping chamber.
- Consider measuring pressure with manometer.
- If no spontaneous flow, aspirate CSF with syringe.
- Send CSF for MC&S, protein/glucose, cell count.

General points

- There is no figure for how much CSF to drain in hydrocephalus—as much is needed . Normal CSF production is 500mL/day. Normal CSF capacity is 150mL. Usually set external ventricular drains at 10cm (i.e. drain if pressure in the ventricle >10cmH_2O). Risk of draining too quickly is CSDH.
- Immaculate sterile technique when caring for EVDs or shunts.
- Follow local guidelines on routine CSF sampling from EVD.
- For shunt-related problems, see section on EVDs, reservoirs and shunts (📖 p267).

Differential diagnosis

- Hydrocephalus ex vacuo—ventricular enlargement 2° to cerebral atrophy.

Brain abscesses

- Alert neurosurgeon immediately.
- Potentially fatal—requires immediate diagnosis and immediate surgical intervention.

Think about

Brain abscess and subdural empyema are mostly 2° to mastoiditis, sinusitis and middle ear infections. Other causes included endocarditis, dental and pulmonary infections.

CT scans show ring-enhancing lesions (often multiple) with surrounding oedema (usually extensive) (Fig. 6.16) and subdural empyema as a thin subdural collection, often along the falx.

It may be difficult to differentiate between abscess and tumour. Patients with intracranial abscesses may be apyrexial and have normal inflammatory markers. Abscesses tend to have shorter history (days/weeks as opposed to weeks/months) and are usually more spherical with more extensive oedema than tumours.

To confirm the diagnosis and identify pathogens, tissue should be obtained. Ideally antibiotics are be commenced until after operative sampling, but this is not always appropriate. The IV antimicrobial course is usually several weeks and long-term lines should be considered.

Ask about

- Duration of symptoms, e.g. headache, fever focal weakness, seizures.
- Previous medical history inc. cranial surgery, penetrating head trauma, immunocompromised states, sinusitis, otitis media and mastoiditis, endocarditis, dental and pulmonary infections.

Look for

- Any neurological deterioration.
- Pyrexia—typically low grade but often absent.
- Source of infection—sinuses, ears, teeth, lungs, heart.

Investigations

- FBC, U&Es, glucose, clotting, group and save.
- Blood cultures.
- CXR and echocardiogram.
- CT/MRI brain—will usually have been done by referring team.
- Do not perform a lumbar puncture!

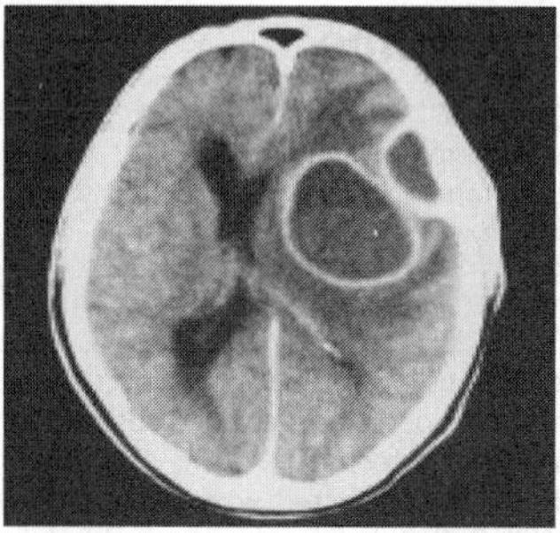

Fig. 6.16 Left frontal abscess. Note ring enhancement and surrounding oedema.

Management

- See ↓ GCS (📖 p224), ICP management (📖 p226) and postoperative management (📖 p252) sections as appropriate.
- Antibiotics as discussed with microbiology—cultures from cerebral abscesses are often sterile.
- Investigate cause, e.g. CXR, blood cultures, urine and sputum cultures, echocardiogram for infective endocarditis, ENT review for sinusitis, otitis media and mastoiditis.
- Arrange long-term IV access.

General points

- Consider gastrointestinal ulcer protection.
- Consider antithrombotic prophylaxis.
- Consider district nurse for IV antimicrobials at home.

Differential diagnosis

- Intracranial tumour.

☠ The acute spine

- Alert neurosurgeon immediately.
- Potentially fatal—immediate diagnosis and treatment can prevent significant morbidity.

Think about

Acute spinal cord and nerve root injury may occur as a result of trauma, disc prolapse, infection (tuberculosis, epidural abscess) or tumour (typically metastases involving the vertebrae).

Spinal injury should be suspected with any trauma; often more than one level is involved. Remember head and spinal injuries often coexist: if the patient has one, consider the other. Significant impairment of motor, sensory and autonomic function may result as a consequence of spinal cord or nerve root compression.

Various patterns of spinal cord injury have been described. Broadly, lesions can be defined as complete or incomplete, e.g. anterior cord syndrome, central cord syndrome, Brown-Séquard syndrome. Patients with complete lesions (no preservation of any sensorimotor function > three segments below the level of injury) are unlikely recover.

Loss of sphincter control is important to elucidate when dealing with any spinal patient. Typical findings include loss of sensation, e.g. no urinary or faecal urgency, with ↓ anal tone → faecal soiling, and urinary retention → overflow incontinence. Patients may have to strain and press on the abdomen to initiate urinary flow. A post-void bladder scan, if available, can be a very useful tool.

Diagnosis and cause of spinal cord and nerve root injury may be confirmed with imaging (usually done by the referring team). Treatment depends on cause and injury sustained, e.g. conservative, discectomy, laminectomy, internal fixation.

High-dose steroids have been given following spinal cord injury. However, the results of the studies (NASCIS 1, 2 and 3) that led to their use being advocated have not been reproduced and steroid use in spinal cord injury may be associated with higher morbidity. The treatment regimen for steroids in acute spinal cord injury is given here but should be administered only after discussion with the registrar.

Terms commonly used in spinal cord and nerve root injury

- Radiculopathy—nerve root pathology.
- Myelopathy—spinal cord pathology.
- Anterior cord syndrome—anterior spinal artery territory infarct, results in paraplegia and dissociated sensory loss (pain and temperature lost whilst posterior column function is preserved).
- Central cord syndrome—usually seen following hyperextension injury, results in motor deficit affecting upper limbs more than lower limbs.
- Brown-Séquard syndrome—spinal cord hemisection, classically results in contralateral dissociated sensory loss and ipsilateral loss of posterior column and motor function.

- Cauda equina syndrome—typically presents with lower back pain, sciatica, disturbance of saddle sensation, bladder and bowel dysfunction, variable lower limb motor and sensory loss. Caused by any lesion that compresses the cauda equina nerve roots.
- Spinal shock—transient loss of all neurological function below the level of the spinal cord injury resulting in flaccid paralysis and areflexia. The cause is physiological rather than anatomical; however, it is a poor prognostic sign.
- Neurogenic shock—disruption of the sympathetic outflow (T1–L2) → loss of systemic vascular resistance and unopposed vagal tone. Classic triad of hypotension, bradycardia and hypothermia may be seen. Most commonly occurs following injuries above T6.
- Autonomic dysreflexia—massive imbalanced reflex sympathetic discharge in response to noxious stimulus; typically urinary infection, bladder or bowel distension, or skin breakdown. Leads to hypertension, headache, bradycardia and potentially death.

Ask about
- Mechanism of injury and length of symptoms.
- Pain, numbness and weakness.
- Bladder sensation.
- Previous medical history inc. previous surgery, vascular disease, any anticoagulant medication inc. aspirin, clopidogrel.

Look for
- Tone—limbs typically flaccid in the acute setting.
- Muscle weakness and paralysis inc. respiratory muscles.
- Paraesthesia and anaesthesia, esp. saddle sensation.
- Reflexes inc. cremasteric, abdominal, anal wink, bulbocavernosus.
- Autonomic dysfunction, e.g. neurogenic shock (hypothermia, hypotension without tachycardia), Horner's syndrome, priapism, sexual dysfunction.
- Urinary retention.
- Anal tone.
- Any other injuries if traumatic.

Investigations
- FBC, U&Es, glucose, clotting, group and save.
- Plain X-rays—may show fractures, dislocations, bony infiltration or osteoporosis.
- CT to elucidate extent of bony trauma.
- MRI to determine soft tissue injury—disc prolapse or cord contusion.
- Absence of fracture does not ensure spinal stability (ligament injury) or rule out spinal injury (spinal ischaemia or haematoma).
- Post-voiding bladder scan—to rule out occult urinary retention.

Management

- ABC.
- ATLS, inc. spinal stabilization, if trauma.
- Analgesia, esp. for the acute disc—consider involving the pain team.
- Maintain normal BP—to ensure adequate spinal perfusion.
- Consider high-dose steroids if within 8hr of injury:
  - Methylprednisolone 30 mg/kg bolus over 15min.
  - 50mL infusion using 5% dextrose or 0.9% NaCl.
  - Leave 45min gap.
  - Methylprednisolone 5.4mg/kg/hr for 23hr.
  - 500mL infusion using 5% dextrose or 0.9% NaCl.
  - Use separate IV site for infusion.
- Does patient need transfer to specialist spinal unit?
- Long-term management and prevention of nosocomial infections, gastrointestinal (ileus, constipation, ulcers), genitourinary (UTI, hydronephrosis) and musculoskeletal complications (osteoporosis, contractures).

General points

- Ensure adequate hydration and nutrition.
- Skin care—prevention of bed sores.
- Consider rotating mattress.
- Consider laxatives.
- Consider antithrombosis prophylaxis.
- Consider gastrointestinal ulcer protection.
- Regular physiotherapy.
- Counselling, e.g. re-sexual dysfunction.

Differential diagnosis

- Peripheral neuropathy.
- Intracranial pathology.
- Munchausen's syndrome.

ⓘ The elective spine

Think about

Back pain is very common and can often be treated/prevented with weight loss, avoiding heavy lifting, good posture, strong core truncal muscles (transversus abdominis), pilates and physiotherapy.

Neurosurgery tends to be reserved for patients with a neurological condition for whom conservative treatment has failed. The vast majority of surgical interventions aim to alleviate or halt the progression of the neurological symptoms rather than treat back pain.

Common terms

- Spondylosis—degeneration of the vertebra at the articular surfaces.
- Spondylolysis—fracture of the pars interarticularis of the vertebrae.
- Spondylolisthesis—slippage of one lumbar vertebra on another.

Ask about

- Pain—is it worse in the back or the limb?
- Neuralgia, e.g. sciatica.
- Leg claudication.
- Bowel or bladder dysfunction.
- Previous medical history, inc. previous surgery, vascular disease, any anticoagulant medication inc. aspirin, clopidogrel.

Look for

- Tone.
- Muscle weakness, paralysis and atrophy.
- Paraesthesia and anaesthesia.
- Reflexes.
- Anal tone.

Investigations

- FBC, U&Es, glucose, clotting, group and save.
- MRI—do the symptoms fit with the scan? Is it up to date?

Management

- Preoperative optimization.

General points

- Consider gastrointestinal ulcer protection.
- Consider antithrombosis prophylaxis.
- Physiotherapy.

Postoperative care of patients with intracranial pathology

Ask about

- Preoperative and operative management.
- Previous medical history.
- Respiratory wean if on support or tracheostomy in situ.
- Feeding.
- Mobility.
- Rehabilitation.

Look for

- Any neurological deterioration.
- Any other injuries, esp. spinal (trauma).
- Cardiovascular or respiratory compromise.
- Drains—remove after 24–48hr; if deep to the dura then *always* stitch.
- Fluid status.
- Infection—wound, chest, line, consider CSF.
- Sutures—remove after 5–7 days (if repeat surgery: 2 weeks).

Investigations

- FBC, U&Es, glucose.
- CT head if neurological deterioration—see ↓ GCS (📖 p224).
- Spinal and other imaging as indicated (trauma).
- Consider further imaging to rule out underlying cause of ICH, e.g. MRI, CTA or angiogram.

Management

- See ↓ GCS (📖 p224) and ICP management (📖 p226) if appropriate.
- Rehabilitation.
- Optimize antihypertensive medication, whilst avoiding hypotension (ICH).
- Referral to specialist stroke team or rehabilitation.

General points

- Consider OG/NG feed—check for base of skull fracture first if trauma!
- Avoid sedation—unless discussed with registrar.
- Consider laxatives.
- Consider gastrointestinal ulcer protection, esp. if on steroids.
- Consider antithrombosis prophylaxis .
- Wean steroids as appropriate.
- Multidisciplinary team approach to rehabilitation.
- Consider neuropsychological referral.
- Risk and management of seizures should be explained to patient and family.
- Patient must be told to inform the DVLA before driving.

Postoperative care of patients with spinal pathology

Think about

Only mobilize the patient who has a stable spine and if it is not contraindicated by intraoperative dural breach. If it is safe, mobilization should be encouraged.

If the dura has been breached, the patient commonly has a gravity drain, and bed-rest is usually indicated.

For trauma patients, always check with your registrar before mobilizing. A brace or collar may be needed. Pain may be an indication of instability; consider this when prescribing analgesia,

Most elective patients should be safe for discharge home within a couple of days of surgery.

Ask about

- Preoperative and operative management—was the dura breached during surgery?
- Previous medical history.
- Pain, numbness and weakness—Is it new? Have preoperative symptoms improved?
- Bladder sensation.
- Low-pressure headache—if dura breached.

Look for

- Any change in neurological findings.
- Any other injuries (trauma).
- Drains—remove after 24–48hr if no CSF; if dura breached intraoperatively discuss with registrar before removal, then always stitch wound.
- Infection—wound, chest, line, consider CSF.
- Sutures—remove after 7–10 days (if redo surgery: 2 weeks).

Investigations

- FBC, U&Es.
- Postop imaging if fixation used.

Management

- Mobilize if safe.
- Physiotherapy.
- See section on Acute spine (📖 p248) for patients admitted as an emergency.

General points

- See sections on the Acute spine (📖 p248) and Elective spine (📖 p251).

☠ Ventriculitis

- Alert neurosurgeon.
- Potentially fatal—requires urgent diagnosis and immediate treatment.

Think about

Infection of the ventricular cavity and ependymal lining is usually iatrogenic in origin, typically following insertion of ventricular catheters. Non-iatrogenic causes include meningitis or cerebral abscess. Ventriculitis may be complicated by hydrocephalus.

The ependymal lining may show strong contrast enhancement on CT and ↑ signal intensity on MRI. A definitive diagnosis is based on the isolation of a high concentration of pathogens in the CSF from successive specimens. If the white cell to red cell ratio is higher in CSF than in blood, this is also indicative of ventriculitis (white:red cell count is normally ~1:500).

Management is with external ventricular drain and antimicrobial therapy.

Ask about

- Previous neurosurgery.

Look for

- Can be subtle, so a high index of suspicion is needed!
- Any neurological deterioration.
- Fever.

Investigations

- Peripheral WBC may not be raised.
- CSF sample.
- Microbiology advice.
- Does ventricular catheter need to be replaced?

Management

- See section on ↓ GCS (📖 p224) as appropriate.
- Send CSF (sample from ventricular catheter).
- Discuss with microbiology re empirical treatment and intrathecal antibiotics.
- Modify treatment once pathogen identified.

Stepwise approach to CSF sampling and administering intrathecal antibiotics in patients with ventricular catheters

- Meticulous asepsis—handwashing, disinfectant, sterile gloves and drape.
- Close distal stopcock.
- Sample EVD via port or Ommaya reservoir, not bag or end of drainage tube.
- Remove 1–2mL CSF for cell count and microbiology.
- Administer intrathecal antibiotics (sign drug chart).
- After instillation, leave drain clamped for 1hr (inform nursing staff).

General points

- Meticulous asepsis (handwashing, disinfection of connection sites before disconnecting, sterile gloves, drapes) for all patients with ventricular catheters.
- Infected skin exit sites need urgent attention—usually it is necessary to remove the ventricular catheter and insert a new one via a new tunnel.
- Regular CSF sampling as advised by neurosurgeon or microbiology.
- Collect culture 2–3 days before shunt surgery.

Meningitis

- Alert neurosurgeon.
- Potentially fatal—requires immediate diagnosis and urgent treatment.

Think about

Although meningism is common on neurosurgical wards, meningitis is not. Meningism is more typically caused by subarachnoid blood than infection. Postoperative meningitis is rare but serious. If there no obvious cause for pyrexia, CSF infection should be considered.

Patients with meningitis typically present with fever, headache, neck stiffness and photophobia.

Lumbar puncture (LP) is the investigation of choice. There is often discussion about CT brain before LP to rule out possible herniation on LP. If there is any sign of intracranial pathology, get a CT first and check for patency of the basal cisterns. If there are no signs of intracranial pathology then CT is unlikely to be helpful.

Treatment typically involves aggressive antimicrobial therapy.

Ask about

- Previous neurosurgery.
- CSF leak.
- Skull fracture.

Look for

- Any neurological deterioration.
- Fever.
- Meningism—headache, vomiting, neck stiffness, photophobia, Kernig or Brudzinski signs.

Investigations

- FBC, U&Es, glucose, clotting (peripheral WBC may not be raised).
- CT—is there focal neurological deficit or raised ICP?
- Urgent LP.

Management

- See section on ↓ GCS (📖 p224) as appropriate.
- Inform neurology/neurosurgical SpR.
- Discuss with microbiology re empirical treatment.
- Modify treatment once pathogen identified.

General points

- Be vigilant for potential complications—seizures, neurological sequelae.

Differential diagnosis

- Meningism 2° to subarachnoid blood.
- Other causes of pyrexia.
- Other causes of neurological deterioration.

Seizures

- Alert neurosurgeon.
- Potentially fatal—requires immediate management.

Think about

Seizures, the manifestation of abnormal hypersynchronous discharges of cortical neurons, are common symptoms of neurological injury and disease. Typically in the neurosurgical wards seizures occur in patients with a known underlying cortical pathology, e.g. after surgery, tumour or haematoma. They may also be caused by metabolic and electrolyte abnormalities, e.g. hyponatraemia, hypoglycaemia. Epilepsy, characterized by the occurrence of at least two unprovoked seizures, is rarely treated surgically—and only after failure of medical therapy.

Seizures are partial onset (beginning in one focus) or generalized onset (onset recorded in both cerebral hemispheres). They should be considered in the comatose patient.

Treatment is control and prevention of further seizures by appropriate anticonvulsants.

Ask about

- Type of seizure.
- Duration of seizure.
- Underlying cerebral injury or disease, inc. epilepsy.
- Previous medical history, inc. seizures, alcohol.
- Anticonvulsants.

Look for:

- Is the airway protected?

Investigations

- FBC, U&Es, glucose.
- Anticonvulsant drug levels—are they therapeutic?
- Consider CT.
- EEG.

Management

- See section on ↓ GCS (📖 p224) if appropriate.
- Maintain airway (oropharnygeal airway).
- Emergency medication to terminate seizure if necessary.
- Inform anaesthetic SpR if unable to terminate seizures—patient will need general anaesthetic and intubation.
- Inform neurosurgical SpR and consider liaising with neurology if first-line anticonvulsant therapy is failing.
- Commence, increase or change anticonvulsant.

Anticonvulsant guidelines

- For generalized tonic–clonic seizures—phenytoin (1g loading dose followed by starting dose 300mg/day in adults).
- For partial seizures—carbamazepine (starting dose 200mg BD in adults).
- Phenytoin has been shown to reduce seizure frequency in the first week after severe head injury, but there is no clear reduction in seizure frequency beyond this. For this reason a 2-week course of phenytoin following severe head injury may be advocated.

General points

- Follow local guidelines.
- Do not restrain patient.
- Prevent trauma during seizure—cot sides up, move objects away.
- Encourage use of helmet to prevent head injury during high-risk activities.
- Patient must inform DVLA (www.dvla.gov.uk).

Abnormal sodium states

- Alert neurosurgeon.
- Potentially fatal.
- Common on neurosurgical wards.
- Presentation is often non-specific—high index of suspicion needed.

Think about

Three types of sodium abnormality (Table 6.7) are commonly encountered on neurosurgical wards:

- Hyponatraemia 2° to syndrome of inappropriate antidiuretic hormone (SIADH).
- Hyponatraemia 2° to cerebral salt wasting (CSW).
- Hypernatraemia 2° to diabetes insipidus (DI).

Other causes of hyponatraemia include excessive administration of hypotonic IV fluids, psychogenic polydipsia and medications (e.g. carbamazepine, gabapentin, thiazides).

Other causes of *hypernatraemia* include burns and diarrhoea, Cushing's syndrome, nephrogenic DI, hypertonic saline and mannitol.

Disturbances of sodium balance can cause loss of consciousness, seizures and death. It is particularly dangerous for sodium levels to change quickly: treatment aim should always be slow correction.

Ask about

- Recent sodium levels.
- Fluid balance inc. polydipsia and IV fluid regimen.
- Pituitary surgery (DI) or SAH (SIADH/CSW).
- Previous medical history inc. heart failure, renal disease.
- Medication, e.g. carbamazepine (low Na^+), bendroflumethiazide (low Na^+), mannitol (high Na^+).

Look for

- Any neurological deterioration.
- Fluid status—dehydration or fluid overload?

Investigations

- Serum and urine sodium and osmolality.
- FBC, U&Es, glucose.
- Urine specific gravity (bedside test).
- Regular monitoring of serum sodium levels.

Management

- See section on ↓ GCS (p224) as appropriate.
- Elucidate cause, e.g. CSW vs SIADH.
- Inform neurosurgical SpR.
- Reversal of hypo/hypernatraemia—slowly! (Table 6.8).

Table 6.7 Sodium abnormalities commonly seen on neurosurgical wards

	CSW	SIADH	DI
Na^+	Low	Low	High
Urine output	High	Low	High
Urine specific gravity	>1.010	>1.010	<1.010
Plasma osmolarity	Low	Low	High
Urine osmolality	High	High	Low
Urine Na^+	High	Normal	Normal

Table 6.8 Treatment of sodium abnormalities

Diagnosis	Treatment
CSW	0.9% NaCl Oral sodium supplements (3% NaCl if severe)
SIADH	Fluid restriction (3% NaCl if severe)
DI	DDAVP®

General points

- Consider discontinuing medications associated with hypo/hypernatraemia.
- Regular serum sodium levels.
- Strict fluid balance charts.

Differential diagnosis

- Other causes of ↓ GCS, e.g. hypoglycaemia, alcohol, drugs.

Lumbar puncture and drain

LP is an important procedure that enables CSF samples to be obtained from the spinal subarachnoid space for analysis.

Indications for lumbar puncture

Diagnostic

- Meningitis.
- Subarachnoid haemorrhage.
- Inflammatory disease, e.g. multiple sclerosis, Guillain–Barré syndrome.
- Leptomeningeal malignancy.

Therapeutic

- Benign intracranial hypertension.
- Spinal anaesthesia.
- Radio-opaque contrast media (myelography).
- Medication, e.g. corticosteroids, antibiotics, chemotherapeutic agents.

Indications for lumbar drain

Therapeutic

- Prevention and treatment of CSF fistulae.
- Shunt infection.
- Normal-pressure hydrocephalus.
- Adjuvant treatment of ↑ ICP.

Contraindications

- ↑ ICP—LP may lead to coning.
- Spinal abnormalities (congenital or acquired).
- Coagulopathy.

Pre-procedure

- Consider CT head to ensure basal cisterns are patent.
- Consider imaging of lumbar spine.
- Check clotting and platelet count.
- Baseline neurological assessment.
- Consent patient.
- Patient in horizontal lateral decubitus position.
- Flat bed.
- Patient lying on their side.
- Fetal position—knees up to chest, and arms around knees to encourage curvature of spine, thus opening the intervertebral spaces posteriorly.
- Expose back from buttocks to scapula.
- Ensure pelvis is perpendicular to bed and aligned with spine.

Procedure

- Maintain strict asepsis.
- Palpate L4 and L5 spinous processes (at level of iliac crests).
- Mark L4/L5 interspinous space.
- Infiltrate local anaesthetic.
- Prep and drape.
- Introduce spinal needle at L4/L5 interspinous space with bevel upwards.
- Introduction of spinal needle.
- Slowly advance needle at slight upwards angle (towards patient's head).
- Slight 'give' and flow of clear and colourless fluid.
- If ↑ is met, consider thickened dura or bone.
- Prevent introduction of blood into CSF samples ('bloodless tap').
- Measure opening pressure using manometer and stopcock if possible (80–180mmH_2O).
- Obtain CSF samples (few mL for basic studies, more for specialized studies).
- Withdraw needle and apply dry sterile dressing.

For lumbar drain

- Gain access is obtained as above, but use bevelled spinal trocar with bevel cranially.
- Then use Seldinger technique to introduce drain.

Post-procedure

- Maintain strict asepsis.
- Nursing care—lumbar drain sign above patient's bed, frequent neurological assessment, hourly assessment of drain and drainage, assessment of insertion site every 8hr to ensure proper drain ing and patient safety.
- Drain can be clamped briefly when moving patient.
- Patient activity restrictions—bed-rest, level of head of bed, assistance with movement, log rolling.
- Patient activities to avoid—sneezing, coughing, straining.
- Patient to report headache, nausea, vomiting, pain at insertion site, stiff neck, any system disconnection, signs of leakage, new onset of leg pain.
- Common problems include occlusion of tubing, e.g. blood clot and absence of CSF in collection chamber.
- Catheter removal is only by physician.
- Suture must be placed following removal of catheter to prevent leak.

CSF analysis

- Send separate sample for cell count , microbiology and chemical pathology.
- Further samples may be sent for serology and nucleic acid amplification.
- Inform laboratory as centrifugation must be done promptly—red blood cells (RBCs) haemolyse within hours.
- If tap is bloody ('traumatic tap'), consider disposing of initial few mL and sending serial samples.
- For traumatic taps, ~1 WBC per 1000 RBCs and 1mg protein per 750 RBCs is normal.
- Normal CSF may contain up to 5 lymphocytes/mL.
- Xanthochroma—SAH or in patients with high serum bilirubin.
- CSF protein level—high in demyelinating polyneuropathies or infection.
- CSF glucose—normally 60% of serum glucose, low in bacterial infection and meningeal carcinomatosis.
- Cytology—need at least three separate samples to rule out leptomeningeal malignancy.
- Microbiology.

Risks

- Post-tap spinal headache—may last up to 1 week.
- Nerve root trauma.
- CNS infection.
- Intraspinal or subdural haematoma.
- Tension pneumocranium.

Intracranial pressure monitors

Cerebral perfusion pressure = MAP − ICP

- Monitors are either fibreoptic (e.g. Camino® Bolt) or hydraulic (i.e. ventriculostomy).

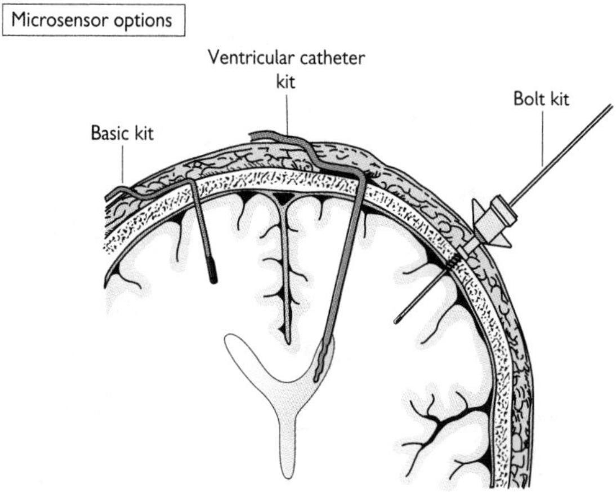

Fig. 6.17 ICP monitor.

Indications

Diagnostic

- Patients with known or possible intracranial pathology in whom neurological assessment is limited, e.g. an anaesthetized patient following head injury.
- Less frequently used to diagnose low-pressure states in patients with shunts in situ, or to differentiate ventriculomegaly (large ventricles) from hydrocephalus.

Contraindications

- Coagulopathy.
- Traumatized skin over insertion site.

ⓘ External ventricular drains, reservoirs and shunts

EVDs are temporary and used in the acute setting, whereas reservoirs and shunts are more definitive means of draining CSF from the ventricles.

Indications

- Hydrocephalus.
- Ventriculitis (EVD only).
- Prevention of hydrocephalus after surgery, e.g. posterior fossa surgery.

Contraindications

- Traumatized skin over insertion site.
- Infection (reservoirs, shunts).
- Intraventricular haemorrhage (reservoirs, shunts).
- Coagulopathy.
- Lack of clinical symptoms.

Risks

- Intracranial haemorrhage.
- Infection, inc. ventriculitis.
- Catheter or shunt obstruction or disconnection.
- Catheter or shunt migration.
- Shunt over drainage, inc. causing CSDH.

If a shunt problem is suspected, the neurosurgical registrar should be informed. Referrals are frequently made of people with long-term shunts with non-specific symptoms. Investigations of choice include CT (to check intraventricular catheter position, under- or over-shunting, and rule out intracranial pathology), shunt series (X-rays following the course of the whole shunt to check continuity, i.e. lateral skull/C-spine, CXR, AXR), shunt palpation (does it pump?) and shunt tap (CSF sampling and manometry to rule out shunt infection and abnormal pressure).

Chapter 7

Ophthalmology

Rob Henderson

Introduction

Ophthalmology is often regarded with fear as a difficult specialty to cover on call. Like every specialty, there are a few basic examinations that are not hard and that, if done well, will cover all eventualities. The slitlamp itself, often found rusting in the corner of an A&E department, is easy to use the basic functions of and will facilitate an exam. It is ∴ advisable, if you are cross-covering eyes on occasion, to find out where the slitlamp is, learn where the on-switch is and which end to look through.

Equally, using a few drops will allow a thorough examination. The perpetual fear that many non-ophthalmologists have is of precipitating an angle-closure glaucoma event post-dilatation. However, this is exceptionally rare, so unless the patient has a history of this—don't worry.

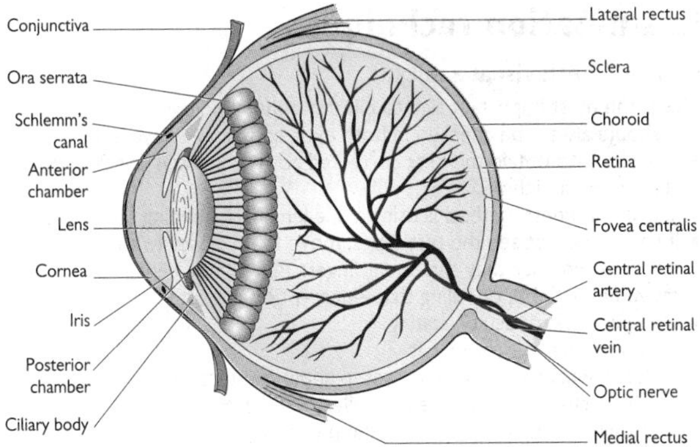

Fig. 7.1 The globe, looking down on the right eye, showing major anatomical structures.

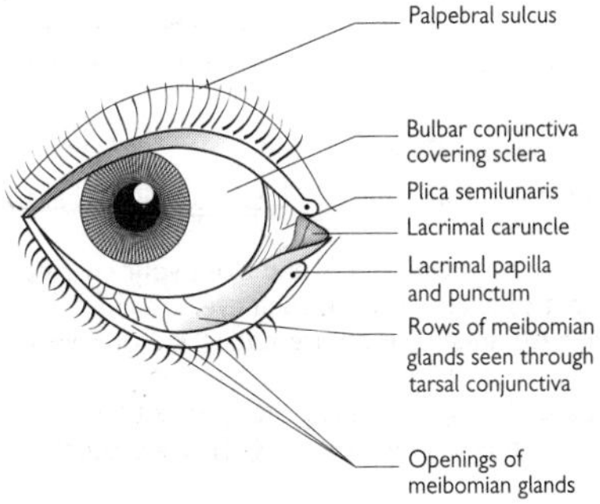

Fig. 7.2 Anatomy of the eye.

Examination techniques

How to check visual acuity

This is the most important sign to elicit in ophthalmology:

- It should always be checked in both eyes, so test each eye in turn.
- The aim is to obtain the best corrected acuity; ∴ always check with glasses and a pinhole.
- The commonest method is using a Snellen chart standing 6m away.
- If patient cannot see the test-types, move them closer to the chart or check whether they can count fingers (CF); if not, sense hand movements (HM), or failing that—perception of light.
- Document visual acuity, stating:
  - Which eye?—right or left.
  - With what visual aid?—glasses, pinhole, contact lenses.
  - What chart is used?—near, Snellen, EDTRS.
  - At what distance?—6m/20ft: the numerator.
  - What line is read?—the denominator.
  - This is recorded as a fraction, i.e. 6/12, 6/18, 6/60, etc.
- If on the ward and no chart is available, use the chart shown in Fig. 7.3 at a distance of 30cm.
- Testing an infant's visual acuities is less exact but should be undertaken nonetheless. Sit the child on an adult's lap and move a small toy from side to side. Assess 'fixing' and 'following'; a pen torch should be used if there is no response to this. Is the child's vision central, steady and maintained?

How to assess visual fields

- Seat the patient at full arm's length opposite you and at the same height.
- Occlude the eye not being tested and close your corresponding eye.
- Ask the patient to fixate on your open eye.
- Test all four quadrants of vision presenting 1, 2 or 5 fingers midway between you.
- With both hands in opposite quadrants, present 1 or 2 fingers simultaneously—this will help detect a relative scotoma.

N48

running off

N36

down cold poor

N24

water sat clamber dye

N18

how superb vile hedgerows sin

N14

twenty batsmen ease the crowd phew!

N12

Cats tea blackmail marquee towel and stuff

N10

One big trailer of course around the sky hitting brambles

N8

The racoon spells mischief on its neighbouring wall; two monks fish

N6

What did postman help the trowel lying in the road when; hence "ahoy" the flies abound

N5

Fall away form the line; fantastic boots the scrambled eggs match. What clowns are reputed to fashion.

N4

Dithering it might be said is always a good pastime: oh to suffer the slings and arrows of outrageous fortune whether tis nobler in the mind.

Fig. 7.3 Near vision test types.

How to perform the swinging flashlight test for a relative afferent papillary defect (RAPD)

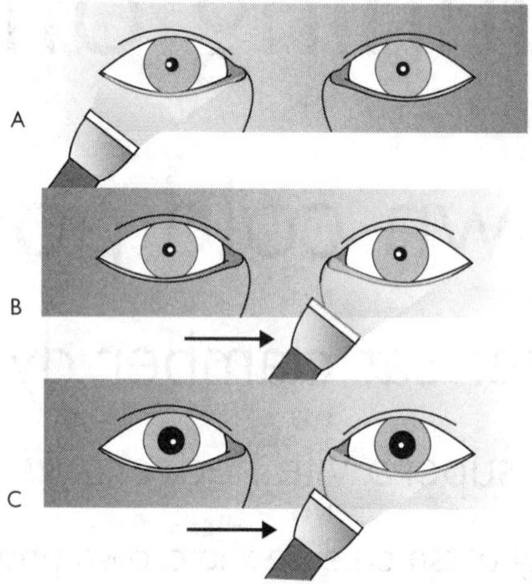

Fig. 7.4 Swinging flashlight test.

- In a dim room ask the patient to fix on a distant object.
- Shine the pen-torch in one eye and note the pupil constriction (A).
- Move the light across the nose to the fellow eye and look for similar pupillary constriction (B).
- Now move the light back again comparing the constriction between the two eyes.
- If one eye does not constrict or even dilates when the light is shone at it there is evidence of a RAPD (C), i.e. the normal pathway from the retina to the lateral geniculate nucleus is damaged somewhere.
- Instil guttate (g) fluorescein 2% into the inferior fornix. Examine under cobalt blue light for evidence of aqueous leakage. Fluorescein may 'pour' like a waterfall.

How to use the slitlamp

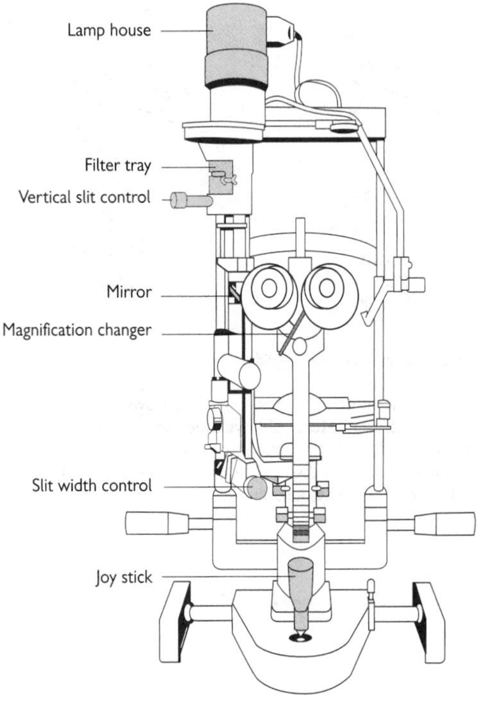

Fig. 7.5 Diagram of a slitlamp.

- Turn on power under table.
- Adjust binoculars for both eyes.
- Move joystick forward and back to bring eye into focus.
- Choose filter for white or blue light in filter tray.
- Left hand on slit width control to move light.

Everting the upper eyelid

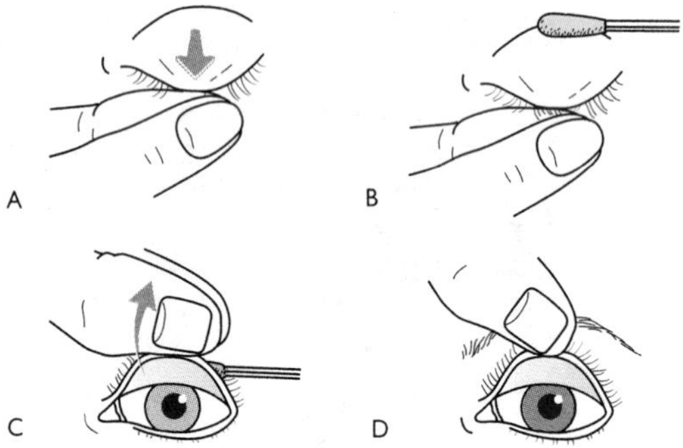

Fig. 7.6 How to evert an upper eyelid.

- Ask patient to look down and keep looking down.
- Using cotton tip applicator, hold eyelashes and pull lid down.
- With other hand put cotton-bud into upper-lid skin crease.
- Pull lid down and round the applicator thus everting the lid.
- Hold lid in position whilst examining.

All images courtesy of Miss Seema Verma, Consultant Ophthalmologist, Moorfields Eye Hospital.

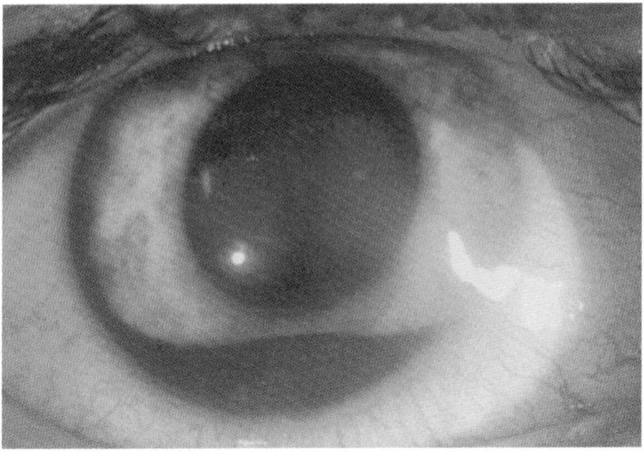

Plate 1 Hyphaemia.

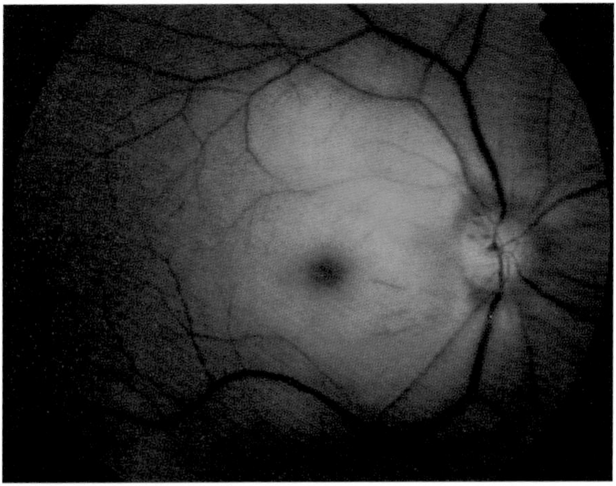

Plate 2 Central retinal artery occlusion. Note the fundal pallor and attenuated arteries.

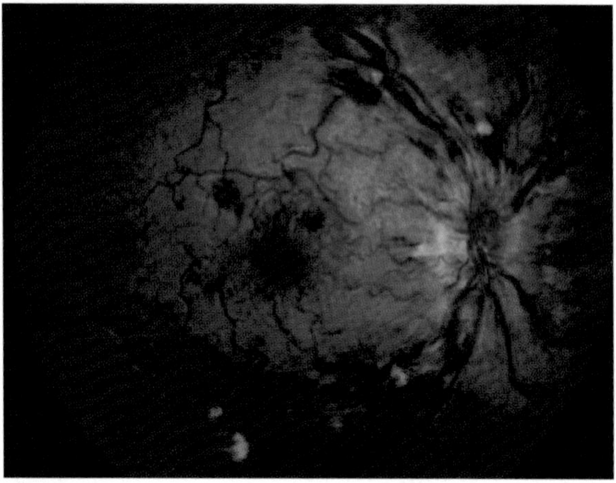

Plate 3 Central retinal vein occlusion—grossly tortuous veins with intraretinal haemorrhage and cotton-wool spots indicative of nerve fibre layer infarcts.

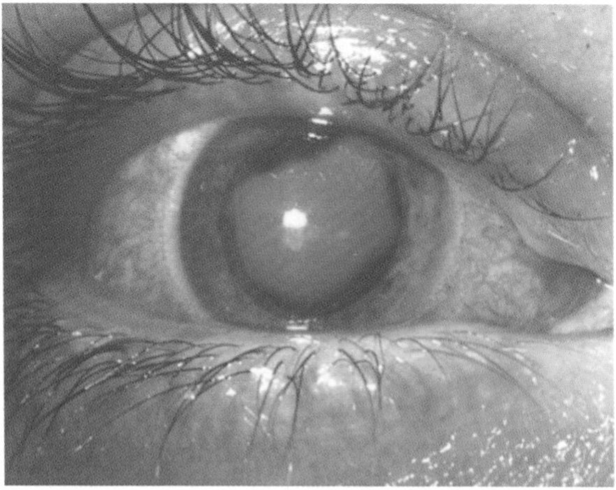

Plate 4 Alkali burn to cornea. Note the large corneal abrasion highlighted by the fluorescein dye. The eye is hyperaemic, but in severe burns the eye may appear white.

Ophthalmic signs not to miss

Call ophthalmologist immediately.

Trauma with distorted pupil, flat anterior chamber—penetrating injury.
Chemical burn—start irrigation immediately.
Sudden painless loss of vision with RAPD and headache in >60-yr-old—think? Giant cell arteritis?
Sudden loss of vision in anybody—get urgent ophthalmic advice vision has already recovered to normal you can wait until mornir
Corneal abscess in contact lens wearer, if white patch on cornea—think ulcer,
Flashes, black floaters, visual field defect or visual distortion—thi retinal detachment.
Pain, vomiting, ↓ vision, cloudy cornea and poorly reactive pupil—think acute angle-closure glaucoma.
Headache, 3rd nerve palsy—think vascular. Call neurosurgery.
6th nerve palsy, mild headache and disc swelling—think raised intracranial pressure (ICP).

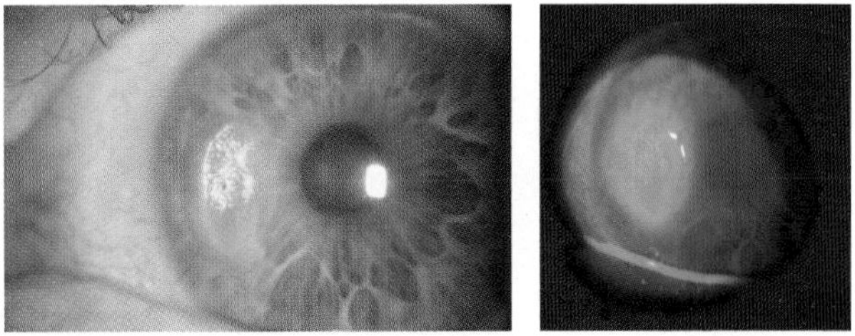

(a) (b)

Plate 5 (a) Corneal abscess of the left eye. (b) Stained with fluorescein.

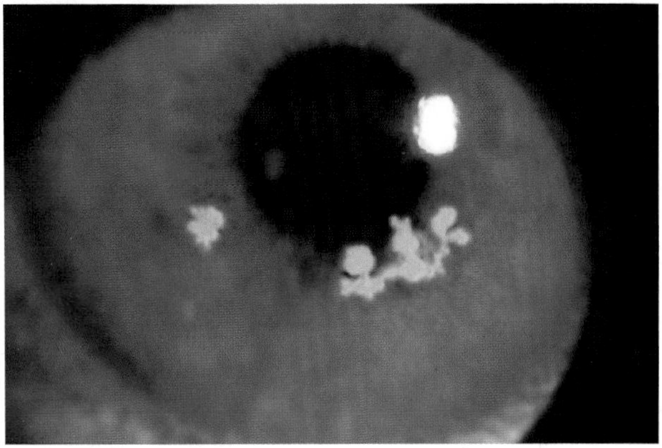

Plate 6 Dendritic ulcer—HSV infection of the cornea. Note the typical branching pattern highlighted with fluorescein.

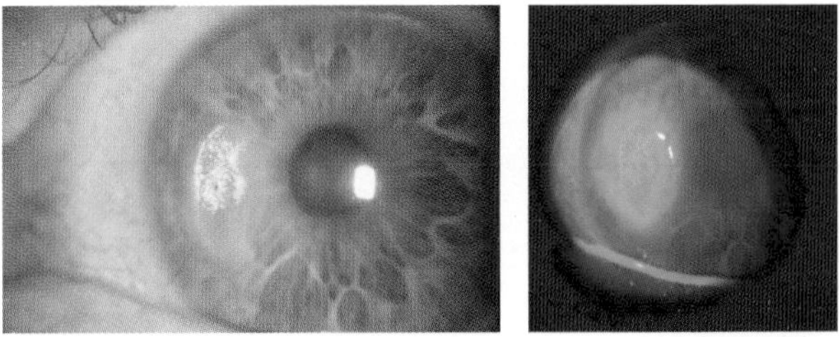

(a) (b)

Plate 5 (a) Corneal abscess of the left eye. (b) Stained with fluorescein.

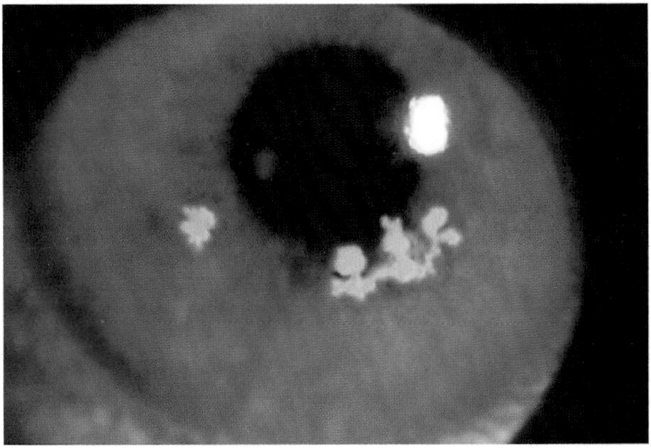

Plate 6 Dendritic ulcer—HSV infection of the cornea. Note the typical branching pattern highlighted with fluorescein.

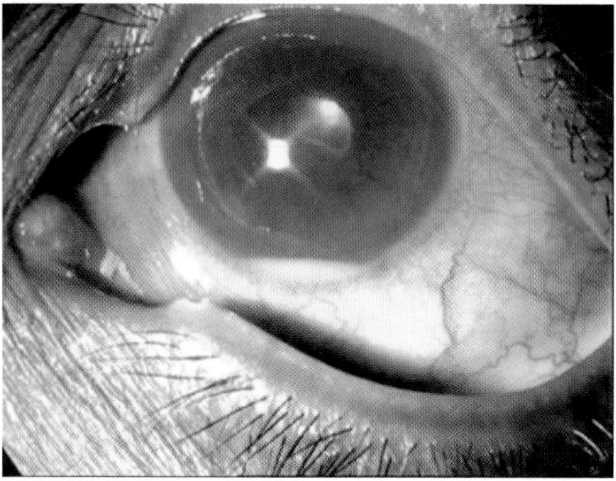

Plate 7 Hypopyon of the left eye.

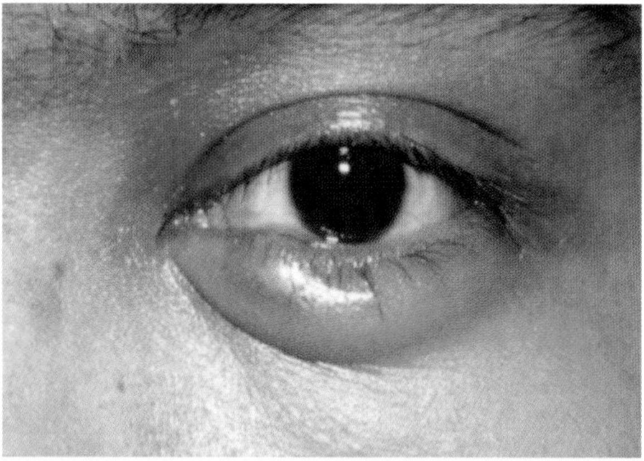

Plate 8 Chalazion—meibomian gland abscess.

Penetrating injury

- Alert ophthalmologist immediately as potentially blinding.
- Patient should be seen within 1hr.

Think about

Any blunt or sharp injury can cause a globe rupture or penetration. If the striking object is small enough to hit the eye directly, a penetrating injury must be excluded.

Ask about

- What was the mechanism of injury?
- What struck the eye? e.g. metal, plastic, wood.
- What was the likely velocity and angle of entry of the object?
- Does the patient report a flow of fluid (aqueous) after the injury?

Look for

- Check visual acuity—a severe reduction in visual acuity is indicative of a severe injury.
- Examine lids—if very swollen, carefully separate lids without putting pressure on the globe. Remember if there is a laceration to the lid a globe perforation must be excluded.
- Eye contents outside the globe—if there is obvious perforation stop the exam, carefully tape a shield across the eye and call ophthalmology.
- Limitation of eye movement—worse in the direction of the rupture.
- Conjunctiva—severe subconjunctival haemorrhage.
- Cornea—if there is no obvious extrusion of ocular contents (e.g. iris plugging corneal wound), perform a Seidel test with a drop of fluorescein instilled in the inferior fornix and examine with a cobalt blue filter.
- Sclera—uveal or vitreous prolapse through the scleral wound.
- Iris—is there deformity of the pupil?
- Are there associated signs—e.g. hyphaemia (blood in the anterior chamber), asymmetrical anterior chamber depth.
- Vitreous haemorrhage—can you see the fundus?
- Check for RAPD (📖 p274).
- Check tetanus status.

Investigation

Computed tomography (CT) of the orbits should be booked prior to theatre if there is any suspicion of an intraocular foreign body.

Management

- Pain management:
  - Carefully instil 1 drop g.amethocaine, a topical anaesthetic.
  - G. atropine 1%—1 drop will dilate the pupil and relieve discomfort by alleviating ciliary spasm.
  - Antiemetic to prevent Valsalva and ↑ intraorbital pressure.
- Tape shield across affected eye (do not pad as this will not protect the globe and pressure may induce prolapse of ocular contents).
- Do not put antibiotic drops or ointment into the eye.
- Nil by mouth and find out when patient last ate/drank.

Differential diagnosis

- Partial-thickness corneal laceration.
- Conjunctival laceration without scleral laceration.

Blunt trauma

High to moderate urgency, depending on extent of injury.

Think about

Blunt injury, e.g. from fight, champagne cork, squash ball, leads to significant periorbital oedema and ecchymosis—a 'black eye'. The ophthalmic disorders not to miss are:

- A posterior globe rupture.
- A blow-out fracture of the orbit.
- A significant hyphaema (Fig. 7.7).

Ask about

- A sudden reduction in visual acuity after the trauma, double vision or numbness of the cheek inferior to the eye or of the brow.
- Non-steroidal anti-inflammatory drug (NSAID) use in hyphaema.

Look for

All require ophthalmology registrar review:

- A significant reduction in visual acuity.
- Squint or double vision on eye movement examination.
- A relative afferent pupil defect.
- ↓ sensation.
- Blood in the anterior chamber.
- Abnormal deviation of one eye relative to its fellow (hypotropia).

Investigation

- Facial views to assess maxillary sinus fracture, a blow-out fracture.
- If globe rupture is suspected an ultrasound should be arranged.
- CT of the orbits and brain (axial and coronal views, 3mm cuts) if diagnosis is uncertain (inform maxillofacial and ophthalmology for review).
- If significant hyphaema, dilate with g.cyclopentolate 1% and discuss with on-call ophthalmologist.

Management

- If blow-out fracture—nasal decongestants, broad-spectrum antibiotics, and instruct patient not to blow nose. Maxillofacial and ophthalmology review.
- Any hyphaemia should always be reviewed by an ophthalmologist upon presentation, particularly after trauma, to exclude globe rupture. May lead to glaucoma.

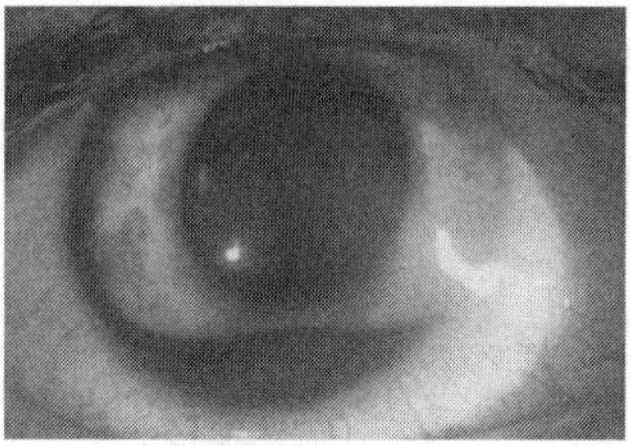

Fig. 7.7 Hyphaema. (Courtesy of Miss Seema Verma, Consultant Ophthalmologist, Moorfields Eye Hospital). Please see Plate 1 for a colour version of this figure.

Sudden painful visual loss

Potentially blinding—should be seen as soon as possible by ophthalmologist.

Think about

Acute angle-closure glaucoma is an ophthalmic emergency: the pressure in the eye is severely raised → rapid retinal nerve cell death within hours.

Think: Does the eye feel hard and is the pupil unreactive?

Ask about

- Was there a sudden onset of rapidly deteriorating vision?
- What is the nature of the pain?—intense with photophobia or frontal headache? (Rarely, pain is not a predominant feature so be aware of this.).
- Are there any vagal symptoms?—vomiting or nausea.
- What were the circumstances when the pain began?—e.g. dark room, stress, mid-level lighting (i.e. early evening).
- Have there been previous episodes of acute glaucoma or recently of uniocular halos around lights or pain that subsides after a period or on going to sleep?
- Is the patient very long sighted?
- Is there any drug history of anticholinergic or sympathomimetic medications?

Look for

- Visual acuity is reduced substantially compared to fellow eye (unless similar event previously in other eye).
- The eye is injected.
- The cornea is hazy (oedematous).
- A poorly reactive or fixed mid-dilated pupil is seen.
- Intraocular pressure is raised >50mmHg—gently ballot both eyes with the lids closed: the eye will feel hard relative to the fellow eye.

Management

- Discuss with the on-call ophthalmologist whether they would like drops administered before their arrival.
- IV access for acetazolamide.
- Oral analgesia/antiemetics.

Differential diagnosis

- Acute anterior uveitis—onset slower and visual loss less severe.
- Corneal trauma—history usually obvious and pain resolves with topical anaesthetic.
- Keratitis, e.g. viral (herpes simplex virus [HSV] dendritic ulcer).

Sudden painless visual loss

Alert ophthalmologist—potentially blinding and should be seen within 1hr.

Think about

The diagnoses not to miss here are a central retinal artery occlusion (CRAO) (Fig. 7.8), which is effectively a 'stroke to the retina', or anterior ischaemic optic neuropathy (AION), effectively a 'stroke to the optic disc'. There are a number of causes but the embolic or vasculitic forms, from giant cell arteritis (GCA), are particularly important not to miss. There is a number of other causes but usually the presenting symptoms are serious enough to warrant an immediate ophthalmic referral.

Ask about

- A sudden painless, unilateral loss of vision →:
  - Completely absent vision (counting fingers to hand movements)—?CRAO.
  - Horizontal hemifield loss or quadrant loss—?branch retinal artery occlusion.
  - Sudden, often extreme, visual loss in one or both eyes with systemic symptoms, most often in patients older than 60yr—? GCA, arteritic anterior ischaemic optic neuropathy.
  - Significantly blurred vision or hemifield loss (frequently noted on arising in the morning) in a patient older than 40yr—? non-arteritic anterior ischaemic optic neuropathy.
- Is there a history of:
  - Atherosclerotic carotid/cardiac disease or embolic phenomenon—transient ischaemic attack (TIA) or cardiovascular accident (CVA), hypertension, diabetes.
  - GCA—scalp tenderness, jaw claudication, etc.
  - Clotting disorders—hypercoagulability.
  - Sickle cell disease.

Look for

- A relative afferent pupillary defect.
- Temporal tenderness with pulseless temporal artery—is this GCA?
- Retinal pallor, narrowed retinal arteries, a cherry-red spot or a calcific embolus within a vessel at the nerve head on ophthalmoscopy—CRAO.
- Unilateral disc swelling with normal-looking retina—?AION.

Investigation

- Check visual acuity.
- Check for RAPD.
- Perform ophthalmoscopy.
- Call ophthalmologist for advice and to review.
- If patient is >50yr, obtain ESR urgently.
- Check BP, blood sugar, clotting.

- Cardiovascular examination for atrial fibrillation (AF), murmur of mitral valve prolapse (MVP), prosthetic valve, carotid bruit.
- If a CRAO, efforts should be made to dislodge the embolus—digital massage can be performed by the clinician.

Differential diagnosis

- Acute ophthalmic artery occlusion—usually no cherry-red spot at the fovea.
- Non-arteritic anterior ischaemic optic neuropathy—optic nerve swelling with a normal retina.
- Central retinal vein occlusion (CRVO)—the fundus appearance is classic with intraretinal haemorrhage, cotton-wool spots, disc swelling and dilated, tortuous retinal veins (Fig. 7.9).

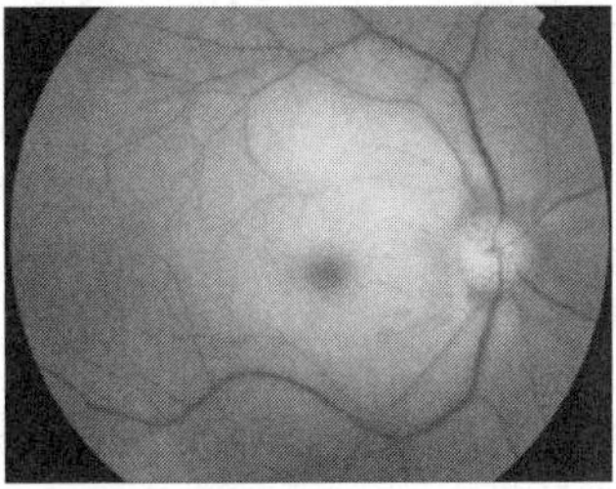

Fig. 7.8 Central retinal artery occlusion. Note the fundal pallor and attenuated arteries. (Courtesy of Miss Seema Verma, Consultant Ophthalmologist, Moorfields Eye Hospital). Please see Plate 2 for a colour version of this figure.

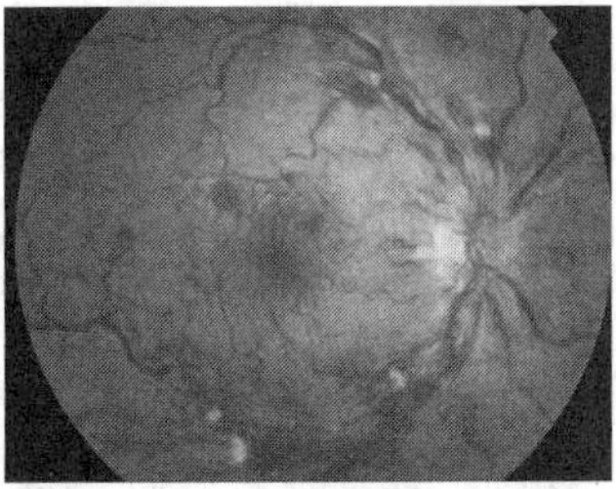

Fig. 7.9 Central retinal vein occlusion—grossly tortuous veins with intraretinal haemorrhage and cotton-wool spots indicative of nerve fibre layer infarcts. (Courtesy of Miss Seema Verma, Consultant Ophthalmologist, Moorfields Eye Hospital). Please see Plate 3 for a colour version of this figure.

Chemical burn

- Alert ophthalmologist as soon as possible—potentially blinding.
- Institute treatment immediately.

Think about

The cornea is exquisitely sensitive to damage from chemical trauma (Fig. 7.10), and the examining physician should be mindful that with any history of exposure careful examination is needs and a low threshold for referral if unsure.

Ask about

If there is any history of alkali (cements, plasters, etc.), acids, solvents or detergent exposure, do not wait to take a further history or examine visual acuity—initiate irrigation.

Look for

- Severe pain,
- Blurred vision,
- Red eye,
- Eyelid spasm.

Critical signs of conjunctival pallor, corneal opacification with no view of the iris, or burns to the surrounding skin may necessitate hospital admission.

Think: Treat first, ask questions later.

Management

- Administer g. benoxinate or other topical anaesthetic.
- Irrigate with normal saline for at least 20–30min (use intravenous tubing connected to solution to facilitate process); ask for nursing assistance while you contact the ophthalmologist.
- Evert upper and lower lids and remove any visible particulate matter by further irrigation and sweep with moistened cotton-bud.
- Measure pH 10min after finishing irrigation using litmus paper in inferior lid fornix—continue irrigation until pH has reached 7.0.
- The volume of saline required varies according to the type of chemical and duration of exposure.
- To reduce discomfort administer g.cyclopentolate 1% to dilate the pupil and reduce ciliary spasm.
- Rarely, if the chemical is thought to be 'tear or CS gas', use of a fan pointed at the face to speed up evaporation of the agent is recommended.
- Do not discharge until discussed with ophthalmologist.

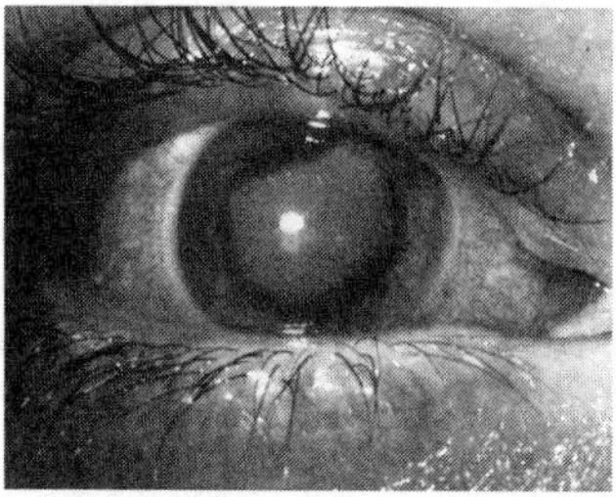

Fig. 7.10 Alkali burn to cornea. Note the large corneal abrasion highlighted by the fluorescein dye. The eye is hyperaemic, but in severe burns the eye may appear white. (Courtesy of Miss Seema Verma, Consultant Ophthalmologist, Moorfields Eye Hospital). Please see Plate 4 for a colour version of this figure.

☠ Infectious corneal ulcer

Potentially blinding—should be seen by ophthalmologist within 4hr.

Think about

Most often seen as a white abscess on the cornea, these ulcers have the ability to perforate or lead to a generalized infection of the globe known as 'endophthalmitis'. Although most abscesses are bacterial in aetiology, viral ulcers (e.g. HSV) are common, and fungi or acanthamoeba are also occasionally causative.

Ask about

- The patient usually complains of a several day history of gradually worsening pain associated with ↓ vision and a red eye.
- Usually associated with previous trauma or contact lens wear, so find out about contact lens-wearing habits:
  - Does the patient wear soft or hard lenses?
  - For how many hours per day are they worn?
  - Has the patient been swimming in their lenses?
  - Find out about what cleaning solutions are used and contact lens hygiene.
- Is there a previous history of HSV infections with cold sores or intercurrent shingles in a V1 or V2 distribution?

Look for

- A deeply injected eye.
- Discharge—ranging from watery to purulent.
- ↓ visual acuity.
- Photophobia.
- Lid spasm.
- Check corneal sensation if suspicious of HSV. Corneal sensitivity is also reduced by contact lens use.
- Instill g. proxymetacaine or g.benoxinate (oxybuprocaine) for temporary analgesia to facilitate examination.
- Look with pen-torch or slitlamp for presence of ulcer on cornea.
- Instil g. fluorescein (a very small drop will suffice) and shine cobalt blue light looking for fluorescent pattern that highlights epithelial breaks.
- A white opacity on the cornea that stains with fluorescein under a cobalt blue light is a corneal abscess (Fig. 7.11) until proven otherwise.
- A 'dendritic' ulcer that has little or no white 'infiltrate' but has a classic branching pattern on fluorescein examination is HSV (Fig. 7.12) or herpes zoster virus (HZV).
- Check for RAPD.
- Instil g.cyclopentolate 1% (if older than 1yr) to dilate pupil and relax ciliary spasm, thereby relieving discomfort, only after discussing with on-call ophthalmologist (who will review to do corneal scrape for microbiology and organize treatment).

Management

If any corneal pathology is seen, call ophthalmologist for review.

Differential diagnosis

- Sterile ulcer, i.e. non-infectious.
- Residual corneal foreign body.

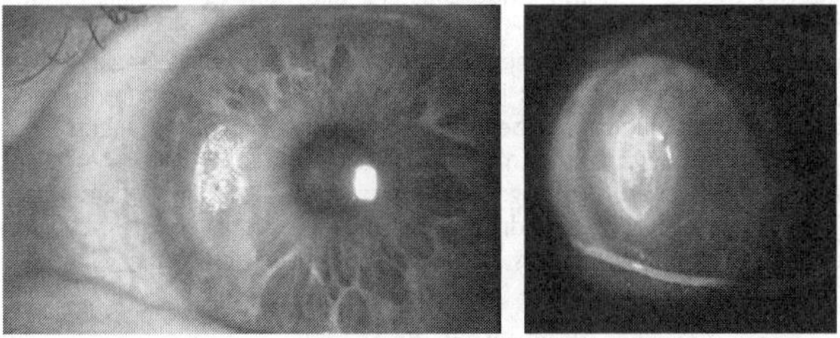

(a) (b)

Fig. 7.11 (a) Corneal abscess of the left eye. (b) Stained with fluorescein. (Courtesy of Miss Seema Verma, Consultant Ophthalmologist, Moorfields Eye Hospital). Please see Plate 5 for a colour version of this figure.

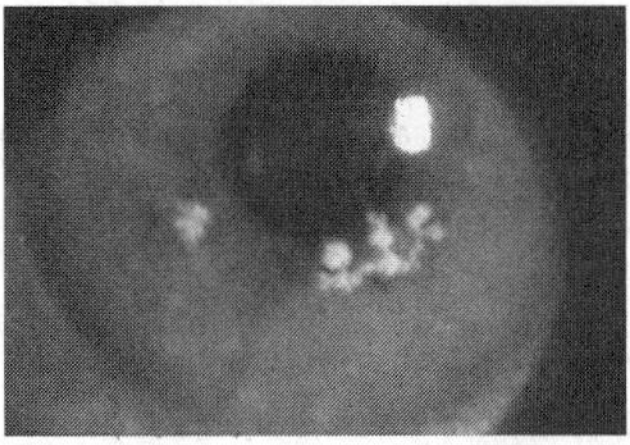

Fig 7.12 Dendritic ulcer—HSV infection of the cornea. Note the typical branching pattern highlighted with fluorescein. (Courtesy of Miss Seema Verma, Consultant Ophthalmologist, Moorfields Eye Hospital). Please see Plate 6 for a colour version of this figure.

⊕ Anterior uveitis (iritis)

Should be seen by ophthalmologist within 24hr.

Think about

Anterior uveitis, iritis and iridocyclitis are all synonyms for inflammation in the anterior chamber of the eye. Under slitlamp examination the ophthalmologist is able to see the individual cells and can ∴ make a diagnosis. For those not trained in the use of this equipment, the diagnosis can be difficult but should be borne in mind as a prolonged untreated episode of uveitis can cause many problems in the long term. The causes are many and varied, including: trauma, ankylosing spondylitis, inflammatory bowel disease, Reiter's syndrome, sarcoid, infections—herpes, syphilis, tuberculosis. Most commonly, however, the cause is idiopathic.

Ask about

An acute red eye, with slightly ↓ visual acuity and photophobia with some tearing. There may have been several previous similar episodes. Chronic anterior uveitis is also seen commonly and has few of the acute symptoms. There may be non-ocular symptoms such as back pain, joint stiffness, bowel symptoms or dysuria.

Look for

- Unilateral or bilateral?
- Visual acuity is usually slightly reduced.
- Conjunctival injection classically 'circum-ciliary', although a moderate to deeply injected eye is most often noted.
- In severe cases, white precipitates are seen on the posterior surface of the cornea ± a hypopyon (Fig. 7.13).
- The pupil is occasionally stuck to the lens in places (posterior synechiae), causing a small or irregular pupil.

Think: Is this red watery eye infective or inflammatory?

Management

- The management for uveitis is topical steroids, although these should never be commenced unless seen by or agreed with the ophthalmologist on call.
- Analgesia until the patient can be seen by the ophthalmologist should be g.cyclopentolate 1% or g.atropine 1%.

Differential diagnosis

- Conjunctivitis.
- Episcleritis/scleritis.
- Keratitis.
- Endophthalmitis—if occurring soon after intraocular surgery.
- Intraocular malignancy—rarely.

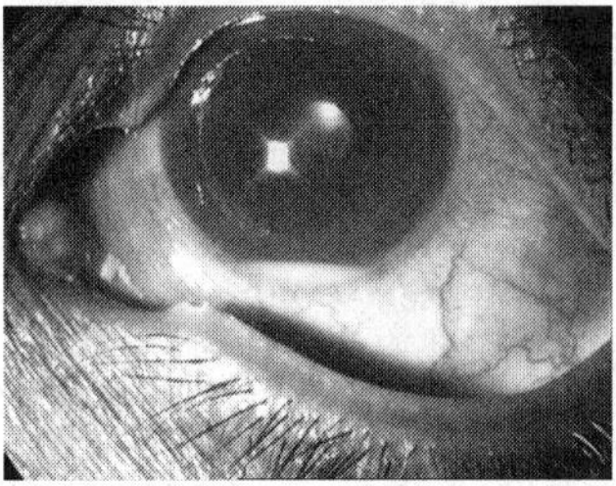

Fig. 7.13 Hypopyon of the left eye. (Courtesy of Miss Seema Verma, Consultant Ophthalmologist, Moorfields Eye Hospital). Please see Plate 7 for a colour version of this figure.

Corneal abrasion/foreign body

Can be treated by resident on-call with follow-up in ophthalmology clinic.

Think about

Any minor trauma to the cornea can result in significant discomfort. Commonly caused by a contact lens, fingernail, plant or tree branch, a scratch on the cornea is easily treated. A foreign body (FB) should be examined closely to exclude any penetrating injury, especially when caused by welding, grinding, etc. If the FB is seen clearly on the front of the cornea, the resident on call can make an attempt to remove it.

Ask about

- Mechanism of injury.
- Wearing protective glasses?
- Type of material.
- Velocity of FB.
- Tetanus status.
- Pain and foreign body ('gritty') sensation is often severe.
- Photophobia.

Look for

- Conjunctival injection.
- Lid spasm and occasional swelling.
- Tearing.
- If the abrasion is central the visual acuity may be reduced.
- Fluorescein staining reveals a hyperfluorescent epithelial defect under cobalt blue light.
- Rust ring or FB visible on cornea.
- Immediate relief with topical anaesthetic.

Management

- Administer topical anaesthetic, e.g. g.proxymetacaine, g.benoxinate or g.amethocaine, for temporary analgesia—do not prescribe for patient to take home as these agents inhibit corneal wound healing.
- Check visual acuity.
- Document size of abrasion.
- Instil one *small* drop of g.fluorescein and inspect lesion under cobalt blue light.
- Evert lids to ensure no FB in lid fornices (📖 p276).
- Analgesia is achieved through cycloplegia, e.g. g.cyclopentolate 1% or g.atropine 1% (warn that drops will blur vision) to reduce iris spasm.
- If FB is seen on cornea, attempt to remove it using a cotton-tip applicator under topical anaesthetic.
- Removal of superficially adherent FB is not difficult under slitlamp viewing using an orange needle held parallel to the cornea and using the bevel to lift the edge and remove the FB. However, this should not be attempted unless supervised initially by someone with previous experience. If the FB is deeply embedded, refer the patient to the ophthalmology clinic for removal.

- All abrasions and FBs should be treated with g.chloramphenicol QID, chloramphenicol ointment (oc) nocte and cycloplegia for the first 48hr, e.g. g.cyclopentolate BD (2–3 days).
- Patching is only rarely necessary; and then only with very large abrasions and significant discomfort. There is no good evidence that it is superior to leaving the eye unpatched in the majority of cases.
- Follow-up in ophthalmology clinic if uncomplicated—in 2–3 days is sufficient. If the abrasion is large, or the FB is not removed, bring back the next day.
- If the injury was sustained via contact lens-related means, ensure no lens wear until 1 week after symptoms resolve.

Differential diagnosis

- Herpes simplex keratitis.
- Recurrent erosion syndrome (pain on opening eyes in the morning that settles during the day and associated with previous significant corneal abrasion).

Orbital and periorbital cellulitis

All cases should be assessed by ENT.

Think about

Periorbital/preseptal cellulitis is infection or inflammation of the eyelids and surrounding skin but with no involvement of structures posterior to the tarsus (collagenous central structure within the lid). Occasionally chemosis is seen (swelling of the conjunctiva) but there should be no involvement of the globe or extraocular muscles. Orbital cellulitis is a sight-threatening infection of the orbit and involvement of both ophthalmology and ENT at an early stage is vital. Ophthalmology should be informed at any stage if vision appears compromised.

Ask about

- Preseptal cellulitis can arise from a number of aetiologies:
  - Sinus disease (especially ethmoid).
  - Nasolacrimal duct obstruction (dacryocystitis) is common, especially in children.
  - Traumatic abrasions around the eye.
  - Lid infections, e.g. chalazion (blocked and infected meibomian ducts) (Fig. 7.14), stye.

In children under 5yr the orbital septum is very thin and thus infections starting as preseptal may migrate posteriorly very rapidly and further progress to become meningitis. The younger the child, the faster this progression can occur.

- Orbital cellulitis arises from:
  - Direct extension from a sinus infection, focal orbital or dental infection.
  - Complication of orbital trauma, e.g. a blow-out fracture.
  - Complicating eye surgery, e.g. following retinal detachment repair.

A history should ∴ include questions regarding trauma, ENT infections.

Look for

- Preseptal cellulitis:
  - The skin of the lids is red, swollen and warm—the patient may not be able to open the eyes because of the oedema.
  - Conjunctival swelling (chemosis) and mild injection may be present.
  - Discharge from the nasolacrimal duct is often seen.
- Orbital cellulitis:
  - A red eye.
  - Pain worse on eye movement.
  - Double vision with restricted ocular motility ± proptosis.
  - Significant chemosis.
  - Blurred vision.
  - Headache.
  - Fever.
  - ↓ periorbital sensation.
  - RAPD.
  - Disc swelling on fundoscopy.

Investigation

- Check mental state, cardiovascular stability and for any neck stiffness.
- Check temperature.
- Check visual acuity.
- Check that eye movements are full and symmetrical with no diplopia or pain.
- Check for presence of obvious proptosis.
- Assess degree of conjunctival injection.
- Check for RAPD.
- Check fundus for disc swelling or vessel tortuosity.
- Inform ENT of findings.

Management

If preseptal cellulitis suspected and the child is <5yr, hospital admission is warranted for intravenous antibiotics (check local guidelines). For those >5yr who are not systemically unwell, oral antibiotics should suffice, e.g. co-amoxiclav and metronidazole (to be discussed, if possible, with microbiology). Bring back to ENT clinic after discussion with on-call registrar.

If orbital cellulitis is diagnosed:

- Inform ENT/ophthalmology.
- Organize CT scan.
- IV access.
- Full blood count.
- Blood cultures.
- Admit.

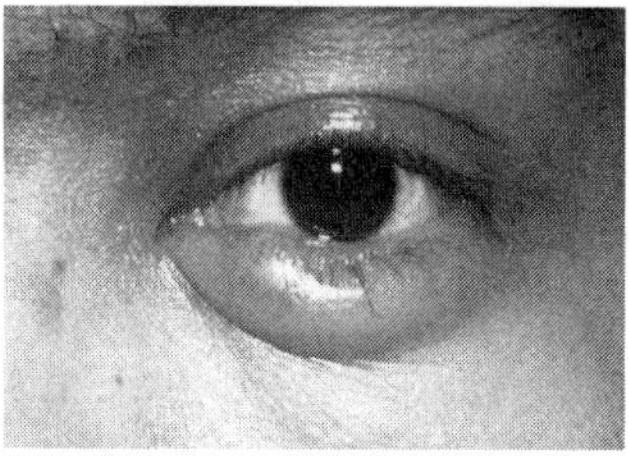

Fig. 7.14 Chalazion—meibomian gland abscess. (Courtesy of Miss Seema Verma, Consultant Ophthalmologist, Moorfields Eye Hospital). Please see Plate 8 for a colour version of this figure.

ⓘ Herpes zoster ophthalmicus

Patient should be reviewed in clinic the following day.

Think about

An acute vesicular rash following the fifth dermatome, usually unilateral. Headaches, fever and malaise with a painful red eye may indicate ocular involvement.

Ask about

- Duration of rash and pain.
- Immunocompromised status.

Look for

- Distribution of rash.
- Check visual acuity.
- Evaluate cornea with fluorescein.
- Dilate to perform optic nerve and retinal examination.

Management

- Adults with a severe rash for less than 3 days—give aciclovir 800mg PO 5 times daily for 10 days.
- If ophthalmic involvement suspected—inform ophthalmologist for review.

ⓘ Bacterial/viral conjunctivitis

Ensure patient has follow-up in 2–3 days unless concerned.

Think about

Particularly common and generally easy to treat, the majority of conjunctivitis does not need to be seen by the ophthalmologist. Occasionally, though, infections with less common organisms cause problems, so if there is a history of prolonged conjunctivitis refractory to treatment don't send away the patient with another course of chloramphenicol. It is particularly important not to miss *Neisseria gonorrhoeae, Chlamydia,* HSV or HZV. In summer months the commonest presentation is allergic.

Ask about

- One eye or both?
- Contact with other affected individuals.
- Pink, itchy, gritty, watery—more likely viral or allergic.
- Whether sticky (esp. in mornings) or purulent—more likely bacterial.
- If no resolution with common topical antibiotics consider Chlamydia and take sexual history.
- Cold sores (HSV).
- If significant pain, consider other causes of red eye, e.g. uveitis, scleritis.
- Associated viral upper respiratory tract infection.
- Associated allergic rhinitis.

Look for

- Check visual acuity.
- Examine and document conjunctival injection and papillae in conjunctival fornices.
- Pre-auricular lymph node—usually viral.
- Fluorescein uptake by cornea under blue light—?dendritic ulcer.
- Small gray subepithelial opacities in cornea—?adenoviral conjunctivitis.
- Corneal thinning or infiltrate.
- Investigation.
- Bacterial and viral conjunctival swabs.

Management

- If you suspect bacterial conjunctivitis, prescribe g.chloramphenicol QID for one week and oc.chloramphenicol nocte for one week.
- Viral conjunctivitis is self-limiting, although it can take 2–3 weeks to resolve fully. Advise careful hygiene and prescribe g.hypromellose PRN for comfort. If corneal opacities present, refer to ophthalmology clinic.
- If repeat attendance for non-resolving conjunctivitis, refer to ophthalmology clinic for early review.
- Allergic conjunctivitis—prescribe g.sodium cromoglycate, g.opatanol, g.rapitil or g.lodoxamide; advise GP referral if no improvement in 1 month.

Flashes and floaters

- Very urgent when retinal detachment.
- Less urgent when posterior vitreous detachment.

Think about

The retina gives symptoms of flashing lights if pulled or distorted. The vitreous becomes progressively more 'liquid' with age—a normal process called 'syneresis'. With this process the vitreous cortex can peel away from the retina to collapse centrally. This is known as posterior vitreous detachment. The floaters that are seen are remnants of the solid vitreous, often where it was previously attached to the retina, e.g. at the optic nerve. This process gives rise to the common symptoms of flashes and floaters.

This must, however, be distinguished from a retinal detachment (RD)—most commonly, a tear in the retina occurs, allowing entry of the vitreous fluid to the subretinal space, thereby → separation of the retina from the underlying retinal pigment epithelium. RD is sight threatening and an urgent opinion should be sort.

Ask about

- Posterior vitreous detachment:
  - Sudden onset and episodic flashes of light in part of the visual field of one eye.
  - Concurrent grey floaters described as 'spider's web' or 'tadpoles' waving in front of vision—'I kept trying to wipe them away.'
  - Normal vision.
- RD:
  - Sudden onset of very bright flashes.
  - Accompanying history of floaters 'like black rain' (blood).
  - 'A curtain hanging in front of my vision.'
  - 'Straight lines look bent.'
  - 'There are bits missing in my vision.'
  - Vision normal or significantly reduced (dependent upon whether macula is 'on' or 'off', i.e. detached).
  - More common in high myopes (ask if patient is very short-sighted).
  - More common if previous history of RD.
  - More common in proliferative diabetic retinopathy.

Look for

- Check best corrected visual acuity in both eyes—visual acuity normal or reduced.
- Look for and document whether presence of RAPD.
- Instil g.tropicamide 1% both eyes.
- Abnormal red reflex—significant RD.
- Perform ophthalmoscopy, looking in all quadrants for presence of blood or retinal detachment. Blood visible in the vitreous cavity—RD.
- If nothing is seen and there are no other suspicious features in history or exam, ask patient to return next day for dilated fundus exam by ophthalmologist in clinic.
- If retinal detachment, retinal tear or haemorrhage is seen, call the ophthalmologist on call to discuss further management and possibly to admit.

ⓘ Dry eyes, blepharitis, lid lumps and bumps

With the right advice, the patient may not require another hospital appointment.

Blepharitis, meibomianitis and dry eye

Ask about

Symptoms of itching, burning, FB sensation, frontal headaches, constant watering, and crusting on the lids—bilateral.

Look for

Crusty lids or lashes, foam in tear film inferiorly, reddened lid margins, punctuate erosions on corneal examination with fluorescein and blue light (pin-prick superficial dots on cornea).

Management

Eyelid hygiene and artificial tears:

- Place hot face-towel across lids for a minute.
- Massage lids—down for top lid, up for bottom lid.
- Take cotton-tip applicator. Dip in solution of previously boiled cup of water mixed with a teaspoon of Johnson's baby shampoo or sodium bicarbonate. Scrub lashes and lid margins.
- After use artificial tear drops.
- Perform twice daily.
- Referral from GP if no improvement after persistent effort.

Styes (hordoleum) and meibomian cysts (chalazion)

Look for

- Painful, red lid lump on lid margin or within lid, occasionally with discharge.
- Blocked meibomian gland or sebaceous gland orifice.
- On lid eversion, red lump apparent under tarsal conjunctiva.

Management

Eyelid hygiene and topical antibiotics. Advise to obtain GP referral if no improvement in a month.

Postoperative cataract care

If cataract surgery is done under local anaesthesia, most patients should be able to go home after 2hr. The eye may be bandaged overnight and the bandages are taken off by the patient the following day. Patients are typically given topical steroid drops and antibiotics (e.g. g.maxidex and g. chloramphenicol) to use for the next 4 weeks.

Pain

This is a common problem and should be relieved with NSAIDs/ paracetamol. If it does not settle, postoperative inflammation is the next most likely cause. This occurs routinely after surgery, but occasionally the routine drop schedule is not sufficient and needs to be ↑ by the ophthalmologist. ∴ if pain is not reducing, bring the patient back to clinic the next day for review.

Visual acuity reduction

Most patients after routine cataract surgery can expect their vision to take several days to improve fully. If it improves but subsequently relapses, inflammation is again likely and the patient should attend the next day for assessment in clinic.

Infection

Pain in conjunction with infection (endophthalmitis) in the eye is rare but must not be missed. The signs are a hypopyon, severely ↓ visual acuity, poor or absent red reflex and a deeply injected eye with severe pain. Contact should be made with ophthalmology on call immediately.

Common drops

Table 7.1 Commonly used eye drops

Drop	Strength	Action	Administration
g.tropicamide	0.5%,1%	Mydriatic, cycloplegic	Stat (lasts 3hr)
g.cyclopentolate	0.5% or 1% lasts up to 12hr	Mydriatic, cycloplegic	BD–TDS (lasts 12–18hr)
g.phenylephrine	2.5%,10%	Mydriatic	Stat (lasts 3hr)
g.atropine	0.5%, 1%, 2%	Mydriatic	BD (lasts 3–7 days)
g.homatropine	2%, 5%	Mydriatic, cycloplegic	BD (lasts 2–3 days)
g.proxymetacaine	0.5%	Short-acting topical anaesthetic	Stat (lasts 10min)
g.benoxinate	0.4%	Topical anaesthetic	Stat (lasts 20min)
g.amethocaine	0.5%	Topical anaesthetic	Stat (lasts 30min)
g.fluorescein		Highlights epithelial breaks	
g.pilocarpine	2% or 4%	Miotic	QID
g.latanoprost (Xalatan®)	0.05%	Anti-glaucoma (prostaglandin analogue)	Nocte
g.bimatoprost (Lumigan®)	0.03%	Anti-glaucoma (prostaglandin analogue)	Nocte
Travoprost (Travatan®)		Anti-glaucoma (prostaglandin analogue)	Nocte
g.betaxolol (Betoptic®)	0.5%	Anti-glaucoma (β-blocker)	BD
g.timolol	0.25% or 0.5%	Anti-glaucoma (β-blocker)	BD
g.Xalacom®	latanoprost 0.0005% + timolol 0.5%	Anti-glaucoma	OD
g.brimonidine (Alphagan®)	0.2%	Anti-glaucoma (sympathomimetic)	BD
g.dorzolamide (Trusopt®)	2%	Anti-glaucoma (carbonic anhydrase inhibitor)	TDS
g.Cosopt®	dorzolamide 2% + timolol 0.5%	Anti-glaucoma	BD

Table 7.1 (*Contd.*)

Drop	Strength	Action	Administration
g.apraclonidine (Iopidine®)	0.5%	Anti-glaucoma (α_2 agonist)	Stat
g.prednisolone (Predsol®)	0.5%	Topical steroid	1–2 hourly
g.prednisolone (Pred Forte®)	1%	Topical steroid	1–2 hourly
g.fluorometholone (FML®)	0.1%	Topical steroid	BD–QID
oc.aciclovir		Anti-HSV	
g.dexamethasone (Maxidex®)	0.1%	Topical steroid	4–6x (if severe, every 15–60min)
g.Maxitrol®		Topical steroid + antibiotic (neomycin)	QID
g.ketorolac (Acular®)	0.5%	NSAID	TDS
g/oc.chloram phenicol		Antibiotic	QID/nocte
g.ofloxacin	0.3%	Antibiotic	4–6x
g.lodoxamide	0.1%	Anti-allergy	QID
g.olopatadine (Opatanol®)	0.1%	Anti-allergy	BD–TDS
g.nedocromil (Rapitil®)	2%	Anti-allergy	QID
g.sodium cromoglycate	2%	Anti-allergy	QID
g. hypromellose		Artificial tear	PRN
g. polyvinyl alcohol (Liquifilm Tears®)		Artificial tear	PRN
g.carbomer (Viscotears®)		Artificial tear	
oc.Lacri-Lube®		Artificial tear	
g.carmellose (Celluvisc®)	0.5% or 1%	Artificial tear	
oc.propamidine (Brolene®)	0.1%	Anti-*Acanthamoeba*	Hourly

Note: a combination of generic and trade names have been used depending upon which is commonest in practice.
Topical steroids should not be used without direction and ongoing follow-up by an ophthalmologist.
g = guttate (drop); oc = ointment.
Minims are disposable, preservative-free drop containers holding about 4 drops each.

Chapter 8

Ear, nose and throat surgery

Isobel Fitzgerald O'Connor

Introduction

It is important to remember that ENT is 95% routine and 5% 'hot sweat inducing and Medical Defence Union phoning' terror. ∴ many of the referrals that come to the non-ENT-trained junior doctor after hours can be dealt with safely the next working day. Hopefully this chapter will set you along the path of deciding which problems fall into each category.

Useful terms

- AC—air conduction.
- BC—bone conduction.
- BIPP—bismuth iodoform paraffin paste, used in ENT for nasal packing, as a postoperative dressing and in wounds.
- EAC/EAM—external auditory canal/external auditory meatus.
- FB—foreign body.
- FESS—functional endoscopic sinus surgery.
- SNHL—sensorineural hearing loss.
- TM—tympanic membrane.

Anatomy

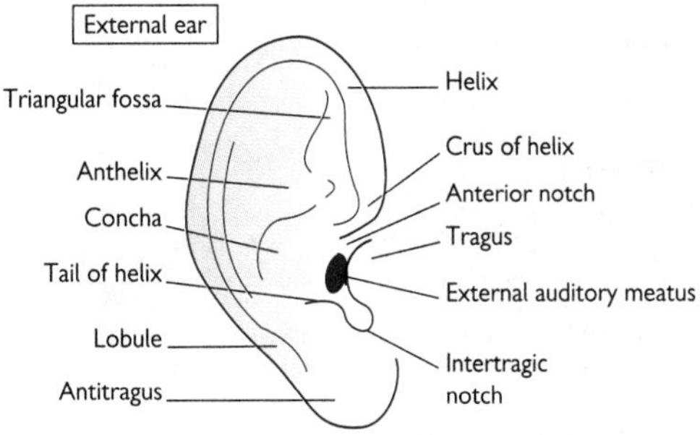

Fig. 8.1 External ear.

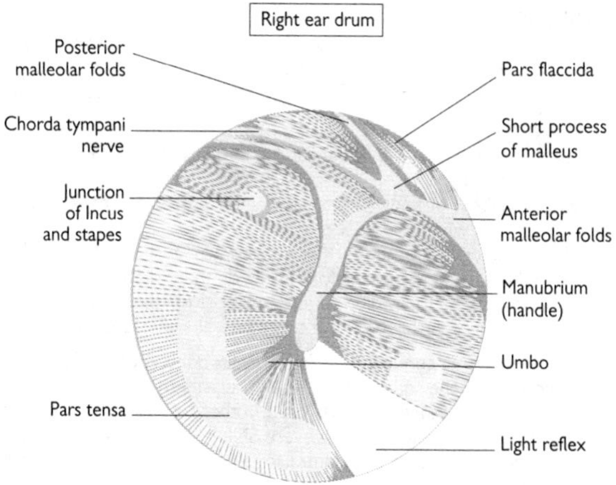

Fig. 8.2 Normal tympanic membrane (right ear).

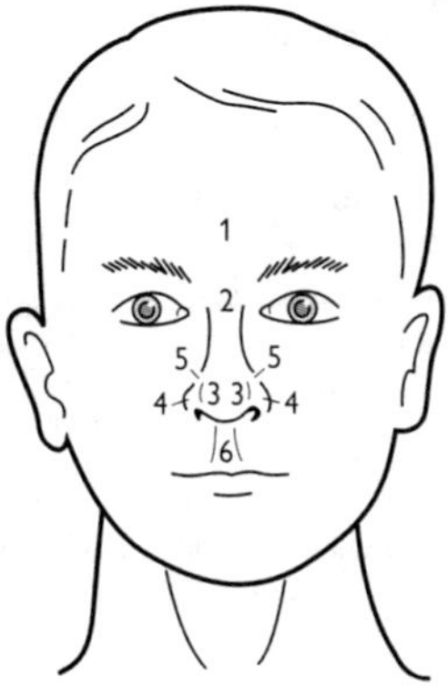

Fig. 8.3 Surface anatomy of the nose. 1, Glabella; 2, nasion; 3, tip-defining points; 4, alar sidewall; 5, supra-alar crease; 6, philtrum.

Hearing tests

Tuning fork tests can appear complicated, but if you can perform them you will be able to impart useful information to the senior on the end of a phone.

Rinne's test

Compares air conduction with bone conduction. Test each ear individually.

- Use a 512Hz tuning fork.
- Strike your elbow or knee (not the patient's) and ask the patient which sound is louder when:
    - Placing the prongs of the fork in line and 2cm away from the EAM.
    - Place the base of the tuning fork firmly on the ipsilateral mastoid process (providing counter-support for this action by resting your other hand on the contralateral side of their face).

In normal hearing, air conduction is better than bone conduction and the patient should hear the sound better when presented to the EAM (Rinne's positive). A negative Rinne's test will occur if there is a conductive hearing loss >20–25dB (true negative) or a severe SNHL (false negative), in which case the auditory nerve of the contralateral ear identifies the sound by bone conduction through the skull.

Weber's test

This test works because a conductive hearing loss causes a relative improvement in the ability to hear a bone-conducted sound.

- Use a 512Hz tuning fork.
- Strike your elbow or knee (not the patient's) and place the base of the tuning fork on the forehead in the midline, providing counter-support for this action by resting your other hand on the occipital region.
- Ask the patient which ear they hear the sound in.

In normal-hearing ears the patient will hear the sound equally loudly in both ears, although if there is a symmetrical hearing loss the patient will also hear the sound equally loudly in both ears. If the patient hears the sound louder in one ear there is a conductive hearing loss >10dB in the louder ear or a SNHL in the opposite ear.

As this book deals with 'out-of-hours' hospital medicine I will not explain audiometry as it is unlikely to be available outside normal working hours. It is also unlikely that out-of-hours you will be expected to use an operating microscope, so its use is not described.

Nasendoscopy

Fibreoptic nasendoscopy allows visualization of the laryngeal structures and aids location of a foreign body.

- Ask the patient if they have one nostril that is more patent than the other. If not, spray both nostrils with 2–3 puffs of co-phenylcaine. Advise the patient that this can lead to a numb tongue and that they should not consume hot drinks for about an hour after the procedure.
- Ask the patient to put the scope under their tongue for 30sec to warm the end up. De-mist the end with a Steret (alcohol wipe).
- Tell the patient that you are going to gently insert the scope into the right nostril first (usually the more patent nostril). Get them to breathe out of their mouth and point their nose forward, and not tilt their head.
- The entire nasal cavity can be visualized. Try to run the scope under the inferior turbinate to the postnasal space.
- Position the scope downwards and the oropharynx can be identified. Identify the soft palate, uvula, posterior pharyngeal wall and the base of tongue.
- As the scope progresses, the valleculae and epiglottis appear, then the aryepiglottic folds, arytenoids and piriform fossae—a common site for foreign bodies to reside in.
- Finally visualize the vocal cords and see whether their movement is symmetrical—ask the patient to say 'aayh' and 'eeyh', to stick out their tongue and to pinch their nose around the scope and blow out their cheeks with their lips pursed. This improves the view of the piriform fossae.

Emergency department

ⓘ Otitis externa

This is one of the most common problems dealt with by ENT surgeons and is an infection of the skin and cartilaginous external ear canal that leads to otalgia (sometimes very severe), aural discharge, ↓ hearing, tinnitus, vertigo and systemic upset.

Think about

Cause: swimming, foreign travel, trauma (foreign body/cotton buds), eczema and narrow EACs.

Ask about

- Is the patient immunocompromised or diabetic—much more likely to progress to malignant otitis externa (📖 p313)?
- Is the infection recurrent (unlikely that previous antibiotics treated the infective cause)—retake swabs?
- Has a superimposed fungal infection developed?

Look for

Ensure there is no mastoid swelling or fluctuance. Use an auriscope to examine the EAM.

Management

If there is a lot of debris, either remove this by microsuctioning or dry-mop it away. If this is not possible, arrange for the patient to be seen in an outpatient clinic the next day for this to happen.

If the canal is too stenotic and the drum cannot be seen:

- Insert a 'Pope Wick' and apply a few Sofradex® or Gentisone® HC drops, allowing the wick to swell and coat the EAM.
- Advise the patient that the wick may fall out but to continue with the drops (2 drops TDS).
- Arrange for follow-up the next day.

If the patient has mastoid tenderness and fluctuance:

- Admit them for IV antibiotics, monitor temperature, blood glucose and neurological signs.
- Give cefuroxime (750mg IV TDS) and metronidazole (500mg IV TDS) in addition to the topical antibiotics.
- Inform the registrar as soon as possible and monitor the patient—they may need urgent computed tomography (CT) of the temporal bones, and surgical intervention.

Malignant otitis externa: alert senior

This is caused by *Pseudomonas aeruginosa* in diabetic patients and must be taken very seriously as it can advance rapidly to intracranial complications and potentially death. The patient usually presents with a painful discharging ear that has proven very resistant to topical and systemic antibiotics, and it may cause a cranial nerve palsy.

- Arrange for microsuctioning of the ear.
- Take a microbiology sample.
- Start on ciprofloxacin eardrops and IV meropenem (you must contact the on-call microbiology services and ask for their recommendations for IV antibiotics) and analgesia (may need opiates).
- Check recent glycaemic control and FBC, U&Es, CRP and ESR—as a baseline, and to monitor whether treatment is working.
- Discuss with the registrar to see whether the patient needs admission—if they do not, they will need very early review.

ⓘ Otitis media

This is not commonly seen as an emergency referral in adults, and presents most commonly in children.

Think about

Bacterial (*Streptococcus pneumoniae, Haemophilus influenzae, Moraxella catarrhalis*) or viral cause.

Ask about

Previous episodes.

Look for

Full, erythematous, bulging tympanic membrane, which may perforate.

Management

- Antibiotics—Augmentin® or erythromycin in penicillin-allergic patients (use BNF for Children for doses).
- Analgesia.
- Can try topical decongestants to aid middle ear ventilation.

ⓘ Traumatic tympanic membrane perforation

This does not need to be seen as an emergency unless the patient has vertigo.

Think about

Penetrating injury, slap to side of face, blast injury.

Ask about

Does the patient have vertigo? This raises the suspicion of a subluxed stapes, in which case the ear should be explored and repaired to avoid a permanent sensorineural hearing loss.

Look for

The site of the perforation—document the position and size of the perforation in the notes so that the next doctor reviewing them can identify any improvement.

Investigations

- Rinne's and Weber's tests.
- If the patient has vertigo, discuss with the SpR whether they need CT of the temporal bones.

Management

Book the patient into an emergency clinic and arrange audiometry over the following 1–3 days to identify a baseline audiogram. If there is no evidence of infection, no treatment will be given, except to arrange a follow-up appointment in 3–6 months to ensure the perforation has healed or, if it hasn't, to assess whether the patient may be suitable for a myringoplasty if they are now more prone to ear infections. Advise the patient to keep the ear scrupulously dry.

Temporal bone fractures: alert senior immediately

Think about

Does the patient have a facial nerve palsy?

Ask about

Have they noticed a hearing loss?

Look for

All head injury patients must have an otoscopic examination—is there blood or cerebrospinal fluid (CSF) in the EAC, or a perforation of the TM?

Investigations

Temporal bone fractures are picked up on CT, not by plain X-ray. Test hearing with tuning forks and audiometry as soon as it is available.

Management

Alert the senior about management. Most situations will be dealt with conservatively, except when there is an immediate facial nerve palsy—it is likely the patient will need to have the facial nerve decompressed surgically without delay, so work them up for theatre and discuss with the senior when they should be nil by mouth (NBM).

Sudden-onset hearing loss

Sudden hearing loss (SHL) is a medical emergency for which definitive diagnosis and treatment is still largely unknown. SHL generally refers to hearing loss of *sensorineural origin*. It has been defined for research purposes and accepted by most authorities as 30dB or more sensorineural hearing loss over at least three contiguous audiometric frequencies occurring within 3 days or less.

Despite taking a full history and examination, many patients have none of the causes of hearing loss described below, and it is thought that the cause is 2° to a viral infection or a vascular episode.

Think about

- Has the patient got a conductive hearing loss 2° to otitis media with effusion?
- Have they recently undergone ear surgery?
- Have they suffered a recent head injury or barotrauma with rupture of the round window due to alteration in cabin pressure during an aeroplane flight or after diving?
- Could the patient have syphilis (rare cause) or an acoustic neuroma?
- Has the patient been exposed to ototoxic drugs?

Table 8.1 Potentially ototoxic drugs

Class of drug	Example
Non-steroidal anti-inflammatories	Salicylates
Antibiotics	Gentamicin topically and systemically
β-blockers	Atenolol
Loop diuretics	Furosemide
Metals	Cisplatin (chemotherapy)

- Is this sudden-onset hearing loss or has the patient got a mechanical obstruction (e.g. impacted wax in the ear)?
- Are audiology facilities available at the time of admission?

Ask about

Details of the circumstances surrounding the hearing loss and the time course of its onset should be elicited. Associated symptoms, such as tinnitus, vertigo or dizziness, and aural fullness should also be asked about. Past medical history of other diseases associated with SHL should also be obtained, such as diabetes, autoimmune disorders, malignancies, neurological conditions (multiple sclerosis) and hypercoagulable states.

Look for

More often than not, the examination will be unremarkable. However, any processes such as middle ear effusions, infections, cholesteatoma and wax impaction should be excluded.

A thorough neurological exam including Weber's and Rinne's tests should be performed. Examine specifically the facial nerve and look in the ear to exclude infection, perforation or vesicles.

Table 8.2 Interpretation of tuning fork tests

Test	Conductive hearing loss	Sensorineural hearing loss
Rinne's	Negative	Positive
Weber's	Will show 'better' hearing on the affected side	Will show 'better' hearing on the unaffected side

If the hearing loss is conductive the patient can be sent home if seen out of hours, but an audiogram should be arranged for the next working day to confirm the diagnosis.

Investigations

An audiogram (pure tone, speech, tympanometry, including stapedial reflex testing) should be performed on all patients with SHL. The audiogram is the foundation of the diagnosis and provides prognostic information. Serial testing provides documentation of the progression or resolution of the sensorineural hearing loss and response to treatment. However, on admission out-of-hours this may not be available, so discuss this with the registrar on call with you, as Rinne's and Weber's tests will be the only tests that a decision to admit a patient can be made on.

The following blood tests should be performed: FBC, ESR, clotting studies, thyroid function tests, glucose, and VDRL.

An MRI scan should be arranged for the near future to exclude an acoustic neuroma.

Management

The treatment of sudden-onset sensorineural hearing loss can be very varied between senior clinicians even in the same hospital, as essentially there is no evidence supporting any one management plan. ∴ talk to the registrar before implementing a treatment regimen and tell the patient that no one treatment option has proven efficacy, most will do anything that could possibly improve their hearing. You must warn the patient of the side-effects of steroids (acute confusion, gastric irritation, altered diabetic control).

If the hearing loss is recent (over the preceding day or two), arrange admission and bedrest. Advise the patient that they may need to stay in for 2–3 days for treatment and serial audiograms.

- Start the patient on carbogen (5min per hr whilst awake), which is a combination of 95% oxygen and 5% carbon dioxide. Studies have shown that carbogen increases the partial pressure of oxygen in perilymph. In addition, carbon dioxide is a known potent vasodilator of the vestibulocochlear vasculature, resulting in ↑ blood flow.
- Prednisolone 0.5mg/kg OD for 5 days.
- Aciclovir 800mg five times a day for 5 days.
- Betahistine 8mg PO TDS.

Other treatment options include anticoagulation and low molecular weight dextran to lower blood viscosity.

If the hearing loss was sudden but happened >7 days previously, the opportunity to treat may have been passed, so discuss the benefits of admission with the registrar.

Vertigo

Vertigo is defined as the illusion of movement. Usually these patients do not need admission to hospital but reassurance that the episode will be self-limiting, as the condition is frightening and all consuming.

Think about

- Is the cause central—stroke, migraine, epilepsy, tumour, multiple sclerosis?
- Is the cause peripheral?
  - Ménière's disease—although the aetiology of the condition is unknown, dilatation of the endolymphatic spaces of the membranous labyrinth is thought to be the cause.
  - Benign paroxysmal positional vertigo (BPPV).
  - Acute vestibular failure/labyrinthitis.

Ask about

Patients with vertigo are often vague. Try to get exact details of when it started, what they were doing and whether they have ever had the symptoms before (Table 8.3).

Look for

Full neurological examination, to exclude a central cause. The absence of nystagmus implies a non-ENT cause for the problem.

Dix–Hallpike test (Fig. 8.4)

This test consists of a series of two manoeuvres:

- With the patient sitting on the examination table, facing forward, eyes open, the doctor turns the patient's head 45° to the right.
- The physician supports the patient's head as the patient lies back quickly from a sitting to supine position, ending with the head hanging 20° off the end of the examination table. The patient remains in this position for 30sec. Then the patient returns to the upright position and is observed for 30sec.
- The manoeuvre is repeated with the patient's head turned to the left.

A positive test is indicated if any of these manoeuvres induces vertigo, with or without nystagmus.

Investigations

If the patient is unwell enough to require admission (so unsteady that they cannot walk or live on their own) an audiogram should be performed during the next working day, and consider an urgent MRI if the dizziness is not settling.

Management

BPPV: perform the Epley manoeuvre; otherwise treatment is largely symptomatic—stemetil and betahistine (SERC) 8–16mg TDS. If the Epley manoeuvre improves the patient's symptoms, they can be taught Brant–Daroff exercises, which they can do themselves.

Table 8.3 Diagnostic features in the differential diagnosis of vertigo

	Ménière's disease	BPPV	Labyrinthitis
Onset	Sudden	Sudden	Sudden
Episode length	Minutes to hours	Seconds to minutes	Hours to days
Related to movement?	No	Yes—usually turning over in bed or looking up to get an object from a high shelf	No
Nausea	Mild	Yes	Yes
Previous episode	Yes	Yes	No
Other features	Tinnitus	Associated with head injuries and ear infection; nystagmus is rotational, not vertical	Recent upper respiratory tract infection (URTI)

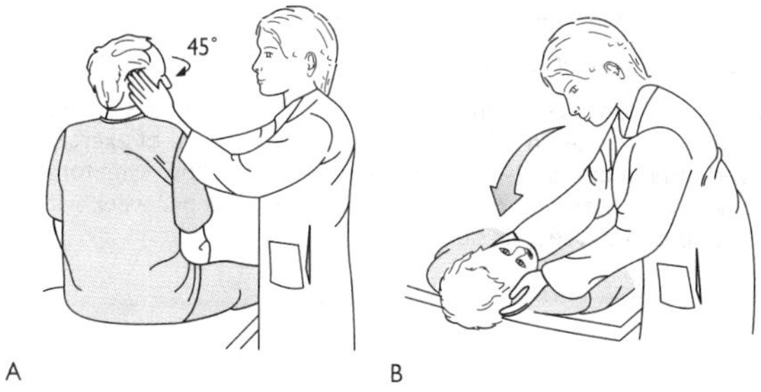

Fig. 8.4 The Dix–Hallpike test—diagnostic for BPPV.

Epley manoeuvre

- The patient sits on the examination table, with eyes open and head turned 45° to the right.
- The doctor supports the patient's head as the patient lies back quickly from a sitting to supine position, ending with the head hanging 20° off the end of the examination table.
- The doctor turns the patient's head 90° to the left side. The patient remains in this position for 30sec.
- The doctor turns the patient's head an additional 90° to the left while the patient rotates their body 90° in the same direction. The patient remains in this position for 30sec.
- The patient sits up on the left side of the examination table. The procedure may be repeated on either side until the patient experiences relief of symptoms.

Brandt–Daroff exercises

These exercises can be given to the patient to perform at home. Ask the patient to sit on the edge of the bed near the middle with their legs hanging over the side. Give them the following instructions (Fig. 8.5):

- Quickly lie down on to your left side and turn your head 45° to the right (toward the ceiling). Hold this position for 30sec or until any dizziness passes (1).
- Return to the upright position, looking straight ahead for 30sec (2).
- Perform same manoeuvre to the right side, with head rotated toward the left. Hold the position for 30sec or until any dizziness passes (3).
- Return to the upright position, looking straight ahead for 30sec (4).

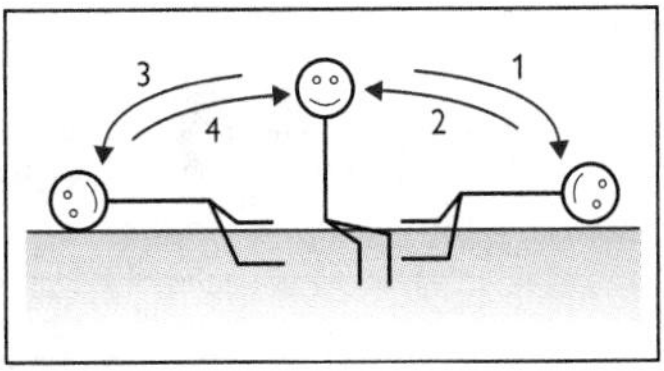

Fig. 8.5 Brandt–Daroff exercises.

The four positions (1–4) comprise one 'set' of the exercises. Complete 5 repetitions of this set in one sitting, for a total of 10min of exercises. Do this 2–3 times a day for 2–3 weeks. If you have no further symptoms after 1 week of exercises, you may decrease to 3–4 times per week with only 2 repetitions of the set per sitting.

ⓘ Sinusitis

This is a relatively common problem, but is not often seen as an out-of-hours referral, as the patient can usually wait until the next day. Patients with sinusitis do not often need admission, although the complications can be severe and need to be contemplated before a decision to admit (or not) is made.

Children progress far more quickly from a cold to the complications of acute sinusitis, so have a much lower index of suspicion.

Think about

Symptoms:

- Does the patient have a recent history of a cold or URTI?
- Do they have an episode of acute or acute on chronic sinusitis?

Ask about

- Is this the first episode?
- Have they had previous surgery (antral washouts or functional endoscopic sinus surgery (FESS)?
- Have they had previous complications associated with sinusitis?

Look for

Evidence of:

- *Periorbital cellulitis*—proptosis, swelling of the eyelid, difficulty opening the eye and painful movements, ↓ red/green colour vision (severe sign).
- A soft boggy swelling overlying the frontal sinus: *Potts' puffy tumour*, osteomyelitis of the frontal bone.
- Intracranial extension—cavernous sinus thrombosis.

Management

Discuss with senior as soon as you decide to admit the patient. Always refer to an ophthalmologist if you are concerned about orbital cellulitis (📖 p296). Start Otrivine® nasal drops, a broad-spectrum antibiotic such as Augmentin® IV and arrange a CT scan to image the sinuses and orbit, and looking for evidence of mucoceles.

Facial nerve palsy

It is important fully to assess a patient before making a diagnosis of facial nerve palsy.

Think about

Site along the facial nerve where the problem could arise:

- *Intracranial*—acoustic neuroma, brainstem tumours, stroke, multiple sclerosis.
- *Intratemporal*—cholesteatoma, otitis media, Ramsay–Hunt syndrome (herpes zoster oticus).
- *Infratemporal*—trauma, parotid tumours.
- *Other*—Bell's palsy (idiopathic facial nerve palsy).

The terms facial nerve palsy and Bell's palsy are *not* interchangeable: a facial nerve palsy can be described as a Bell's palsy only when all other causes have been excluded.

Ask about

- Has this happened before?
- When was the onset?
- Is the facial nerve palsy worsening or improving?

Look for

Examine the ear for signs of infection or vesicles (Ramsay–Hunt syndrome) and perform a full neurological examination, as this may be a stroke.

- Is the patient able to wrinkle their forehead on the affected side?
  - Lower motor neurone lesion—forehead involved.
  - Upper motor neurone lesion—forehead spared due to contralateral supply to lower motor neurone.
- Grade the facial nerve palsy using the House–Brackmann grading system (Table 8.4).

Investigations

These depend on the examination findings. If there is evidence of infection in the ear, consider otitis media or malignant otitis externa, and follow the investigation and management plan detailed above, contacting the registrar soon after seeing the patient. Take into consideration that the patient may need to undergo surgical decompression after a CT scan of the temporal bone.

Arrange for the patient to have an audiogram and stapedial reflexes as soon as possible (if seen out-of-hours this should be during the next working day) as these may give an indication of the level of the palsy.

Table 8.4 House–Brackmann grading system for facial nerve palsy

I	Normal facial function
II	Mild dysfunction, moderate to good forehead function, complete eye closure, slight asymmetry of mouth
III	Moderate dysfunction, slight to moderate movement of forehead, complete eye closure with effort, mouth slightly weak
IV	Moderately severe dysfunction, no forehead movement, incomplete eye closure, mouth asymmetrical
V	Severe dysfunction, asymmetrical at rest, no forehead movement, incomplete eye closure, slight mouth movement
VI	Total paralysis

Management

As with sudden-onset hearing loss discuss the management plan with the patient. Evidence that steroids alter the course of the palsy is minimal, especially if the palsy has been present for more than 48hr. However, most patients will try anything that could improve this disfiguring condition.

If the neurological examination is normal except for the facial nerve palsy, and the ear appears normal or has vesicles, treat with:

- 0.5mg/kg prednisolone for 5 days.
- Aciclovir 400–800mg 5 times per day for 5 days.

The most important structure to protect is the eye and it is vital that the patient is given Lacri-Lube® or hypromellose eye ointment or drops (2 drops at night) and taught how to tape their eye shut with an eye patch and tape at night. If the eye is not taped, corneal ulceration may develop. It is vital that the patient is referred and seen by the ophthalmologist as soon as possible after being seen by you, as they may need to be offered operative intervention.

Epistaxis

Alert the senior if you are unable to stop the bleeding rapidly.

Epistaxis is potentially fatal—it must be taken seriously and seen rapidly.

Think about

- Airway, breathing, circulation (ABC).
- On which side did the bleeding start?
- Did the patient first notice blood in the throat or from the nose?
- Duration of bleed—has it stopped spontaneously?
- Has it happened previously? If so, how was it treated? Did it need surgical intervention?

Ask about

- Aspirin, warfarin or other anticoagulation use.
- Hypertension—treated or untreated
- Recent surgery to nose or epistaxis following trauma, nose-picking or foreign body.
- Neoplasia or systemic disorder—liver disease, thrombocytopenia, haemophilia, hereditary haemorrhagic telangiectasia.

Management

- Well recorded, regular observations.
- IV access, FBC, U&Es, clotting, group & save.
- Attempt to localize site of bleeding using adequate lighting, nasal speculum, suction and protection from the patient's blood.

Stepwise approach to stopping the epistaxis

1. *Simple first aid measures*

- Sit upright, protect the airway, stop patient from swallowing blood.
- Ice to nasal bridge (protect skin to prevent thermal burns).
- Pinch the nostrils together over the fleshy part, not the nasal bridge. Most bleeds occur in Little's area.

2. *Cautery*

Soak topical vasoconstrictor (co-phenylcaine) on to a small pledget of cotton wool and gently insert it into the affected nostril. Re-apply pressure to the outside of the nostrils for 2–3min. Warn the patient they may develop a numb lip.

To visualize Little's area use a Thudicum's speculum and, with a silver nitrate cautery stick, dab (for 1–2sec) around the bleeding point in a circle from the outside inwards; this cauterizes the vessels feeding into the main bleeding point. The aim is for the mucosa to develop a grey residue after the cautery has been applied. If this residue drips out of the nose, clean it away as it can stain the skin with silver nitrate burns, and advise the patient to do this when they leave the clinic room if it continues to dribble from the nose. Persevere with cautery as it will often work and prevent the need for hospital admission. However, if it does not work or the bleeding point is too posterior, nasal packing will be needed.

Do not cauterize both sides of the septum as this can lead to a septal perforation.

If cautery is successful, discharge the patient with an epistaxis advice sheet (no hot or cold drinks, no alcohol or strenuous exercise, and stay inside) and Naseptin® cream (except in those with peanut allergies, as it has a peanut oil base), one application BD to both nostrils.

3. Nasal packing

Pack affected side with a Merocel® nasal tampon. Swiftly insert the tampon fully into the nose, so that only the threads are visible. Inflate with ~10mL water or co-phenylcaine and secure threads to the side of the patient's face (diagram). A second Merocel® can be inserted into the contralateral nostril for tamponade effect.

4. It epistaxis is not halted by anterior packing.

Insert a post-nasal pack using a BIPP pack or in combination with a Foley catheter.

5. Senior review

This is required if epistaxis continues, as the patient may require surgical intervention, particularly if they become haemodynamically unstable.

General points

If the patient is admitted, ensure they are adequately hydrated, do not consume hot food or drinks, and are put on bedrest (with TED stockings). Consider mild sedation to help with anxiety-induced high blood pressure (BP), but beware of respiratory problems and nasal packing-induced hypoxia.

If the patient is discharged, consider Naseptin® nasal cream (1 application to both nostrils BD—check the patient is not allergic to the peanut oil base), 1% ephedrine nasal drops (2 drops TDS both nostrils) and an outpatient appointment in the ENT clinic if nasendoscopy has not been performed as an inpatient. Ensure adequate follow-up for undiagnosed hypertension.

Hypertension in epistaxis

Resuscitate the patient using the Advanced Life Support (ALS) protocol and ABC,

Important points in assessment of the patient

- History of hypertension, diabetes or cardiovascular disease?
- Family history of hypertension? History of asthma or renal failure?
- Normal medications—any regular antihypertensive medication or drugs contributing to high BP or anticoagulants/antiplatelet therapy (check indication, don't just stop it).
- Have they taken their normal prescription for their high BP or are they NBM?
- Is the BP measurement 'real'—check the measurement yourself manually twice.
- Essential investigations:
  - Full blood count (platelets).
  - Group and save/cross-match (as appropriate).
  - Urea and electrolytes (renal failure can result from hypertensive medication and can cause clotting problems).
  - Clotting (also check drug card for heparin, warfarin, aspirin, clopidogrel. **Clopidogrel must not be stopped without checking the indication—if it is for a coronary stent, establish date of intervention and if possible the type of stent, then *check with cardioldogist.***
- Dipstick the urine, looking for blood and protein (signs of renal failure).
- Examine fundi with ophthalmoscope.
- Perform ECG.

Treatment

URGENT: Requires immediate referral to medical team

- If BP >200mmHg systolic or 120mmHg diastolic, *or*
- Any signs of hypertensive encephalopathy (headache, confusion, fits, nausea and vomiting, *or*
- Blood in urine, *or*
- Fundal changes.

Acute management

- If BP persistently >150mmHg systolic, start 2.5mg bendrofluazide OD before discharge and refer to general practitioner (GP).
- In patients who are thiazide intolerant or who are already taking a thiazide (and have definitely taken that day), start amlodipine 5mg OD. **Do not start more than one agent.**

Non-urgent management of hypertension

- If BP >130mmHg systolic, refer to GP on discharge for management of BP control.

Top tips

- If you are worried, inform your seniors.
- Too rapid a reduction in BP may precipitate 'watershed' cerebral infarction.
- **Do not use nifedipine**—this can cause a rapid and unpredictable reduction in BP.
- Angiotensin-converting enzyme (ACE) inhibitors should be avoided because of the risk of first-dose hypotension, especially in elderly patients.
- **Do not stop clopidogrel without checking the indication**—if it is for a coronary stent, discuss with cardiologist before stopping.
- Oral therapy with 2.5mg bendrofluazide will lower BP smoothly in most patients.
- Always inform patient's GP about the hypertension.
- Do not try to lower BP too much in patients with ischaemic heart disease as they may be relying on the perfusion pressure to supply the myocardium.
- Always give lifestyle modification advice (salt, exercise, weight, alcohol and smoking) and make an assessment of cardiovascular risk.
- If you are worried, inform your seniors or seek help.
- *Dr Lucy Hudsmith, Cardiology SpR, Oxford.*

Tonsillitis

Tonsillitis is a common ENT referral. Treatment as an inpatient is, despite starting IV antibiotics, generally supportive by using IV access for fluids and giving regular analgesia.

Think about

- Does the patient have glandular fever?
- Does the patient have a quinsy (peritonsillar abscess)?
- If the patient is older than 40yr, could this be a tonsillar tumour—especially if the history is not acute.

Ask about

Can the patient eat, drink, swallow their own saliva? Admission is reserved for patients who cannot swallow their saliva.

Look for

- Deviation of the uvula—indication of a possible quinsy.
- Does the patient have lymphadenopathy, exudative tonsils or other signs of glandular fever?
- Could the patient have a parapharyngeal abscess?
- Is there trismus?

Investigations

FBC, CRP, U&Es and Paul Bunnell (glandular fever/infectious mononucleosis screen); throat swabs can be taken, but the results usually come back after the patient is discharged so in practice are often not taken.

Management

Admit the patient if they are not able to swallow liquid or their own saliva. Start them on IV fluids but encourage them to keep drinking liquids; unless there is a contraindication, give the first litre very quickly as the patient will be dehydrated and this will make them feel considerably better.

- Start IV antibiotics—1.2g benzylpenicillin QDS IV unless allergic (give erythromycin) and 500mg metronidazole TDS IV. Do not prescribe amoxicillin or Augmentin® as the patient may have undiagnosed glandular fever and a rash will develop that can potentially scar.
- If there is significant trismus, 4–8mg IV dexamethasone can be given as a once-only dose and repeated as necessary, but if you are worried about the patient's airway ensure they are closely monitored and are in a bed near the nurses' station.
- Analgesia—try Difflam® spray or gargle, 1 spray or 5mL to tonsils every 2hr. Paracetamol 1g PO QDS, codeine phosphate 30–60mg PO QDS and diclofenac 50mg PO QDS can be used, but make sure that the patient has started eating or can drink something like milk.

The above management plan is the same for the treatment of a quinsy after the abscess has been drained.

Post-tonsillectomy bleed

1° haemorrhage occurs in the first 24hr after surgery, and 2° haemorrhage usually occurs 5–10 days postoperatively.

Think about

- Is this related to infection?
- How much blood has the patient lost for their bodyweight? Small children have less to lose and ∴ need to return to theatre at an earlier stage than adults, who can usually be managed conservatively.

Ask about

- Bleeding problems,
- Non-steroidal anti-inflammatory drug (NSAID) use.
- Duration and volume of the bleed.

Look for

Active bleeding points, blood in the tonsillar fossa and erythema around the palatal arches (indication of infection).

Management

- Admit the patient.
- Discuss these patients urgently with a senior as they may need to return to theatre (especially if the haemorrhage is 1° or the patient is a small child).
- Gain IV access and send full blood count and group and save samples.
- Start IV fluids and antibiotics (e.g. Augmentin®).
- If the patient will tolerate it, an adrenaline (epinephrine 1:1000)-soaked gauze swab can be applied to the tonsillar fossa with sponge forceps.
- Hydrogen peroxide gargles can be given.

Epiglottitis

Call your senior as soon as you get the referral.

This is a medical emergency as complete respiratory obstruction can occur, classically caused by *H. influenzae* type b. Epiglottitis is fortunately rare in children in the UK because most are vaccinated.

Treatment of epiglottitis in a child should be dealt with by the ENT and paediatric registrars. The child should not be examined until in theatre, with a senior anaesthetist present and a doctor who is able to establish a surgical airway. This is because the child may become distressed, precipitating airway obstruction.

Think about

Is the patient using accessory muscles of respiration, or drooling?

Ask about

- Has the patient been stridulous—the noise produced during inspiration through narrowed upper airways.
- Have they complained of a recent URTI or sore throat?

Look for

Examine the oropharynx, Is there lymphadenopathy or neck swelling?

Investigations

- FBC, CRP, U&Es and possibly a lateral soft tissue X-ray of the neck.
- Fibreoptic nasendoscopy can be performed in adults (**not children**), but is best left to the ENT registrar.

Management

Start IV antibiotics—1.2g benzylpenicillin QDS IV, unless allergic (give erythromycin), and 500mg metronidazole TDS IV.

Oesophageal foreign body

This could be more urgent, depending on the age of the patient, the foreign body and its site.

This is a common presentation in A&E, and the adult patient will already have tried to shift the foreign body with bread, coke or coughing.

Think about

- Type of FB:
  - Adults—fish or meat bones; in young men (who eat too quickly) or elderly patients: pieces of meat.
  - Children—coins.
- Could the patient have pathology that predisposed them to this episode—previous stricture or stenosis, carcinoma, oesophageal web, neurological disease?
- **Has a bone been swallowed** or other sharp FB (psychiatric patients)—this determines whether the patient needs to go to theatre or whether the treatment can be conservative.

Ask about

- Airway compromise.
- Was the onset of symptoms immediately after ingestion had occurred?
- Is the patient drooling or regurgitating food?
- Has this happened before? Was the patient hospitalized? Did they need surgical removal of the FB?
- Does the patient have any condition that might predispose to a delicate oesophagus?

Look for

- If the patient takes a sip of water, how long does it take for it to regurgitate?
- Perform a full examination of the oropharynx and palpate the tonsils and tongue base. Try, if you can, to perform a nasendoscopy and see whether the FB is near or obstructing the larynx.

Investigations

Soft tissue neck X-ray (anteroposterior and lateral)—make sure that you don't mistake the hyoid bone or a calcified larynx/cricoid cartilage for the FB.

Some fish bones are radiolucent and will not be seen on a plain X-ray. You can try to get the patient to swallow a piece of cotton wool, and then contrast.

Patients find it difficult to identify the location of a FB in the oesophagus, so if they feel it is retrosternal a contrast swallow is a helpful investigation. If the FB is past the cricoid, the patient may need flexible oesophagogastroduodenoscopy (OGD) performed by the gastro enterologists, as the risk of perforation by a rigid scope is much higher than when using a flexible scope for more distal FBs.

Management

- FB: caustic or containing bone—the patient will need to go to theatre today. Call the registrar.
- FB: meat—put the patient NBM, try Buscopan® IV, and consider the need for a contrast swallow and for theatre during the next available list if the FB doesn't pass and is in the oesophagus and not the larynx. Call the registrar about this.

Common ENT procedures

Table 8.5 Common ENT procedures

Operation	Risks	Inpatient stay	Time off work/away from school
Tonsillectomy	Infection, bleeding (in first 24hr & day 7–10), sore jaw, damage to teeth	Occasionally home the same day, usually overnight	2 weeks, to minimize catching infection
Adenoidectomy	Infection, bleeding, nasopharyngeal regurgitation, damage to teeth, sore jaw, hypernasal voice	Home the same day	2 weeks
Grommets	Infection, permanent perforation or need for removal	Home the same day	Back as soon as they recover from anaesthetic
Manipulation of nasal fracture	No improvement cosmetically, the need for further surgery/septorhinoplasty, nasal cast	Home the same day	Back as soon as they recover from anaesthetic
Septoplasty	Infection, bleeding nasal packs, no improvement in nasal obstruction	Overnight or day case	1 week
Functional endo-scopic sinus surgery	Infection, bleeding nasal packs, CSF leak, damage to eye/cribriform plate	Overnight or day case	2 weeks
Mastoidectomy	Infection, bleeding, hearing loss, damage to chorda tympani and facial nerve, second operation, dizziness	Overnight or day case	2 weeks (until packing removed)
Myringoplasty	Infection, bleeding, failure of graft, worsening of hearing or no improvement, damage to chorda tympani and facial nerve, graft not taking	Overnight or day case	1 week
Thyroidectomy	Infection, bleeding, scar, altered voice (recurrent laryngeal nerve damage), drain, need for medication	2 days (until drain removed)	2 weeks

☠ Carotid blow-out/catastrophic haemorrhage

Call the ENT registrar.

This occurs in patients who have a cancer of the head and neck, or have undergone surgical excision of one.

Think about
- What is the patient's diagnosis? Is the patient being treated palliatively?
- Get a senior there as soon as possible ± an anaesthetist.
- Stay with the patient—they will be terrified, as will the ward staff.

There is very little time for any other action, so management consists of resuscitation (ABC) and ensuring the patient is as calm as possible—so sedation should be readily available:
- Benzodiazepine—preferably midazolam 5mg IV, SC or buccal, repeated as necessary to maintain drowsiness.
- Diamorphine injection 2.5–10mg SC every 2hr max.

Postoperative thyroidectomy problems

Haemorrhage after thyroid surgery

Think about

- *Airway*—if the patient bleeds into the wound, the airway can become compromised by external compression.

Ask about

- When was the operation performed?
- Has the patient been started back on anticoagulation?

Look for

- *Airway*—is the patient stridulous or short of breath?
- Is the drain full of blood or not working?

Investigation

Check the Hb and that there is an up-to-date G&S or cross-match, depending on the severity of the bleed.

Management

- If the neck is increasing in size before your eyes, open the wound by releasing the clips or removing the sutures while reassuring the patient.
- If it is gradually increasing in size, contact your senior and arrange for the patient to return to theatre.

Hypocalcaemia after thyroid surgery

Hypocalcaemia can occur for a number of reasons, but in a surgical patient it occurs most commonly as a result of parathyroid or thyroid surgery.

Parathyroid hormone is crucial to the regulation of serum calcium. In patients undergoing parathyroidectomy, the inadvertent removal or damage to the other parathyroid glands results in hypocalcaemia; the more extensive the surgery, the more common this problem.

Another patient group in which hypocalcaemia is a potential problem is those with chronic hyperparathyroidism. The dominant parathyroid may have suppressed the remaining normal glands, resulting in temporary hypocalcaemia following surgery.

During thyroid surgery damage, devascularization or inadvertent removal of the parathyroids can also potentially cause hypocalcaemia.

Think about

The main feature of hypocalcaemia is neuromuscular irritability. This can be subtle with mild symptoms including paraesthesia of the extremities or muscle cramps, although in severe cases seizures and laryngeal spasm can occur.

Clinical features of hypocalcaemia

- Paraesthesia.
- Fatigue and irritability.
- Muscle cramps.
- Tetany, e.g. carpopedal spasm.
- Seizures.
- Laryngeal spasm.
- Prolonged QT interval.

A useful bedside test is to attempt to elicit Trousseau's or Chvostek's sign (Table 8.6).

Table 8.6 Examination of patients with hypocalcaemia

Trousseau's sign	Induction of carpal tunnel spasm upon inflation of a BP cuff 10mmHg above systolic BP for 3–5min
Chovostek's sign	Tapping the facial nerve in the preauricular area and observing for facial contractions (this test can be positive in a small proportion of normal individuals)

Investigations

- If hypocalcaemia is suspected, check calcium (2.12–2.65mmol/L), magnesium (0.75–1.05mmol/L), phosphate, U&Es and albumin.
- If magnesium is low this needs correction before hypocalcaemia will resolve.
- Check ECG for prolonged QT interval (normal <0.44sec/ 11 small 1mm squares).

Management

Patients who have *symptomatic hypocalcaemia* (e.g. seizures, positive for Trousseau's or Chvostek's sign)in the early postoperative period, or whose calcium levels continue to fall, require treatment:

- 10mL 10% calcium gluconate (8.9mg calcium) IV diluted with 100mL sodium chloride 0.9% and infused over 10min. This can be repeated up to three times to control symptoms.
- Patients then need to be commenced on a slow infusion of calcium to maintain normocalcaemia via a cannula in a large peripheral vein or central access:
  - 100mL 10% calcium gluconate (89mg calcium) added to 1L sodium chloride 0.9% and infused via a volumetric pump over 24hr.
  - Titrate to maintain serum calcium in the low normal range.
- **Monitor the calcium level regularly, at least 6 hourly**.

Cardiovascular monitoring

- Monitor BP and pulse.
- Patients with existing cardiac disease must be placed on a cardiac monitor.
- Slow or stop infusion if bradycardia, hypotension or peripheral vasodilatation occurs.

- When the patient is stable and tolerating oral fluids, start on oral calcium replacement:
  - calcium 1g QDS, which is equivalent to Calcichew® 2 tablets QDS.

If hypocalcaemia is likely to persist, oral vitamin D should be started with endocrinology advice.

- *Dr Neil Walker, Endocrinology SpR, Oxford.*

Practical procedures in ENT

Foreign body in the nose

Alert senior if you are unable to remove the FB.

Think about

If a child presents with a foul-smelling unilateral nasal discharge, they have a FB in the nostril until proven otherwise. Epistaxis and nasal obstruction may also be presenting symptoms.

- Will the FB be inhaled because it's small enough to travel through the nasal passage?
- Is the FB a magnet or small battery that will erode the septum? If so, the senior must be informed if you are unable to remove it, as the patient must be admitted and have it removed under general anaesthesia (GA) as an emergency.

Ask about

What is the FB? Is it a pea, piece of tissue paper or a bead?

Look for

The site of the FB in the nose:

- Look into the nose with an auroscope, gently pushing the tip backwards, and make sure the inferior turbinates have not been mistaken for the FB.
- With the parent or an assistant to help you steady the child, try removing the FB with Tilley's or crocodile forceps if it is soft or has an edge to grab. However, if the FB is smooth (e.g. a bead), hook a slightly bent Jobson–Horne over the top and drag the instrument and FB forward.

The removal of FBs from children's noses is incredibly stressful for all involved. When you reach a point at which you feel the child will not tolerate the procedure any more, arrange for removal under GA, after discussion with your senior.

Foreign body in the ear

Alert senior if you are unable to remove the FB.

Think about

Adult or child—attempt removal in a child only once (and quickly) as if you don't get the FB out and traumatize the patient in the process you will hinder the chances of the next person getting it out.

- Is the FB composed of natural fibres—as it may swell in size if left for any length of time and become painful.
- Insect—can be drowned in mineral oil and then removed by microsuctioning.
- FBs do not need to be removed urgently unless there are other extenuating circumstances (e.g. the FB is a small battery). Take the patient's details and arrange for them to be seen in an emergency clinic in the next 1–3 days. Consider arranging an early appointment and bringing the patient in starved if you feel that they are unlikely to tolerate removal in the outpatient clinic.

Using a microscope there are a number of instruments to help remove FBs:

- Suctioning—try this first, using a small suction end and if the FB is not occluding the EAM.
- Crocodile forceps—useful if the FB is soft and won't be pushed further in.
- Wax hook or Jobson–Horne probe—use if the FB is smooth. Pass the instrument over the top the FB and gently drag it out of the EAC.

Arrange follow-up if you suspect damage to the TM and start an antibiotic drop (e.g. Sofradex® 2 drops to affected ear TDS) if there is evidence of infection after FB removal.

Drainage of a quinsy

Alert senior if you are unable to drain the quinsy or you are concerned about airway compromise .

The treatment of any abscess is incision and drainage, and quinsy is a peritonsillar abscess that develop 4–5 days after an initial sore throat. The patient will have a 'hot potato voice' and on examination a unilateral fullness in the soft tissue lateral to the tonsil with uvular deviation.

Think about

Quite often, when you see the patient for the first time, they will have a degree of trismus and will not be able to open their mouth to allow a full view of the oropharynx. Try 4–8mg dexamethasone to reduce the trismus and inflammation; review the patient an hour later and attempt aspiration or incision and drainage of the quinsy.

Ask about

The patient will be very nervous about having a needle or scalpel in their mouth. Explain the procedure, then spray the oropharynx with co-phenyl caine (4–6 sprays over the area to be drained).

Look for

The area of greatest fluctuance. Insert a white needle or the trocar needle of a large cannula about 5mm into the abscess. It is important to draw back on the plunger of the syringe at the same time, as the negative pressure exerted will help to draw out the pus. Patients will feel relief from the aspiration of relatively small volumes of pus.

It is really important to make a determined movement to insert the needle, as not piercing the mucosa is uncomfortable and the patient knows that you will have to attempt this again.

Some ENT surgeons suggest that needle decompression is not adequate and that formal incision and drainage with a scalpel should be performed to prevent the re-accumulation of pus. This is almost as stressful for the doctor as it is for the patient the first time you attempt it, and I would recommend doing it with senior support initially.

Investigations

As for tonsillitis.

Management

Admit the patient and start them on IV penicillin 1g QDS, metronidazole 500mg TDS, using erythromycin if penicillin allergic. IV fluids should be used if the patient is unable to eat and drink, and a short course of dexamethasone (4–8mg TDS for 1–3 doses) if the oropharynx remains very swollen. Adequate analgesia is important and should be prescribed regularly (see Analgesia in tonsillitis, p332).

Pinna haematomas

This is a common injury seen on Saturday after the rugby match has ended.

Think about

Delayed drainage can lead to fibrosis of the cartilage of the pinna and leads to a cauliflower ear.

Ask about

- What the ear looked like previously?
- Has it been injured previously?

Look for

A fluctuant purple swelling.

Management

- Insert a white needle into the area that is most fluctuant.
- Drain as much blood off as possible and then pack BIPP or proflavin-soaked ribbon gauze into the contours of the ear.
- Place a sterile piece of gauze over this to protect the ear, and dress the whole head with a pressure dressing. Ask a nurse to help you with this.

Arrange review in the next emergency ENT clinic (i.e. 1–2 days) and ask the patient to come back if the dressing slips off or feels too tight.

Displaced tracheostomy tubes

If a tracheostomy falls out, PUT IT STRAIGHT BACK IN. Don't wait for the registrar to arrive.

Ask an experienced nurse to help you.

- Put the introducer back into the tracheostomy tube.
- Put some Aquagel® on to the end and, using a pronating movement of your wrist, slip it back in.
- Remove the introducer and suction any secretions, as this whole episode will have made the patient cough.
- Hold on to the tube until you can suture it in place or apply ties—**do not use ties in patients with a free flap as this can affect the vascular supply**.

If the tracheostomy is *not* the only airway (i.e. the upper respiratory tract is patent), put an oxygen mask on the patient to increase their oxygenation before the procedure starts.

Calls from GPs or A&E SHOs

Some 30% of an average GP's workload is ENT based, and if you didn't get much ENT teaching at medical school, neither did they. Consequently, a proportion of your workload after hours will involve calls from GPs. Sometimes the non-ENT trainee won't be expected to take calls, but occasionally they will. The 1° principle of this is: if you don't know the answer, call the SpR then call the GP back with the answer or with the SpR's contact details.

Always ask for the GP's mobile number to call them back on—getting the out-of-hours service or an automated receptionist can be very frustrating.

My patient has a discharging ear with pain, reduced hearing and

- **Nothing else**—see them over the next 1–3 days. Advise the GP about pain relief and topical ± systemic antibiotics.
- **They are an elderly diabetic with poor glycaemic control**—see them that day. You need to exclude malignant otitis externa, or stop it from developing.
- **Mastoid tenderness**—see them that day. You need to exclude mastoiditis.

My patient has an episode of sudden-onset acute nausea and vertigo, and can't get out of bed

Ensure there are no symptoms to suggest the patient has had a cerebellar stroke. Advise on antiemetics and arrange an outpatient appointment for the next 1–3 days.

My patient has had three episodes of epistaxis in the last week, which have stopped now

Ask about anticoagulation, hypertension and book an appointment for nasal cautery for within the week. Consider asking for the patient to be prescribed Naseptin® nasal cream.

My patient ate cod at lunch and now says it feels like there is a bone stuck in his throat

See the patient that day. He needs to have direct visualization of the area with a nasendoscope.

My patient has felt for a few weeks that there is something in her throat, but she doesn't remember eating anything that got stuck

Ask the GP to write a referral letter to an ENT consultant. The patient is likely to have globus pharyngeus.

My patient has a sore throat

- Can they eat and drink?—if not drinking and spitting saliva, arrange admission.
- And has not responded to antibiotics—consider glandular fever. Admit if not drinking for supportive treatment, or consider a quinsy. Ask the GP what the oropharynx looks like.
- And a hoarse voice with otalgia/weight loss/lymphadenopathy—consider malignancy. Arrange for a 2-week cancer wait appointment

My patient, aged 2yr, has put a bead in her ear
Arrange to see the child the next morning and ask for her to come to the appointment starved in case she does not tolerate removal and needs a GA.

FB in the ear can be left for a few days without causing harm, unless it is of a natural material that will expand or is likely to be corrosive, e.g. a small battery. If this is the case, bring the patient to the outpatient department or the treatment room in the ward and, using the microscope and suction ± forceps, attempt to remove the FB.

My patient has a foreign body in his nose
- Is it a small watch/camera battery?—needs to come out as soon as possible.
- Is it a bead/toy?—see the patient, preferably starved, in daylight hours when a senior will be nearby.

Initially try to get the child or parent to occlude the unaffected nostril and snort the FB out. If that doesn't work, spray the affected nostril with co-phenylcaine, position the child with good light (microscope or headlight) and use either a small sucker (e.g. if the FB is a pea), a pair of crocodile forceps (if its a sticker, piece of sponge or bit of wool) or a bent Jobson–Horne probe (if it's a bead or plastic toy). Advise the parents that the child will find the process distressing, especially if they are little. Make firm, decisive attempts at this as you have a finite number of attempts before the child completely refuses to co-operate. If the FB is smooth and/or plastic, aim to get the Jobson–Horne probe behind the object and drag it out of the nose.

There may be a small amount of traumatic epistaxis, but this usually resolves very quickly and, if the FB has been there for a long time, the parents may have noticed that it was present by a foul-smelling unilateral nasal discharge. The child can be prescribed a course of Naseptin® nasal cream, 1 application to the affected nostril twice daily for 1 week to combat any infection that may have or potentially will develop.

If, by the time you review the patient, you are unable to visualize a FB and there is a good history for it being present at some stage, make sure that the referring doctor/ENP wasn't thinking that the inferior turbinates were a FB—which frequently happens—and question whether it may have been swallowed, sniffed out or is further back in the nasal cavity.

If the child will let you, the best option is to use a nasendoscope. If there is an unobstructed view to the nasopharynx, the FB is no longer there. If this is not tolerated, discuss the patient with a senior as, depending on the object, the patient may need to be examined under anaesthetic, or can be discharged with the advice to return if they develop a unilateral nasal discharge.

My patient has eaten a big piece of meat and now it's stuck
Arrange for the patient to be transferred to you. See whether the GP can give them some Buscopan® IM before they arrive.

My patient has poked his ear with a cotton-bud and perforated the eardrum

The patient needs to be seen at some point over the next few days to assess the extent of conductive hearing loss. If there is no evidence of infection, no treatment will be given, except to arrange a follow-up appointment in 3–6 months to ensure the perforation has healed or, if it hasn't, to assess whether the patient may be suitable for a myringoplasty if they are now more prone to ear infections. Ensure that the patient does not get water in the ear.

Two hours ago my patient suddenly noticed that they can't hear anything out of one of their ears

Consider a number of points:

- Getting water in the ear or impacting wax against the TM with a hearing-aide mould or cotton-bud will cause a sudden hearing loss. Ask the GP whether there is wax occluding the EAM—if there is, arrange follow-up for removal over the following week.
- Is there a history of barotrauma, e.g. aeroplane flight or scuba diving?
- Has the patient recently been given an ototoxic drug? e.g. salicylates, beta-blockers, loop diuretics, chemotherapy (e.g. cisplatin) and antibiotics such as gentamicin.

My patient was in a fight last night and now has a broken nose, which looks very swollen, but I'm not sure whether the nose is deformed

Arrange to see the patient 5 to 7 days after the injury. Nasal fractures can be manipulated immediately they occur (in the UK this is usually done only by rugby trainers on the pitch or A&E consultants watching the medical school team playing) or within 2 weeks of the injury with a quick GA.

Ask the referring A&E F2/ST1 or GP whether the patient has a septal haematoma or abscess—if so, the patient will need to be seen in the next 12hr. A septal haematoma is a red swelling that obliterates the nasal passage, is red and soft to the touch, and needs to be drained to avoid damage to the septum. An abscess generally occurs when a haematoma gets infected—admit the patient as they will need incision and drainage.

Do not arrange X-rays for a nasal fracture (unless you suspect other facial fractures) as the findings will not alter your management of the patient.

Oral and maxillofacial surgery

Alistair Cobb

Oral and maxillofacial language

Facial fractures are described in the same way as any fracture elsewhere in the body together with their anatomical location—these are covered under each bone below Fig 9.1. The exceptions to this are the Le Fort fractures. Keep it simple. Describe what you see.

You should also familiarize yourself with the basics of how the system of dental nomenclature works so that you can work out the name of each tooth and how to record this in notes.

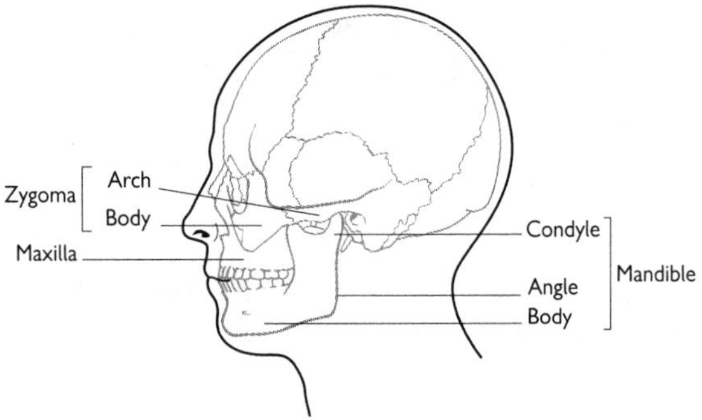

Fig. 9.1 Facial bones.

Dental nomenclature

The tooth

Each tooth has a crown and one or more roots. The bumps on top of the crown are called 'cusps' (Fig. 9.2). The crown sticks out from the gums; the root normally lies buried underneath unless there is periodontal disease present or local trauma.

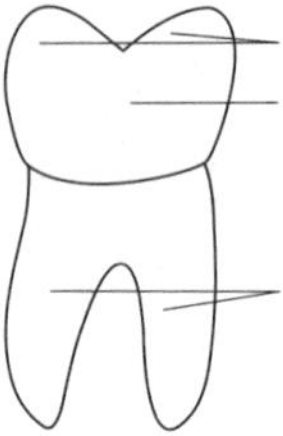

Fig. 9.2 Diagram of a tooth.

The mouth can be divided into four quadrants:

- Upper and lower dental arches, each of which has a left and a right counterpart.
- When all the teeth are present, each quadrant has the same complement of teeth, and of type of tooth.
- Working from the middle ('mesial') round the arch to the posterior ('distal') aspects, these are:
  - Two incisors—one central and one lateral.
  - A canine—'eye tooth', because its long roots point up to the eye.
  - Two premolars—referred to as the first and second premolars (these may have one or two roots).
  - First, second and third molar teeth—these molars have two or more roots. The third molars are more commonly called the wisdom teeth.
  - Any additional teeth are called 'supernumerary' teeth.

It is not uncommon for teeth not to be present in the mouth: either they have not erupted or they may not have formed in the first place.

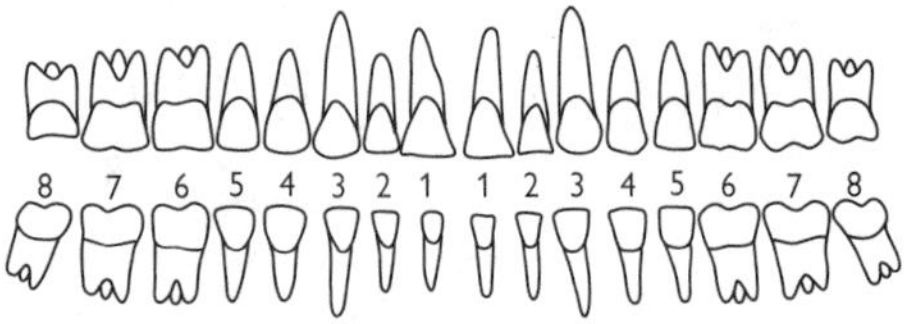

Fig. 9.3 Upper and lower dental arches.

Children are a bit different as they have fewer teeth which usually all wobble out (exfoliate). The deciduous, or 'milk', teeth are:

- A central and lateral incisor.
- A canine.
- A first and second molar.

In the Zsigmond system, teeth can be notated or referred to by a shorthand system based on their position in the quadrants:

87654321	12345678
87654321	12345678

- Thus an upper right wisdom tooth becomes: UR8 or 8|.
- Just remember that upper left is L-shaped and start from there—upper left third molar is UL8 or |8.
- The deciduous dentition is referred to by letters rather than numbers:

EDCBA	ABCDE
EDCBA	ABCDE

Maxillofacial examination

Consider the face as divided into thirds plus the inside of the mouth:

- The upper third is from the top of the nose, between the eyebrows to where the hair line starts. Examination of the cranium is then added.
- The middle third runs from under the supraorbital rims to the tip of the upper front teeth.
- The mandible represents the lower third.
- Inside the mouth is the fourth area to examine.

For each area check the soft tissues for lacerations and bruising, hard tissues (the underlying bony skeleton) and nerve function. Sensation is conveniently conveyed by a branch of the trigeminal nerve for each of the thirds of the face. Motor function is via the five branches of the facial nerve. Any lacerations that cross the path of these nerves may cause a nerve injury. Finally, each area has special features unique to itself which you should note have been checked. All of these are summarized in Table 9.1.

- Start your examination from in front of the face, looking at the injuries and symmetry of the face.
- The three thirds should be equal in vertical height.
- Swellings may indicate underlying injury.
- If any laceration passes over the path of the parotid duct (tragus of the ear to the angle of the mouth), check that saliva is milkable from Stensen's duct, which opens opposite the upper second molar tooth, and is not evident through the laceration.
- The upper third is best examined from above and behind the seated or supine patient.
- Check over the cranium for depressions and bruising.
- Palpate the frontal bones and supraorbital rims.
- Look at the eyes from above—is one sticking out or in more than the other?
- Lay your index finger around the zygomatic bones. Are they symmetrical? If not, the depressed one may be fractured. A dent of the zygomatic arch indicates a fracture here.
- Ask the patient to open and close their mouth while your fingers feel the temporomandibular joints in front of the tragus of the ear. If there is pain, this may indicate a mandibular condyle fracture.
- Now stand in front of the patient. Assess the level of the eyes—are they equal? Do the zygomas look symmetrical? What bruising is there. Is there any subconjunctival or periorbital bruising? Is the middle third of the face lengthened? This would indicate a Le Fort fracture.
- Grasp the front of the maxilla between finger and thumb placed above the incisors in the mouth. Gently see if the maxilla moves.
- Look at the nose. Is there epistaxis?
- Ask the patient to bite their teeth together. Assess the occlusion—the way the teeth bite together. Does it look even or are there any step defects or gaps? Ask the patient if it feels different when they bite together.

Table 9.1 Specific signs to note on examination

	Soft tissues	Hard tissues	Nerves	Special features
Upper third and cranium			Va VII temporal	Battle's sign External ear CSF otorrhoea
Middle third			Vb VII temporal, zygomatic, buccal	Eye movements and acuity CSF rhinorrhoea Stensen's duct (parotid)
Lower third			Vc VII marginal mandibular	TMJ
Intraoral			XII, lingual nerve	Dental occlusion Saliva flow from parotid duct

CSF, cerebrospinal fluid; TMJ, temporomandibular joint.

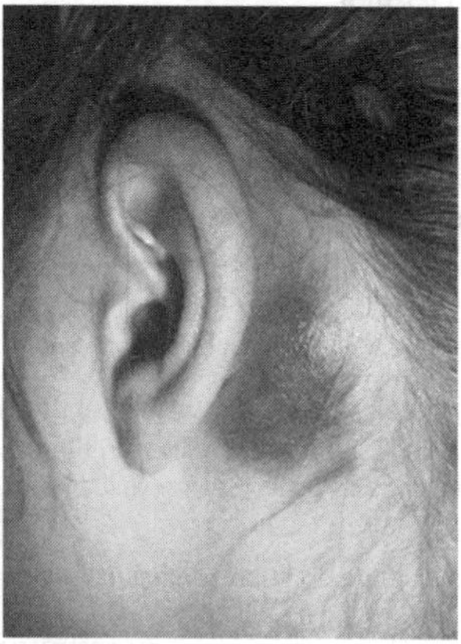

Fig. 9.4 Battle's sign—suggestive of a base of skull fracture.

- Then look in the mouth for bleeding, bruising, broken teeth and step defects between teeth.
- Check the facial and trigeminal nerve function. Then assess visual acuity, pupillary light reflexes and check for any diplopia, especially on upward gaze—characteristic of an orbital blowout fracture. If any suspicion of globe injury, discuss with ophthalmologist.

Middle third fractures of the face

This covers fractures of the maxilla, naso-orbito-ethmoid (NOE) complex and zygomatic spaces.

Maxillary fractures

These result from high-force blunt trauma to the middle of the face. Typically this was seen in road traffic accidents (RTAs), but seat belts have reduced their frequency. They are also caused by interpersonal violence.

Le Fort classified them into three types:

- The Le Fort I—the lower part of the maxilla which contains the teeth and forms the floor of the maxillary antrum is fractured from the rest of the midface.
- In Le Fort II and III fractures, the face and cranial base are separated. In both the fracture line runs across the bridge of the nose and across the orbit. In Le Fort II, the fracture then runs *under* the zygoma, whereas in Le Fort III it runs *over* it.
  - Le Fort II fracture—subzygomatic craniofacial dysjunction.
  - Le Fort III fracture—suprazygomatic craniofacial dysjunction.

Midfacial fractures are usually more complicated and asymmetrical than these simple lines. However, these are good to use to describe the general pattern and level of fracture.

Presentation

Usually as part of a bigger picture of injuries such as an RTA or particularly nasty assault.

Think about

- Airway and eyes.

Look for

- Lengthening of the midface, panda eyes (circumorbital ecchymoses), deranged occlusion of the teeth, CSF rhinorrhoea or otorrhoea, epistaxis, palatal haematoma.
- Gently grasp the bone above the upper central incisors in the mouth with the thumb and place the index finger on the back of this in the palate. Gentle pushing and pulling may reveal a mobile maxilla.

Investigations

- Plain film X-ray should be done on admission, but can wait until the morning.
- Definitive imaging will require CT ± 3D reconstruction—this can wait.

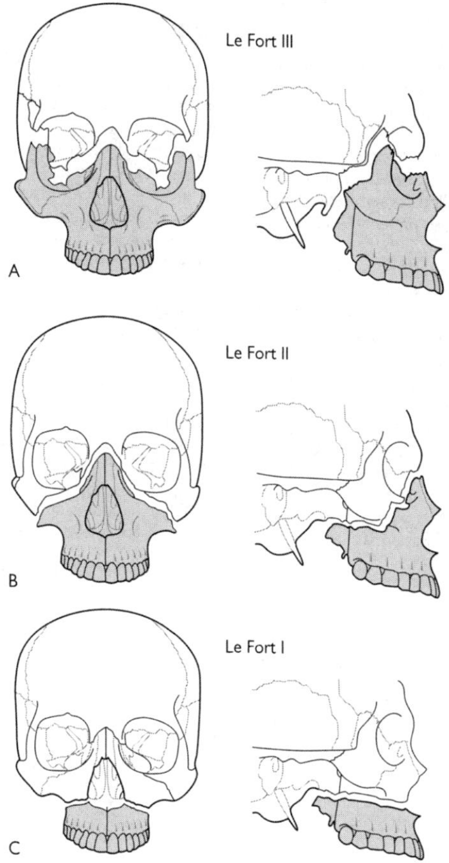

Fig. 9.5 Le Fort fractures. Reprinted from Ward-Booth P, Hausaman J-E, Schendel S (1999) Maxillofacial Surgery. Churchill Livingstone, Edinburgh, © 1999, with kind permission from Elsevier.

Management

- Ensure a clear airway and support if necessary—surprisingly this is not usually a problem. Junior anaesthetists often push for a tracheostomy, but airway obstruction is rare in the absence of significant head injury. This can occur if the midfacial complex is pushed down and back along the cranial base. The soft palate then snags on the tongue. A Guedel airway should provide immediate support, but, if not, two fingers pushed into the mouth, hooked on to the back of the hard palate and pulled up and forward will reduce this. This is not tolerated in a conscious patient. Here the patient needs to sit forward to maintain an airway. Otherwise perform a cricothyroidotomy. This is rarely required and specialist airway management skills should be sought from anaesthetic colleagues.
- Check no cervical spine involvement. These may occur particularly in high-impact, blunt trauma, maxillofacial injuries, e.g. RTA and falls from height.
- Admit the patient for head-injury neuro-observations under the care of either orthopaedic or general surgical teams, and hand over to maxillofacial team in the morning or when other more important injuries have been dealt with. Surgical correction will take place after the swelling has subsided and the aesthetic deformity can be assessed more accurately.
- Meanwhile start co-amoxiclav 1.2g IV TDS. Humidified air nebulizer via oral and nasal mask will help clear the blood-encrusted upper airways.

ⓘ Zygomatic fractures

Types: body or arch.

Presentation

Usually assault or sports injury.

Think about

Associated eye injury.

Look for

- Dimple in skin over zygomatic arch.
- Bruising and/or swelling.
- Trapping of coronoid process of mandible limiting lateral jaw movement to that side.
- Flattened face over cheekbone or under eye.
- Epistaxis.
- Bloody injection into white of eye lateral to pupil—subconjunctival haemorrhage.
- Paraesthesia of the infraorbital nerve distribution.
- Step at infraorbital margin or frontozygomatic suture.

Investigations

A pair of occipitomental (OM) radiographs. A submentovertex (SMV) view can be useful for arch fractures.

Management

- Check for eye involvement—diplopia, visual acuity loss or injury to the globe. If you cannot rule this out, seek ophthalmic review.
- Antibiotics against sinus bacteria—oral amoxicillin 500mg TDS 1/52 or equivalent.
- Analgesia.
- Instruct the patient not to blow their nose if you suspect a zygomatic body fracture as this may cause a periorbital surgical emphysema.
- Maxillofacial outpatient review within next few days.
- Treatment—simple closed reduction; open reduction, internal fixation (ORIF).
- Be sure to record postoperative eye observation in the chart.

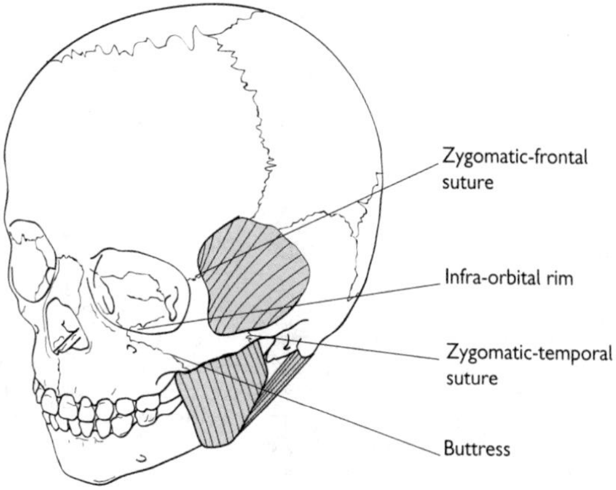

Fig. 9.6 The four sites where the zygomatic body may fracture: the zygomatic-frontal (ZF) suture, the infra-orbital rim, the buttress, and the zygomatic-temporal suture.

Orbital fractures

Internal orbital 'blowout' fractures occur with blunt trauma to the globe or orbital rim. This produces a fracture of the weakest part of the orbit—the paper-thin medial wall (lamina papyracea) or the orbital floor.

Look for
- Diplopia.
- Enophthalmos.
- Paraesthesia of the infraorbital nerve.
- Globe injury.

Classically with orbital floor fractures there is diplopia on upward gaze, with a 'tear drop' sign of muscle, fat and/or bone bulging down into the antrum on occipitomental radiographs. Sometimes there is surgical emphysema around the eye when the patient blows their nose: the ↑ intranasal pressure forces air through the maxillary antrum osteum into the antrum and then through the blowout fracture into the soft tissues around the eye.

Management
- Ensure no globe involvement and no visual acuity loss. Record a visual acuity (Snellen chart assessment).
- Start amoxicillin 500mg TDS or equivalent.
- No nose blowing.
- Adults require maxillofacial outpatient review in the next few days. If the diplopia persists, or there is an enophthalmos or telecanthic deformity, corrective surgery will probably be required. Meanwhile a CT with reconstructed coronal views through the orbital floor will be obtained.
- BUT—patients <20yr need prompter management including immediate CT scanning and possibly surgical correction that day before permanent damage is done. Contact the on-call registrar straight away.
- Ephedrine nose drops help ease the nasal congestion, although any patient involved in competitive sports (even at amateur level) may be in trouble with their sport's governing body for use of this—so check before you prescribe.

Other orbital fractures
The orbits may be involved in other facial fractures—the lateral walls or a nose fracture may both be seen in heavy blunt trauma to the face. However, these can be managed in a similar fashion to other fractures with some common sense. If the patient has marked facial injuries, treat as a Le Fort fracture and admit for head injuries. If not, check the eyes and acuity, and treat as per an orbital floor fracture.

☠ Retrobulbar haemorrhage

Presentation

After orbital surgery, including orbital floor repair, or trauma to the face or eye.

Look for

- Proptosis.
- ↓ Visual acuity.
- Retrobulbar (i.e. retro-orbital) pain.

Management

- This is medical and surgical.
- Speed is of the essence to avoid permanent visual acuity loss.
- Call the maxillofacial registrar and the on-call ophthalmologist urgently.
- Ask whether CT is required and, if so, get it urgently.
- Ask the on-call maxillofacial registrar regarding local protocols for medical treatment. This may include:
  - Acetazolamide 500mg stat IV.
  - Mega-dose IV corticosteroids.
  - Mannitol 200mL 20% IV over 20min.
- Prepare patient for urgent surgical decompression under general anaesthesia (GA).
- Some units practice lateral canthotomy and cantholysis under local anaesthetic in the emergency department. Discuss this with the on-call maxillofacial registrar.

Mandibular fractures

Typically, the patient will have fallen or sustained a hit to the jaw from a punch, kick or blunt implement through assault or sport.

Look for

- Sensory loss of the lower lip.
- Teeth not meeting properly ('deranged dental occlusion').
- Blood and/or gaps around individual teeth.
- Step defects along the plane of the tops of the teeth.
- Movement of the mandible between teeth—passive and active on examination.

Investigations

PA mandible and either an orthopantomograph (OPG) or, less usefully, two mandibular oblique radiographs.

Management

Any fracture with a deranged occlusion or an unstable fracture will need reduction and fixation. Any fracture that runs between teeth or touches teeth (typically an unerupted third molar or 'wisdom tooth') will need antibiotics.

- First match up the fracture(s) with Fig. 9.7.
- Patients with fractures a–d need to be admitted and given IV antibiotics (typically amoxicillin and metronidazole or Augmentin). Instruct the patient to remain nil by mouth from midnight as they may have surgery the next day.
- Patients with fractures e–h can go home on soft diet and no antibiotics if undisplaced, or be admitted on no antibiotics if displaced and there is a deranged occlusion.
- Surgery involving open reduction and internal fixation should happen in the next 24–48hr.

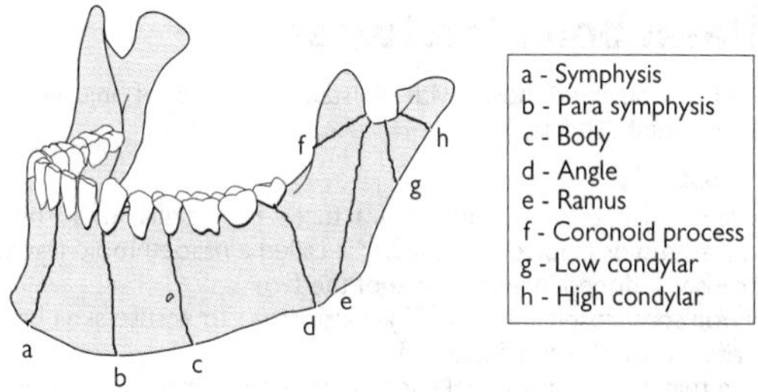

Fig. 9.7 Mandibular fracture sites.

Nasal bone fractures

Flattened or deviated nose with epistaxis at time of injury—usually assault or contact sports.

Think about

- Ensure not part of more complex fracture—i.e. maxilla, infraorbital rim or ethmoids involved. The latter is called a nasoethmoid fracture and causes a dished in appearance of the face.
- Look for cerebrospinal fluid (CSF) rhinorrhoea to ensure skull base (cribriform plate) is not fractured.
- Ensure that there is no septal haematoma—seen as a purple bulging of the medial wall of the nasal vestibule. The bleeding strips the perichondrium from the septal cartilage and will progress to necrosis of the septum if not decompressed. Aspirate the haematoma or make a small incision and squeeze or suction out the blood. The nose then needs to be packed to press the perichondrium back on to the cartilage. You may need to call for help from the maxillofacial registrar for this.

Management

Simple nasal fractures should be reviewed in a maxillofacial (or ENT) clinic within a week.

Complex facial trauma

Inform senior

These are multiple combinations of any of the above fractures. Usually these people have initially been managed through a trauma call and their maxillofacial injuries are of 2° importance to their other injuries.

Think about

- Advanced trauma life support (ATLS).
- Airway.
- Breathing.
- Circulation—blood loss through lacerations.
- Neurological deficits—head and eye injuries.
- Other injuries.

Management

- Hourly neurological observations, admitted under appropriate surgical team.
- Address orthopaedic, general surgical and neurosurgical needs first.
- Close (suture) or apply pressure dressings to lacerations.
- Saline nebulizers will help clear respiratory mucosal dried blood and ease respiration.
- Start appropriate IV antibiotics, e.g. co-amoxiclav 1.2g TDS.

Dislocated temporomandibular joints

Think about

- The anatomy of the TMJ and how this may help you relocate the mandibular condyle.
- Ensure that there is no history of trauma as a fracture dislocation is quite a different problem.

Ask about

- How did it happen? Typically this occurs when yawning too wide.
- Previous similar episodes and how it was reduced—did the patient require GA or sedation?

The TMJ is made up of a mandibular condylar head and a glenoid articular fossa on the skull base on which the condyle articulates. The joint has two movements: first it hinges around a fixed point in the condylar head, which remains in the glenoid fossa. Then, for wider opening of the mouth, the condylar head slides forward out of the glenoid fossa. The forward slide is limited anteriorly by an articular eminence, which forms a physical block to further excursion. If the patient forces the jaw opening beyond this point, or lax ligamentous support allows further opening, the mandibular condyle will pass over the top of the eminence and can become stuck on the other side of it. This then physically restrains the condyle from returning to the glenoid fossa.

Look for

The patient will have an abnormally widely opened mouth that is firmly fixed open. It is *not* a closed mouth that is difficult to open—this is trismus and is quite at the other end of the spectrum and yet is often referred as a dislocation.

Management

- Obtain an OPG radiograph to check that there is no fracture if in any doubt about trauma. If so, refer on to the maxillofacial registrar.
- To relocate the dislocation, first find a quiet room. The patient needs to be relaxed. Reassure them that this is not a painful process. It is uncomfortable, but this subsides the moment the condyle is back in place.
- Lie the patient flat on an examination couch with a pillow under the head.
- Is only one condyle dislocated? Or, as is much more common, are both out?
- With gloved hands insert the index finger into the mouth behind the most posterior lower tooth on to the mucosa overlying the retromolar bone. Do this on both sides if both condyles are dislocated. Make sure that your fingers lie *around* the cheek side of the back teeth and not over them, or you will get bitten when the jaw goes back into place!

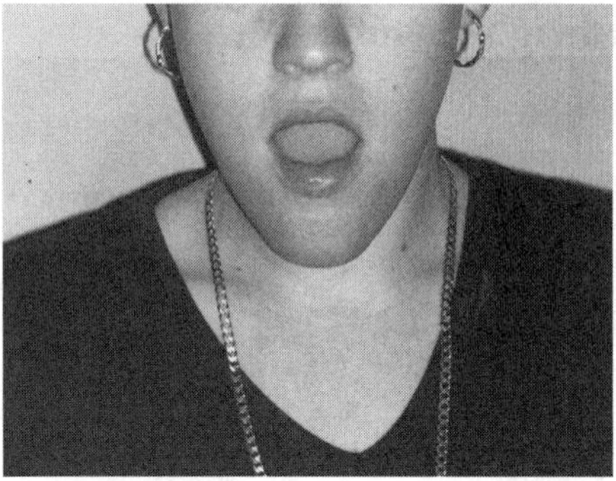

Fig. 9.8 A fixed open mouth with abnormally prominent chin point—typical of TMJ dislocation.

- Then curl the thumbs under the chin on each side. Your aim is not to push the mandible straight back as this just pushes the condyle back on to the articular eminence. Instead you have to push the condyle down and back, *over* the articular eminence before it returns to the glenoid fossa.
- Press down and back with the index fingers and push the chin up with the thumbs. This rotates the mandible, making the condyle move down and back more easily. It is not a sudden relocation but instead is a slow sustained pressure for up to several minutes. Usually one condyle returns before the other. Obviously in unilateral dislocation that is enough, but most are bilateral and require a little more effort. However, once one side is in, the other usually swiftly follows.
- Once the jaw is relocated make sure the patient bites the teeth tightly together for a few minutes. Often the thrill of being able to move the jaw means that the uninformed patient gleely wiggles their mouth open and promptly redislocates!
- Then advise the patient to rest the jaw joint for a few weeks by stifling yawns, preventing wide mouth opening with a hand underneath the chin, and having a soft diet.
- Recurrent dislocations need maxillofacial outpatient review as some cases require surgical intervention.
- Cases that cannot be relocated easily may need IV sedation, local anaesthetic injections to the muscles around the joint, or a short GA to relocate them—in which case you should contact the on-call maxillofacial registrar.

Ludwig's angina

Alert senior

Ludwig's angina is usually defined as a rapidly progressive cellulitis or abscess involving bilateral sublingual and submandibular spaces. It is potentially fatal. and must be taken seriously and seen rapidly.

Think about

AIRWAY, AIRWAY, AIRWAY, breathing, circulation.

Ask about

- Previous episodes of facial swelling associated with dental pain or tonsillar abscesses that have recurred if not treated. This helps guide specific treatment.
- Check causes of bleeding problems—diatheses, medication, hepatic disease, etc., and possible causes of immunocompromise.

Look for

- The patient will present with the neck swollen like a bullfrog, and the floor of mouth pushed up so as to make speech difficult and breathing laboured.
- It can rapidly worsen by tracking round the tissue spaces of the neck.
- It usually stems from untreated rampant dental infection or progression of tonsillar abscess.

Management

- Sit the patient up and provide high flow O_2 via mask with reservoir bag. Consider heliox.
- Call maxillofacial registrar and on-call anaesthetic registrar.
- Patient requires IV access and start IV co-amoxiclav 1.2g TDS.
- Send FBC, CRP, glucose and blood cultures as minimum.
- Move straight to theatres—will require specialist airway management and may require fibreoptic intubation.
- Maxillofacial registrar to meet you in theatres—patient will require surgical decompression of sublingual and submandibular spaces, or possibly conservative management intubated on ITU.
- Ensure that you have a cricothyroidotomy kit with you for transfer—just in case.

Other orofacial infections

Inform senior if you need to admit

Think about

- Possible causes using an anatomical sieve:
  - Skin.
  - Dental.
  - Bone.
  - Salivary glands.
  - Sinuses, etc.

Dental infections can surprise the unwary A&E SHO in the degree of facial swelling they can cause. Salivary glands, particularly the parotids and submandibular glands, are prone to infections especially if stones have caused stasis of saliva. Then all the usual suspects apply: folliculitis, infected sebaceous cysts, fractures, etc.

Investigations

- If teeth are thought to be involved, get an OPG radiograph.
- Ensure FBC, CRP and glucose are sent for.

Management

- If swelling is not too great and there is no obvious pus to drain, then send home on penicillin V 600mg QDS and metronidazole 500mg TDS, or the single agent co-amoxiclav 625mg TDS. Advise the patient to see a dentist the next day.
- If pus can be drained simply, or aspirated, then do so. If the patient is pyrexic or needs GA for drainage, or the swelling is just quite large, admit for IV antibiotics and keep nil by mouth. Put on the emergency list for the next day.
- If there is any difficulty in swallowing or breathing, then admit, start IV antibiotics immediately and call for an urgent anaesthetic assessment. Inform the maxillofacial registrar and prepare to go to theatres. The patient may need to stay intubated on ITU after surgery, or instead of incision and drainage.

Facial and oral lacerations

The key to managing these lacerations is assessment and cleaning.

Ask about

- Whether any sharp or contaminated objects were involved in the injury.

Look for

- Clearly relate the history of the injury to the wounds—could glass, metal or wood foreign bodies be present? If so, a tangential view radiograph of the soft tissues may reveal these.
- Also check that the facial nerve branches or the parotid duct are not involved—these will require GA to repair properly, the next day.
- Explore the wounds thoroughly—they may run much deeper than you think and may overlie bony fractures.
- Clean with saline under local anaesthetic (LA). Some departmental protocols do not permit the use of adrenaline (epinephrine) in LA on the nasal tip or ears.
- Determine whether there is skin loss—this is less common than you may think. The interconnected muscles of facial expression stretch a tight plane over the face. Any breach of this tends to be exaggerated by the tension of the muscles. Thus there may be the appearance of skin loss. If there really is skin loss, contact the on-call maxillofacial registrar.

Management

- Any bleeding can be stopped successfully with a cautery device, if available.
- Ensure you have cleaned the wounds very thoroughly with saline. Then close neatly in layers: 4/0 resorbable sutures deep to the skin surface, and monofilament nylon on the skin. 5/0 nylon is fine, but use 6/0 on the lips and eyelids.
- Take care to match up the tissues—in the deep layers, ensure the same depth of the suture on either side of the wound. On the skin surface the suture should be the same distance away from the wound on either side, and emerge the same depth into the laceration itself on its way through. Always take time to ensure the vermillion border of the lip is *exactly* matched up when suturing lacerations that cross this. There is no magic to this. You simply must be absolutely accurate with the first suture that you place there.
- Sutures should be removed in 5 days. Most facial lacerations do not require antibiotics.
- Any more complicated or heavily contaminated lacerations should be managed under GA. IV antibiotics should be started (e.g. co-amoxiclav 1.2g IV TDS), exposed bone covered with saline-soaked dressings, and the patient kept nil by mouth and put on to the emergency list.
- Intraoral lacerations are closed with resorbable 3/0 or 4/0 sutures. Explore them well using suction. If the labial mucosa is involved, ask for help from a colleague to pull the lip tightly away from the teeth to give you a flat surface to suture. Again, if they are too difficult to close, bring the patient back in the morning to a maxillofacial clinic.

Facial dogbites

Inform senior

The saliva of dogs is second only to that of humans in terms of the infective potential of the microbacterial flora it contains.

Think about

Take these injuries seriously—they will need a thorough cleaning, which may warrant GA, especially in children.

Management

- Unlike elsewhere on the body, facial dogbite wounds *are* sutured and are not left open. Check immunization status and start antibiotics such as co-amoxiclav 1.2g TDS.
- Be aware of the potential for medicolegal issues from such injuries. Clearly document your history and the injuries with a diagram that you can refer back to later if required—even better is to take photographs.
- Smaller lacerations can be cleaned thoroughly with Betadine® or chlorhexidine under LA. However, deeper lacerations should be cleaned thoroughly under GA and the patient admitted for IV antibiotics meanwhile.

Dental avulsion

This is one of the simpler presentations to deal with, but feared by most non-dentists.

The most common teeth to be knocked out are the front ones—the incisors. Typically this will be young children or sports injuries.

Think about

- The teeth should be kept in milk or in the mouth down in the buccal sulcus by the cheek while patient travels to hospital. They should absolutely never be scrubbed as this will remove the soft tissue ligament on the root that will heal and hold the tooth back in place.
- Deciduous ('milk' or 'baby') teeth should never be reimplanted.
- Closely examine a tooth before reimplanting—it should not be broken. A small chip off the crown (the part seen in the mouth) is alright, but the root and root tip (apex) should be complete. Bear in mind that the root is not fully formed at the tip until ~12yrs of age—it should be even and smooth, though.

Management

Time is of the essence: the longer the tooth is out of the socket, the less chance it has of 'taking':

- Wash the tooth with saline squirted from a 20mL syringe. Make sure all dirt has been removed.
- LA may be required for this. If so, use a 2mL syringe of lidocaine with adrenaline (epinephrine). Lift away the lip and inject into the loose gum up in the sulcus in line with the root of the tooth.
- Suction the blood clot from the tooth socket.
- Hold the tooth by the crown.
- Gently but firmly push the tooth back into place, making sure it is facing the front.
- Check the level compared with adjacent teeth.
- The patient should not bite on the tooth at all and should be seen in a dental clinic the next day to have the tooth splinted. Meanwhile stabilize the tooth with tissue adhesive glue, sticking it to the teeth on either side, or with the foil from a suture packet folded several times and then finally folded once more into a U-shaped cross-section to form something like a sports mouthguard. This can be easily snugged around the teeth of that arch until the morning.

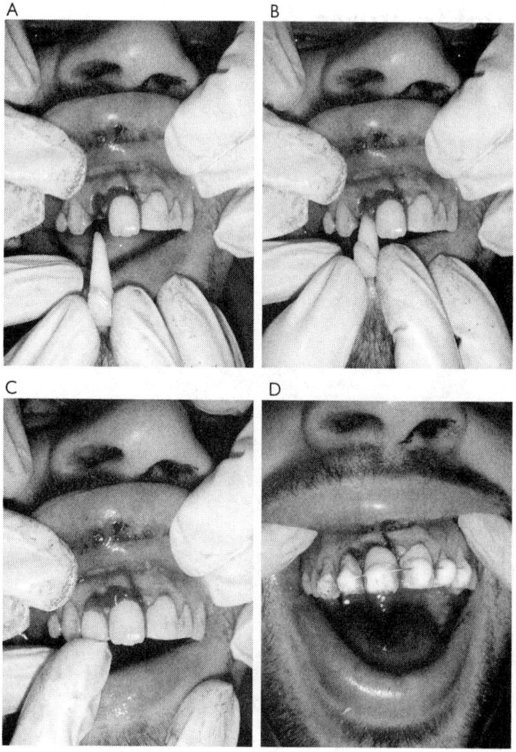

Fig. 9.9 Correct handling and orientation of the tooth (A, B). The tooth is firmly pushed into the socket (C). The splint is applied (D).

ⓘ Dental fractures

If a tooth is broken, leaving a big chip missing, it needs dressing with some white filling material such as a glass ionomer cement mix. If the red nerve ('pulp') is evident in the middle of the tooth, this is definitely needed.

The patient should see a dentist as soon as possible. An emergency dental service is provided by many primary care trusts and A&E departments. Otherwise, the patient should see their dentist in the morning.

ⓘ Dental subluxation

Occurs after a blow to the front teeth, one or more may be pushed back or slightly out of the socket.

Management

- Examine the patient and ensure that the bone around the teeth is not broken—a dentoalveolar fracture.
- Get a radiograph (OPG) and check that there are no fractures of the roots of the involved teeth—this might mean that the tooth will be lost.
- Anaesthetize the tooth by injecting lidocaine above the apex of the root into the sulcus by the tooth, if required.
- Firmly grip the tooth between finger and thumb and push it back into line with the other teeth—it will often click back into position.
- The tooth will need splinting as for an avulsed tooth (see 📖 p376).

Orthodontic problems

Occasionally fixed braces can become partially unattached and a sharp wire sticks into the cheek or lip. Have a commonsense approach to managing the problem:

- If you can get to it and cut it off close to the bracket (little block stuck to a tooth) at which it is still attached, then do so.
- If it is virtually hanging off, see whether you can get the whole wire off easily.
- At worst, find a piece of wax or elastoplast and cover up the end.
- The patient will have to see their orthodontist the next morning.

ⓘ Restorative dentistry problems

This includes fractures or loss of all manner of dental restorations, including fillings, crowns (same thing as 'caps'), bridges (caps stuck to other teeth, usually next to the gap they fill) and dentures.

These are not an emergency but can seem so to some patients who will pressurize an inexperienced A&E SHO into calling you. The patient needs to see their dentist in the morning—no debate!

Bleeding socket

Think about

Pressure stops nearly all bleeding, but make sure it is sustained and uninterrupted pressure with a gauze swab bitten down on to for at least half an hour. This does not mean that someone can lift up the pack and have a look every 5min—half an hour, no peeking!

Management

If this does not work, make your way up a hierarchy of measures, stopping to allow each one to work before thinking about moving on to the next:

- Check no bleeding diathesis; consider FBC and clotting studies. Change the pack for one soaked in hot water and then wrung out. The patient should bite down on this for another 30min, but ensure the pack is making contact with the socket.
- Local anaesthetic with adrenaline (epinephrine) can then be injected into the gingivae next to the tooth. Place a 3/0 horizontal mattress suture across the socket using either black silk or a resorbable material.
- Suction out the socket and place a piece of surgicel pack. Suture over this as above.
- Remove the Surgicel® and get a new piece. Soak this in tranexamic acid IV solution and then pack this into the socket. Bite on gauze for half an hour after this.
- Give up and call for help.

Infected extraction socket

After a tooth has been extracted the dental socket can become infected. This local osteitis is called a 'dry socket'. It is extremely painful and may present with a whitening of the surrounding gum (try to call the gums 'gingivae'—it sounds more professional!).

The treatment is metronidazole 200mg TDS for 1 week—and to stop smoking.

Any trapped food debris can be irrigated out with a syringe, and a local dressing of a proprietary product (e.g. Alvogyl®) can be placed, but this can wait until a dentist can do this in the morning.

On the ward before surgery

Patients having oral and maxillofacial surgery have no real differences to general surgical patients prior to elective surgery. By the very nature of their complaints they tend to be easier to look after, and to have less demanding medical and clinical chemistry issues. The exception are the patients with head and neck tumours, who may be more taxing in the postoperative critical care issues they present. Preoperatively, check whether they are to have a free flap reconstruction. If so, no cannulae should be inserted into the donor limb prior to a free flap procedure.

- Unlike the bowel, mouth surgery requires no special preparation.
- If the notes state the surgeon requires plaster study models of the teeth, check that these are on the ward.

Orthognathic surgery is the correction of facial skeletal deformity by controlled fractures of the mandible and/or maxilla. These are fixed in a similar fashion to traumatic fractures using titanium miniplates and screws.

- 'BSSO' refers to a bilateral sagittal split osteotomy of the mandible. Maxillary osteotomies usually follow the Le Fort I or II fracture lines. Other osteotomies exist, but these are the most common.
- 'Bimax' refers to a bimaxillary osteotomy, which combines procedures on both jaws. 'Wafers' or 'splints' are the hard plastic bite-plates that are required for orthognathic surgery on the jaws. These record the matrix of movement when fracturing the jaw and refixing in a new position. They are fabricated in the lab after the surgery is undertaken on models of the teeth first. They are then fixed on to the teeth during the operation.

Facial radiographs are required for simple trauma and orthognathic work. Complex trauma and head and neck cancer surgery requires CT or MRI. 3D skull models may be required for extremely complex craniofacial surgery, but these are usually brought in by senior team members on the day of surgery.

Appropriate thromboprophylaxis should be observed for all surgical patients.

Failing free flap

Signs

Grey, mottled free flap, turgid to feel, poor capillary refill, with worsening or absent Doppler arterial signal.

Management

- Go to see the patient immediately.
- Check the signs listed above yourself, and compare with what you observed earlier yourself—ideally the patient would have been handed over and you would have seen the healthy flap. A pale and cool flap suggests arterial compromise. A blue and distended flap suggests venous drainage is impaired. Heparin or leeches may be called for, but check with the maxillofacial registrar.
- Check the patient is warm (blankets and Bair Hugger®) and well filled (good urine output and mean arterial pressure [MAP] of 80–100mmHg) to prevent vasoconstriction. If you feel the flap is at all at risk, call the maxillofacial registrar immediately.
- A patient with a failing flap may need to return to theatre. Prepare them and inform theatre and anaesthetic staff.

A guide to free flap care

Adapted from the St George's Maxillofacial Head and Neck Surgery Guidelines by kind permission of Mr Nicholas Hyde.

Microvascular free tissue transfer flaps are used to reconstruct soft and hard tissue defects by moving tissue from one part of the body to another. The attachment to local structure is cut and they are re-anastomosed to local blood vessels to provide their blood supply. They may comprise various combinations of skin, muscle, fascia and bone depending on source of harvest and type of reconstruction required. They are susceptible to ischaemia in their early stages and are observed closely for the first few days.

The patient should be kept sitting up at 45° and warm. The flap should have a healthy colour—i.e. not grey or blue, blanch to finger pressure, and have a capillary refill time of 2sec or less. It should be soft to touch and warm. A Doppler probe should always to be available to assess the arterial pedicle and the patient should maintain a hyperdynamic circulation. This is ensured by a positive fluid balance aiming for at least +2000mL per 24hr, urinary output assessed with a catheter at least 1mL per hr per kg bodyweight, normotensive with a MAP of 80–100mmHg.

These observations should be carried out quarter-hourly for 2hr, half-hourly for the next 4hr and then hourly for 48hr.

If you have any doubt whatsoever, call the maxillofacial registrar or consultant at any time of the day or night. Any delay in dealing with an ischaemic flap will hasten its failure and that would be a disaster.

Key points to check on reviewing patient:

- Patient's head should be in neutral position or turned to the side of the anastomosis to prevent any pressure on the flap or tension on the microvascular anastomosis.
- The patient should be sat up at a 45° angle to help minimize swelling.
- Maintain haemoglobin at 8–10g/dL (patient should not be overtransfused above 10g/dL).
- Maintain MAP at 80–100mmHg.
- Keep pH 7.36–7.44 (acidotic conditions will affect perfusion). Keep PaO_2 above 10kPa.
- Liaise with the critical care team regarding optimum central venous pressure (CVP)—keep well filled, usually positive balance of 2000mL.

Flap observations

As a guide, flap observations should be carried out:

- Quarter-hourly for 2hr.
- Half-hourly for 4hr.
- Hourly for 48hr.

Observations should always be 'handed over' when starting or leaving the on-call period:

- COLOUR: Paleness may indicate an arterial occlusion–the surgeons should be contacted. However, it should be stressed that most flaps, especially intraorally, will appear a little pale compared with normal oral mucosa. A blue flap signifies venous obstruction. This is the most frequent cause of flap failure. Call the maxillofacial registrar immediately if in doubt. The early diagnosis of a failing flap is crucial. If a flap is failing then an early return to theatre can result in flap salvage following re-anastomosis.
- TEMPERATURE: Ideally the flap should be of a similar temperature to the surrounding normal tissue. Test by putting one finger on the flap and one on the surrounding tissue.
- CAPILLARY REFILL: This is assessed by applying gentle pressure to the flap. No blanche may indicate a congested flap. A slow refill >5sec shows venous congestion. A quick refill <3sec indicates good arterial flow. No refill indicates an arterial occlusion. 3–5sec can be considered 'normal'. DO NOT stab the flap with a needle. If this is indicated then it should be performed by the surgeon who will return the patient to theatre—usually the consultant in charge.
- DOPPLER: A Doppler probe should be placed on the flap hourly to listen for the arterial signal. If no Doppler signal is audible then call the maxillofacial registrar immediately.
- TEXTURE: A flap should feel soft to the touch. Any oedema or tension may indicate kinking of the vascular pedicle and be a sign of impending flap failure.

Types of free flap typically used

A number of different flaps can be used to repair the 1° defect left within the oral mucosa and/or facial skin. Most will be slightly paler in appearance than the surrounding tissue. The 2° defect caused by the removal of the flap is ideally closed by direct suturing but may be covered by a split or full-thickness skin graft.

Radial forearm

This is the commonest free flap used in head and neck reconstruction. It can be used as a skin flap, a fascia-only flap or may incorporate a segment of radius as a composite vascularized bone graft. The donor arm should be kept in a Bradford sling for 48hr postoperatively and will have Plaster of Paris (POP) for 6 weeks if bone has been taken. The viability of the hand must be checked with the flap obs. There will be no radial pulse, but the ulnar artery will be palpable, the fingers should be warm and a pulse oximeter will record saturation at the periphery.

Deep circumflex iliac artery (DCIA)

Provides a large bulk of vascularized iliac bone. It can be taken with abdominal wall muscle—usually the internal oblique. It is a painful donor site and appropriate analgesia is required, particularly when mobilizing the patient. If this site has been used then an epidural catheter will have been placed into the wound for the administration of LA. The patient may feel more comfortable with the donor site knee flexed over a pillow—to flex the hip.

Latissimus dorsi

This is used as a muscle-only or a muscle and skin flap. It is used to reconstruct large defects and the donor site can usually be closed primarily. Bleeding into the donor site is occasionally a problem, showing as either high drainage from the wound or haematoma formation.

Fibula flap

This is a bone or bone and skin flap raised from the lateral aspect of the lower leg. The leg may be splinted and will be elevated on several pillows postoperatively. The viability of the foot must be checked, as with the fore arm flap. This flap is generally used for large mandibular reconstructions.

Rectus abdominis

This is a skin or skin and muscle flap. The skin will be the colour of the abdominal skin. The donor site can be closed primarily. The surgery is all extraperitoneal but watch for ileus.

Scapula flap

This is usually used as a skin-only or a skin and bone flap. The donor site is usually closed primarily with a suction drain.

Bleeding

Call senior if haematoma, circulatory compromise or if simple measures do not stop the bleeding.

Postoperative bleeding is something that must always be taken seriously and you must assess the patient clinically quickly.

Haematoma collection can compromise overlying skin and reconstruction, or even compress important head and neck structures such as the trachea. Blood loss can be very great, especially after neck surgery.

Think about

Bleeding within 24hr of surgery is reactive. It usually represents ↑BP, dislodged clips or sutures, or possible relaxation of previous arterial contraction. There may not be escape of blood externally. The only indication may be a gross swelling at the surgical site.

Management

- Apply pressure with gauze swabs to the likely bleeding site and check that the drains are vacuumed and working.
- Resuscitate the patient, depending on the size of the problem.
- Assess the patient for hypotension, anaemia and tachycardia.
- Remember that oxygen saturation may be high but there will be less circulating haemoglobin, so that oxygen supplementation may be required to optimize oxygen delivery. Free flaps are especially vulnerable to a drop in oxygen availability.
- Ensure that you have venous access and obtain FBC, G&S and clotting screen if you feel appropriate. LFT is useful, especially as excess alcohol is an aetiological factor in oral cancer. You should find a pre-operative result for this if it were felt relevant.
- Cross-matched blood may be required.
- Consider IV fluids.
- Call for senior help. If local measures are unsuccessful or the bleeding is anything more than small, the patient may need to return to theatre for exposure of the surgical site and surgical control of the haemorrhage.

Postoperative zygomatic and orbital floor fractures

Zygoma reductions and fixation of orbital floor fractures will require eye observations for the initial period after surgery:

- 1st hour—every 15min.
- 2nd hour—every 30min.
- Then hourly overnight.

These should include the following:

- Pupillary light response—direct and consensual.
- Acuity.
- Pain.
- Proptosis.

Any problems found may indicate a retrobulbar hemorrhage and the patient may require decompression (see 📖 p365). Call the maxillofacial registrar urgently.

Maxillofacial radiology

The basic rules of orthopaedic radiology apply for all maxillofacial trauma: two views.

- For the mandible this is an orthopantomogram, or 'OPG', and a posteroanterior (PA) mandible. Don't be put off by anyone who says otherwise: you need two views. Lateral obliques of the mandible are harder to read than an OPG, but sometimes the only available alternative.
- The same applies for the midface and zygomas. Occipitomental views at 10° and 30°, and a PA face, are required. A submentovertex (SMV) view is particularly useful for looking at the zygomatic arch.
- Complex facial trauma and orbital blowouts require CT, often with 3D reconstruction. This can wait until daylight hours.
- MRI is usually reserved for TMJ assessment and salivary gland disease.

Orbitozygomatic fractures

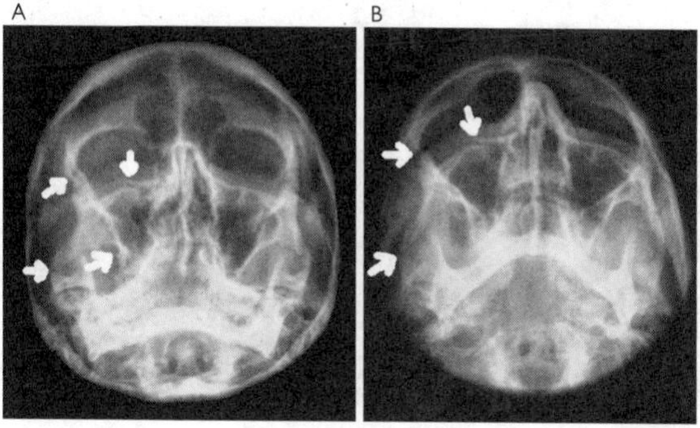

Fig. 9.10 This pair of occipitomental (OM) views at 10° (A) and 30° (B) clearly show a typical right zygomatic body fracture. Often called a 'tripod' fracture, this actually has four lines of fracture evident on plain films. Find them by comparing one side with the other. They are at the junction of the zygoma with the temporal and the frontal bones—the ZF and zygomaticotemporal sutures, and with the maxilla at the infraorbital rim and the 'buttress' above the maxillary teeth.

Mandibular fractures

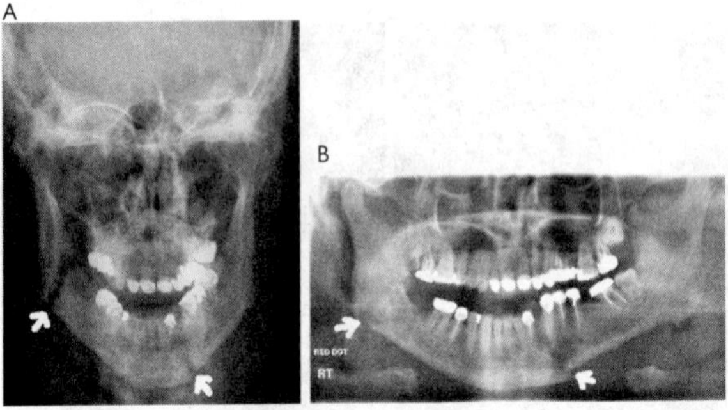

Fig. 9.11 Left mandibular parasymphysis and right-angle fractures.

Le Fort II fractures

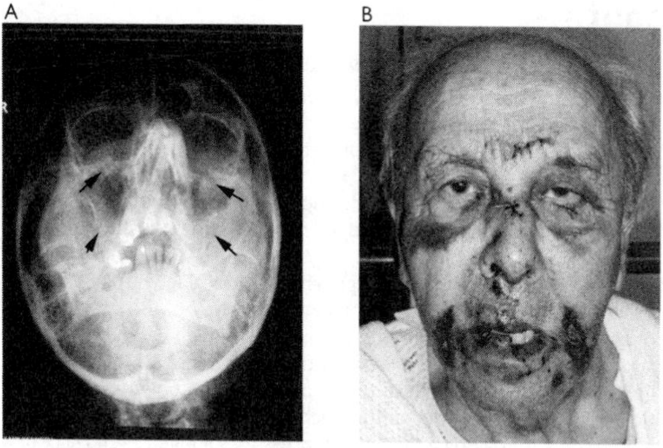

Fig. 9.12 The OM view (A) shows bilateral fractures of the infraorbital rims and zygomatic buttresses. The patient's face is clearly lengthened in the middle third. He has also fractured his nose, which is deviated (B).

Local anaesthesia for the face and mouth

Inferior alveolar (dental) block and lingual block

This is used to anaesthetize all lower teeth on that side of the mandible.

- With the patient's mouth wide open, palpate the external oblique ridge of the mandible from the posterolateral aspect of the most posterior lower molar tooth.
- Place your thumb along this while supporting the mandible on that side with the fingers of that hand. Curl the thumb tip just over the medial edge of the bone.
- Using a dental hypodermic syringe with 2% lidocaine with 1:80 000 adrenaline (epinephrine), approach with the body of the syringe over the contralateral premolar teeth. The needle will then be at approximately 45° to the AP axis of the molar teeth.
- Penetrate the mucosa medial to the point midway up your thumb tip and advance until you gently touch mandibular bone.
- Withdraw very slightly and gently depress the plunger, then relax to check no blood is aspirated. The cartridges are self-aspirating.
- Then deposit ¾ of the 2.2mL cartridge of LA solution. Withdraw almost all the way out and deposit the rest of the solution to block the lingual nerve if required.

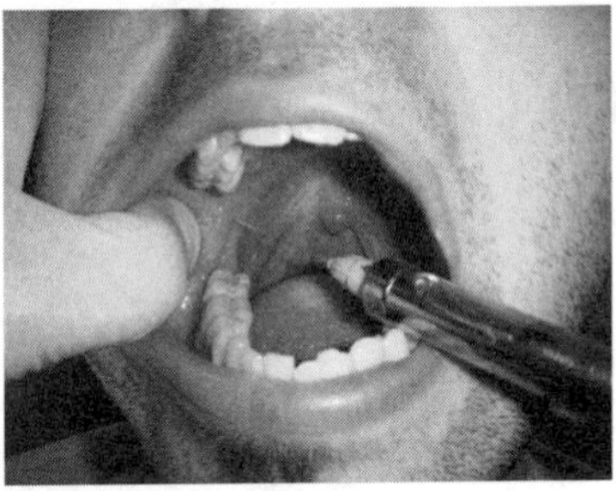

Fig. 9.13 Inferior alveolar dental block.

Intraoral dental infiltration

This is used to anaesthetize individual upper teeth. The upper lip or cheek is gently but firmly pulled away from the teeth to reveal the sulcus. The dental syringe is used to deposit LA solution to the apex of the sulcus immediately above the required tooth.

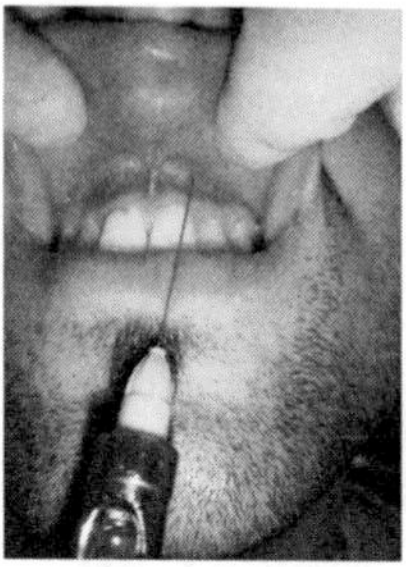

Fig. 9.14 Intraoral dental infiltration.

Plastic surgery

Christine Johnston

Introduction

The word plastic originates from the Greek *plastikos*, which means to mould or give form. Plastic surgery is concerned mainly with reconstruction of congenital defects and defects following trauma and cancer surgery. On calls for plastic surgery can be very busy, depending on the department you work in. There are fortunately few emergencies in plastic surgery, but when they do occur they need to be dealt with appropriately. This chapter aims to advise and guide the junior covering plastic surgery 'on call' so that they can initiate correct management of common problems and know when urgent senior help is needed.

Hand fracture/dislocation

Think about

Open fractures need urgent attention. Call for senior help.

Ask about

- Age, hand dominance, occupation, hobbies.
- Mechanism of injury and time since injury.
- If dislocated, did anyone relocate it?
- Whether open or closed.
- Pre-existing disease—osteoarthritis (OA), rheumatoid arthritis (RA), osteoporosis.
- Previous injuries.
- Steroid use.
- Smoker?
- Last time ate/drank.

Look for

- Compare to other hand.
- Obvious deformity, swelling, discoloration.
- May need to perform a ring block as too uncomfortable to examine without.
- Assess movement—active and passive. Assess stability during movement. If displaces during active movement, major ligament at site of displacement is likely to be ruptured. Passively stress proximal interphalangeal joint (PIPJ) laterally to test collateral ligaments and anteroposteriorly (AP) to stress the volar plate.
- Normal range of movement: metacarpophalangeal joint (MCPJ) 90°, PIPJ 100°, distal interphalangeal joint (DIPJ) 80°.

Investigations

X-ray—AP and true lateral.

Management

- Elevate all hand injuries.
- Allow all uninjured fingers to be free to mobilize.

Terminal phalanx fractures

Associated with nail-bed injuries, usually following fingertip crush. Need to wash out and repair nail-bed under local anaesthesia (LA). Can use fingertip as composite graft if completely severed. Keep tip wrapped in a moist gauze in a sealed bag. Put the bag in a bag of water/ice.

Metacarpal and phalangeal fractures

Acceptable 10° angulation, 20° on the lateral at the metaphysis, 45° at the neck of the 5th metacarpal, and at least 50% contact between the two bony fragments. (Look for scissoring of fingers when they are extended, and overlapping/rotation when they make a fist.) If acceptable position with no scissoring or rotation, put in metacarpal fractures in a Colles' cast for 3–4 weeks. Buddy-strap phalangeal fractures.

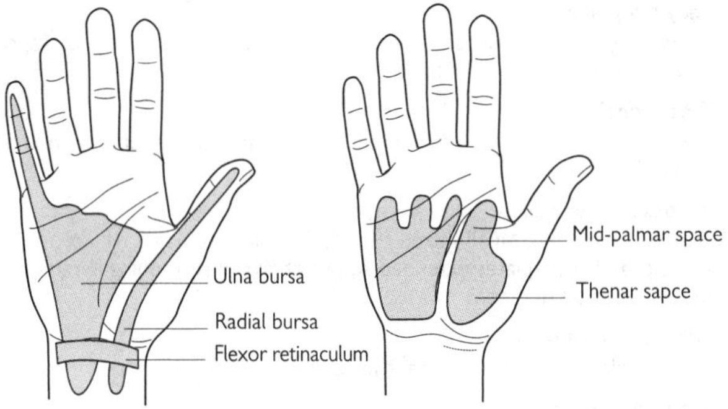

Fig. 10.1 Bones of the hand and wrist.

Unstable fractures

Multifragmentary, multiple, neck of proximal phalanx, displaced articular fractures.

Hyperextension/dorsal dislocation PIPJ

- Common injury after catching a ball.
- Relocate into normal anatomical position and buddy-strap.
- Fracture/dislocation of PIPJ fracture of the volar lip of middle phalanx base—stability depends on % articular surface involved, >40% is unstable. Stable injuries can be buddy-strapped and mobilize. Unstable injuries need to be put in an extension blocking splint, 10° flexion beyond point of instability.

Avulsion fracture

Fracture at site of tendon or ligament insertion.

Pilon fracture

2° to axial force applied to an extended finger. Fracture of the middle phalanx base, intra-articular, comminuted, unstable, need fixation.

Bicondylar fracture

2° to axial load applied to finger while flexed. Again intra-articular, comminuted, requires fixation.

Bennett's and Rolando fracture

Fracture of the base of the first metacarpal. Intra-articular, needs fixation.

Gamekeeper's thumb

Rupture of the ulnar collateral ligament. 2° to forcible abduction. Complain of pain ulnar side of 1st MCPJ. Test for laxity by stressing the joint in abduction. May need scaphoid cast for 6 weeks or, if a Stenner's lesion, open repair of the ligament.

Carpal dislocations

Need reduction under general anaesthesia (GA).

Buddy strapping

For two fingers of similar size. Felt/wool between the two fingers. Tape around proximal and middle fingers.

POP/bandaging

Wrist extended 30°, MCPJs flexed at 90°, PIPJ and DIPJ extended, thumb abducted.

Safe position for hand

Wrist 20° extended, MCPJ flexed to 70°, IPJs fully extended. All collateral ligaments and volar plates extended so not at risk of shortening if immobilized for a period of time.

Fracture healing risks

Mal/non/delayed union, infection, shortening, avascular necrosis.

Long-term complications

Chronic pain, stiffness, early-onset arthritis, deformity, reduced/loss of function.

Hand infections

Alert senior

Hand infections can be devastating if not managed appropriately early, resulting in destruction of tendon/bone joint and may lead to amputation as only definitive treatment.

Think about

- Most common pathogen—*Staphylococcus aureus.*
- Cat/dog bite—*Pasteurella multocida.*
- Human bite—*Staphylococcus aureus* and *S. epidermidis*, streptococci, peptostreptococci, *Bacteroides.*

Ask about

- Hand dominance, occupation, hobbies.
- Diabetes, steroids, immunosuppression, history of penetrating injury—including tooth during punch, tetanus status.
- Allergies.
- Last time ate/drank.

Look for

- Where is the infection?
- Pain, swelling, erythema, pus.
- Look at the hand posture—may be partially flexed if infected.
- Signs of systemic illness—pyrexia, dehydration, tachycardia, tachypnoea.

Investigations

- Temperature, pulse, respiratory rate.
- Blood glucose.
- Baseline bloods—FBC, U&Es, CRP, blood cultures.
- Swab any pus/discharge.
- X-ray of affected hand—look for signs of osteomyelitis.
- ECG ± CXR if indicated for GA.

Management

- See below, depending on type of infection.
- Nil by mouth (NBM) until discussed with registrar or there is obvious paronychia.
- Consider IV fluids if systemic signs of sepsis.
- Consider sliding scale if diabetic.
- Do not give antibiotics until specimen sent for microbiology or have discussed with registrar.
- Elevate and splint all hand infections.
- Analgesia as needed.
- Most infections will need drainage, washout and IV antibiotics.

Acute paronychia

- Proximal to the nail fold.
- Erythema, obvious pus collection, nail itself may appear normal.
- Treat by removing the nail gently and washout under LA using ring block.

Felon

- Finger pulp.
- Usually 2° to penetrating wound.
- Drain over area of maximum fluctuance.
- May go on to develop osteomyelitis, flexor sheath infection, septic arthritis.

Herpetic whitlow

- Finger tip.
- Superficial infection of the fingertip with herpes simplex virus.
- Small clear vesicles seen early.
- Not for drainage, risk of bacterial superinfection.
- Conservative management, usually resolves within 3 weeks.

Flexor sheath infections

- Along volar surface of finger.
- Usually 2° to penetrating injury.
- Four signs described by Kanavel:
  - Fusiform finger swelling.
  - Pain on passive extension.
  - Finger held semi-flexed.
  - Tenderness over flexor sheath.
- Needs to be drained, flexor sheath irrigated open or closed under GA.
- Little finger flexor sheath communicates with the ulnar bursa.
- Thumb flexor sheath infection communicates with the radial bursa.
- Often (70% of cases) these bursae communicate with one another. Swelling is seen in the palm and in the wrist proximal to the flexor retinaculum.

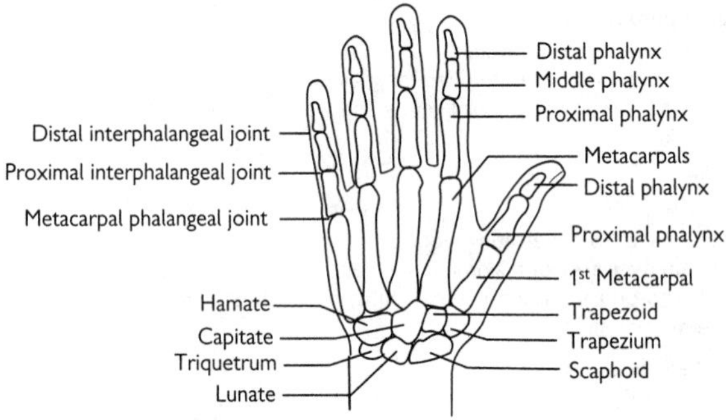

Fig. 10.2 (a) Dorsal hand spaces, (b) Palmar hand spaces.

Palm infections

- Three potential spaces:
  - Thenar space—over thenar eminence to third metacarpal.
  - Mid-palmar space—over fourth metacarpal.
  - Hypothenar space—rarely involved in hand infections, over hypothenar eminence.
- Flexor sheath infections can rupture into the thenar or mid-palmar space.
- Collections in these spaces need to be drained surgically under GA.

Dorsal hand infections

- Dorsal subcutaneous space—dorsum of the hand.
- Palmar infections may spread to this space via communications at the fingerwebs.
- Dorsal subaponeurotic space—lies below extensor retinaculum.

- Is the infection extending into the forearm?
- If so, immediate treatment is needed—call senior.

Nerve injury

Nerve structure

Axon central for nerve conduction. Surrounded by endo-, peri- and epi-neurium (outermost).

Neuropraxia

Temporary, axon intact, but conduction impaired for variable amount of time. Full recovery expected.

Axonotmesis

Axon ± perineurium and endoneurium divided. Epineurium intact. Some recovery expected. Risk of neuroma.

Neurotmesis

Nerve trunk completely divided—no recovery unless surgical intervention and then only partial recovery at best.

Think about

Associated injuries. Vulnerable areas where nerves are superficial/near bone, so at risk if fractured. Radial nerve at mid-shaft of humerus, dorsal wrist, snuff box. Ulnar nerve at cubital tunnel, posterior elbow and volar wrist. Median nerve at cubital triangle, medial to brachial artery anterior elbow and volar wrist. Digital nerves over heads of metacarpals, lateral fingers.

Ask about

- Age, hand dominance, occupation, hobbies.
- Mechanism of injury—if laceration, thickness of blade and edge of blade (smooth, serrated).
- Time since injury.
- Loss of sensation/paraesthesia—progressive or improving.
- Weakness—difficulty performing certain tasks.
- Pre-existing disease—OA, RA.
- Previous injuries.
- Steroid use.
- Tetanus status.
- Smoker?
- Have the patient had any LA yet—will alter examination.
- Last time ate/drank.

Look for

- Record positions, lengths of wounds.
- Test the three main nerves to the forearm/hand as below.
- Test sensation—C5 radial upper arm, C6 radial forearm, C7 hand, C8 ulnar forearm, T1 ulnar upper arm. Record findings accurately in notes.

Median nerve

- Lateral and medial cords of the brachial plexus—C5–T1.
- Supplies all flexors of forearm except flexor carpi ulnaris and ulnar half of flexor digitorum profundus (FDP).

- Supplies 'LOAF' in the hand—Lumbricals 1 and 2, Opponens pollicis, Abductor pollicis brevis, Flexor pollicis brevis. Sensation to radial 3½ digits, palmar side.
- Test motor—abductor pollicis brevis. Hand flat on table, palm side up, ask patient to point thumb to the ceiling against resistance at 1st MCPJ radial side. Feel APB contract at same time.
- Sensory—radial side of index fingertip.

Ulnar nerve
- Medial cord—C8 and T1.
- Supplies flexor carpi ulnaris and ulnar half of FDP in forearm.
- Supplies small muscles of the hand except for LOAF.
- Sensation to ulnar 1½ digits.
- Test motor—1st dorsal interosseus. Ask patient to abduct index finger against resistance, feel muscle contract in 1st dorsal web space.
- Sensory—ulnar side of little fingertip.

Radial nerve
- Posterior cord—C5–T1.
- Supplies extensors of forearm and hand.
- Test motor—wrist/finger extension.
- Sensory—dorsal hand, dorsal radial 3½ fingers. Consistently over 1st web space dorsally.

Digital nerves
- Two per finger/thumb, run along mid-lateral border of digit, run more anterior along the thumb.
- Test either side of finger/thumb pulp.

Investigations
- As with any hand injury, X-ray if fracture/foreign body suspected.
- Baseline bloods if needs GA or suspect infection.
- ECG, CXR again if indicated for GA.

Management
- If nerve injury suspected, usually needs exploration under GA. Direct repair or occasionally a nerve/vein graft needed.
- Nerve grafts—sacrifice nerve, usually sensory, to repair more important nerve.
- Sural—runs behind lateral malleolus; loss of sensation to lateral side of foot.
- Lateral cutaneous nerve of forearm—adjacent to cephalic vein along ulnar border of brachioradialis; loss of sensation along radial side of forearm.
- Medial cutaneous nerve of forearm—between triceps and biceps along basilic vein; loss of sensation along ulnar border of forearm.
- Terminal branch of posterior interosseous nerve—radial side of extensor digiti communi at the wrist; supplies joint.

Tendons

Flexor and extensor tendon injury

Think about

Associated fracture/neurovascular injury.

Ask about

- Age, hand dominance, occupation, hobbies.
- Mechanism of injury—if with blade, thickness of it, type of edge (smooth, serrated).
- Time since injury.
- Risk of infection.
- Tetanus status.
- Pre-existing disease—OA, RA.
- Previous injuries.
- Steroid use.
- Diabetes?
- Smoker?
- Last time ate/drank.

Look for

- Swelling, deformity.
- Movements—active and passive. Pain on active movement indicates partial tear/rupture.
- Weakness.
- Sensation.
- Capillary refill.
- Palmaris longus—may be needed for graft.

FDS injuries

Test each finger individually, holding the other fingers in extension. Ask patient to flex the finger. When finger flexed, flex fingertip to check that DIPJ is relaxed. If tip flicks back easily then FDP is relaxed and is not being used to flex the finger.

Extensor terminal slip injuries

Test each finger individually. Ask patient to extend the fingertip. If not able to extend, the patient has a mallet finger due to rupture of the lateral bands and distal tendon or avulsion from its bony attachment.

FDP injuries

Fix PIPJ/hold middle phalanx to test FDP. Ask patient to flex distal phalanx.

Extensor central slip injuries

Flex PIPJ over table edge. Ask patient to extend finger. May have boutonnière deformity.

Proximal extensor tendon injuries

Flex finger at MCPJ, extend finger at PIPJ and DIPJ. Ask patient to extend finger at MCPJ.

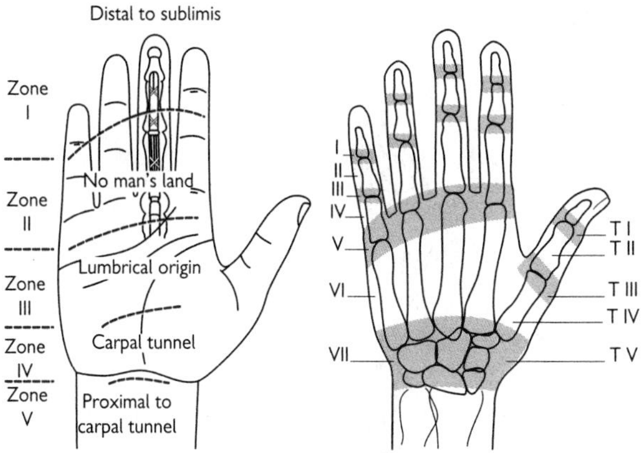

Fig. 10.3 (a) Flexor and (b) extensor tendon injury zones. (T = Thumb).

Flexor zones:
- Distal to insertion of flexor digitorum superficialis (FDS) (1).
- Between proximal end of flexor sheath and insertion of FDS (no man's land) (2).
- Between distal edge of flexor retinaculum and proximal end of flexor sheath (3).
- Under flexor retinaculum (4).
- Proximal to flexor retinaculum (5).

Extensor zones:
- Over DIPJ (1).
- Between PIPJ and DIPJ (2).
- Over PIPJ (3).
- Between MCPJ and PIPJ (4).
- Over MCPJ (5).
- Between MCPJ and extensor retinaculum (6).
- Under extensor retinaculum (7).
- Proximal to extensor retinaculum (8).

Flexor/extensor pollicis longus
Hold proximal phalanx and ask patient to flex/extend thumb tip.

Mallet finger
Unable to extend DIPJ. Occurs after forcible flexion against resistance of fingertip. Distal extensor tendon is torn from its attachment to the distal phalanx or an avulsion fracture is associated. If more than 20% of the articular surface of the distal phalangeal base is associated, formal repair may be needed. Can normally be treated with 6 weeks in mallet splint, holding DIPJ in extension, leaving PIPJ free to flex/extend. Temporary splint can be made from a tongue depressor and tape.

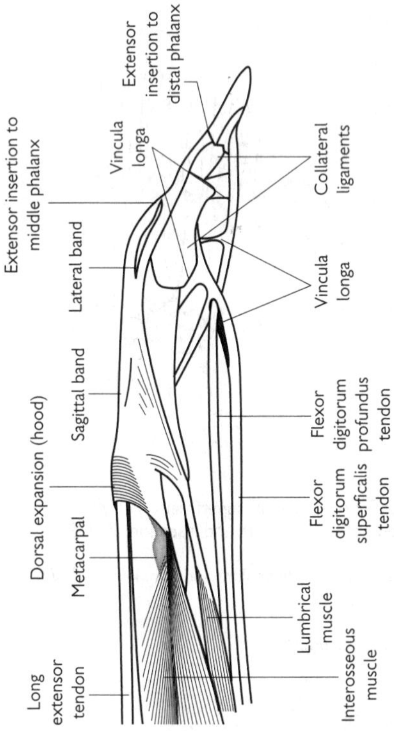

Fig. 10.4 Flexor and extensor tendons of the finger.

Boutonnière deformity

Flexion of PIPJ, hyperextension of DIPJ, due to detachment of the central slip of the extensor tendon attached to the base of the middle phalanx. Seen in wounds over PIPJ.

Swan neck deformity

Extension of PIPJ, flexion of DIPJ. Seen after rupture of FDS.

Investigations

- X-ray—look for fractures, especially avulsions, foreign bodies, underlying disease (OA, RA).
- Baseline bloods.
- CXR.
- ECG if indicated for GA or suspect infection.

Management

- Proximal extensor tendons can normally be repaired under LA. Flexors need to be repaired under GA. Elevate, splint hand. Repairs are usually placed in a splint (dorsal for flexors, volar for extensors) after surgery to protect the repair.
- Tetanus booster if needed.
- Need hand therapy after repair.

Tendon grafts

- Palmaris longus—10% of population don't have this superficial tendon, which is seen running into the palmar fascia when wrist is flexed in the midline between flexor carpi radialis and FDS.
- Plantaris—tendon found in the calf. Runs between soleus and gastrocnemius; inserts into Achilles tendon. No functional use, so good for grafts.

Lower limb trauma

Think about

- Airway, breathing, circulation (ABC).
- Any other injuries.
- Don't be distracted by the obvious injury and miss a more subtle yet equally important fracture, dislocation or soft tissue defect.

Ask about

- Mechanism—high energy (road traffic accident, fall from significant height, missile, crushing).
- Occupation.
- General health.
- Medications.
- Smoker?
- When last ate/drank.

Look for

- A large soft tissue defect suggests a high-energy injury.
- May be much more extensive than evident on simple inspection.
- Associated injuries.
- Check neurovascular status.
- If distant pulses absent, call senior.
- Dirt/tyre imprints.
- Donor sites for free/local muscle or fascia flap—gracilis from inner thigh; gastrocnemius from calf; latissimus dorsi from back. Will usually need split skin graft from thigh to cover muscle flap.

Investigations

- Routine bloods—FBC, U&Es, clotting, cross-match if free flap needed.
- ECG if cardiac disease or >50yr.
- CXR if indicated before GA.
- Suspect pneumo/haemothorax.

Management

Soft tissue defects over metal work need a fasciocutaneous or muscle flap, ideally within 5 days of injury. Liaise with microbiology re antibiotic therapy. Tissue samples should be sent at operation. May need 6 weeks of intravenous antibiotics if infected or not covered within 5 days.

Orthopaedics normally fix any associated fracture first. Ask them about weight-bearing status and follow up.

Deep vein thrombosis prophylaxis, e.g. Fragmin® 5000 units OD.

☉ Pre-tibial lacerations and degloving limb injuries

Usually found in elderly people following a fall.

Think about

- Has the patient got an underlying medical condition that caused the fall?
- Mechanical or medical—syncope? Does this need to be investigated before or after surgery, as an inpatient or outpatient/with the GP?
- Is the patient coping at home or do they need extra help that could take a long time through social services, so the earlier the referral the better.

Ask about

- Age.
- Mechanism of injury.
- Time of injury.
- Any other injuries.
- Normal health status—diabetic, bleeding disorders.
- Medications—steroids, anticoagulants, immunosupressants; grafts may fail if infected or be lifted off by a haematoma.
- Allergies—mesh boards are made out of latex.
- Home set-up, mobility.
- Smoker?
- Last time ate/drank.

Look for

- Skin discoloration—devascularized skin will be discolored and not salvageable.
- Abnormal movement of skin over underlying layers—degloving.
- Layers of soft tissue lost—skin, subcutaneous fat, fascia, muscle, bone. Grafts will not survive on cartilage, tendons or bone unless they are still covered in their perichondrium, tendon sheath or periosteum.
- Surrounding skin—diabetic or venous changes, oedema.
- Donor site—usually anterior or lateral thigh.
- Look for general quality of skin, scars, radiation, naevi.

Investigations

- Baseline bloods—FBC, U&Es, INR if indicated.
- ECG if cardiac disease or age >50yr.
- CXR if asthma/smoker/COPD.
- X-ray if associated fracture or foreign body in wound suspected.

Management

- Good wound toilet to remove debris and foreign bodies.
- Lacerations/wounds need to be excised to healthy tissue with the potential to granulate—fascia/muscle/periosteum.
- Skin graft then applied to the defect—usually performed under GA, so patient needs to be worked up for this.
- Any concerns need to be discussed with the anaesthetist as early as possible.
- Small defects can be done under LA; need Emla® ideally on donor site 2hr preop.
- Patient needs to be starved for a GA if the LA may need to be supplemented with sedation.
- Antibiotics not normally needed.
- Explain to patient the possibility of surgical debridement, skin graft and donor site.

Split skin grafts

- Epidermis and variable amount of dermis.
- Also used in burns management.
- Mesh to variable ratios; fishnet stocking appearance.

Donor sites

- Ideally discrete sites—buttock, upper thigh, but anywhere in desperate cases.
- Can overgraft donor wound to reduce donor site morbidity in patients over 60yr.
- Dressing on graft site usually removed at 5 days.
- Donor site dressing (e.g. Mefix®) usually left to fall off by self.
- Graft may shear if not secured well enough.
- May need splint/bed-rest.

☠ Burns

Call senior immediately if significant burn, child, significant risk of injury, any concerns.

Think about

Non-accidental injury (NAI) in adults and children.

Ask about

- Type of burn—thermal, chemical, electrical, radiation.
- Mechanism and time of injury.
- Action taken and treatment so far.
- If associated with smoke, length of time subjected to smoke.
- Loss of consciousness.
- Other casualties and extent of their injuries.

Look for

- Burn depth:
  - Superficial—red, good capillary refill, sensate, no blisters.
  - Deep—dark pink, slow capillary refill, sensate, large blisters.
  - Full thickness—white/yellow, insensate, no refill.

Wallace rule of nines

- Head and neck 9%, arm 9%, anterior trunk 18%, posterior trunk 18%, leg 18%, genitalia 1%.
- Children as above, but head and neck 18% and leg 14%. For each child above the age of 10yr, take 1% off the head and neck and add it to the combined leg score.

Investigations

- Pulse.
- Temperature.
- RR, BP, Sats, BM, urinary output (UO).
- Baseline bloods—FBC, U&Es, LFTs.
- Arterial blood gas (ABG).
- Carboxyhaemoglobin.

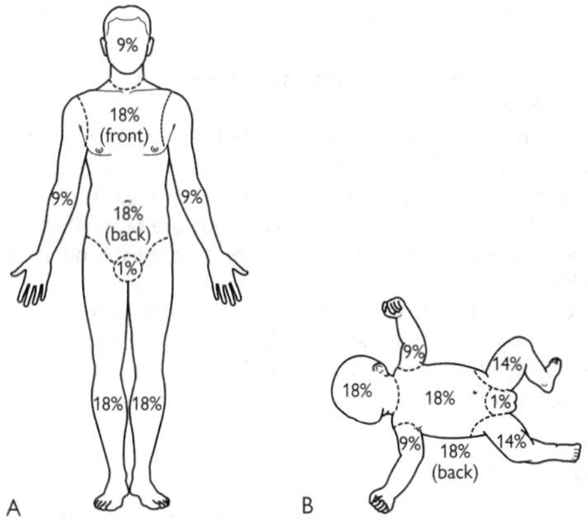

Fig. 10.5 Wallace rule of nines: percentages of total body area in (A) adult and (B) infant.

Management

- ABC.
- Airway is the prime concern, discuss with senior ± anaesthetist.
- Oxygen, analgesia.
- Need to ventilate—inhalation injury with high respiratory rate, stridor, confusion, distress, ↑ tiredness, extensive head and neck burns, supraglottic oedema, high levels of carboxyhaemoglobin.
- Need anaesthetic review prior to transfer to the burns unit.
- May need immediate escharotomy if extensive chest wounds or circumferential limb burns.
- May need immediate tracheostomy if supraglottal oedema.
- Fluid resuscitation—adults with >15% total body surface area (TBSA) involved; children with >10% TBSA involved.
- Cover burns with cling film.

Parkland formula

- 3–4mL/kg/% burn of Ringer's lactate or Hartman's in first 24hr. Give half of the fluid in the first 8hr, in addition to maintenance fluid for children (see below).
- Urine output >0.5mL/kg/hr in adults; >1mL/kg/hr in children.
- Haematocrit should be 0.35–0.45 in adults, 0.28–0.35 in children.
- Children maintenance fluid—5% dextrose and 0.45% saline. 1st 10kg, 4mL/kg/hr; 2nd 10kg, 2mL/kg/hr; 3rd 10kg, 1mL/kg/hr.

Refer to burns unit if

- >10% TBSA involved in adults, >5% in children.
- Full-thickness burns >5% of TBSA in adults and children.
- Face, hands, feet, perineum, major joints involved.
- Significant chemical or electrical burns.
- Extremes of age.
- Associated major trauma.
- Suspicion of NAI.
- Significant pre-existing illness.

Calorific requirements

- Adults—25kcal/kg + 40kcal/% burn/day.
- Children—40–60kcal/kg/day.
- Calorie : nitrogen ratio 150 : 1.

Thermal

- Fluid loss from circulation into interstitial space.
- Systemic effects if >20% of body surface affected; >10% in children.
- Hypovolaemia, immunosuppression, catabolism, loss of protective function of the gut, pulmonary oedema.

Inhalation injury
- Fire in an enclosed space; patient unconscious in fire.
- Hoarse/weak voice, stridor, brassy cough, restlessness, respiratory distress.
- Soot around nose/mouth, singed facial/nasal hair, swollen upper airway, hypoxia, pulmonary oedema, acute respiratory distress syndrome (ARDS).

Subglottic
- From products of combustion.
- May need humidified oxygen, intubation, intermittent positive pressure ventilation (IPPV) and steroids.

Systemic
- Carbon monoxide (CO) poisoning.
- Half-life of CO in patients breathing 100% oxygen is 40min, on air it is 250min.
- Symptoms include headache, confusion, hallucinations, ataxia.
- Treat with 100% humidified oxygen, at 8L/min through a non-rebreathing reservoir mask for at least 8hr.

Chemical
- Alkali—liquefactive necrosis, deep; household bleach, oven cleaners, fertilizers, cement.
- Acid—coagulative necrosis. Irrigate with water or diluted sodium bicarbonate. If hydrofluoric acid, apply calcium gluconate repeatedly.
- Phosphorus—fireworks, firearms, insecticides, fertilizers. Irrigate. May reignite on drying; often military.
- Remove clothing and causative agent.
- Irrigate for 1–2hr. Do not water for lithium, potassium and sodium as may reignite. Use fire extinguisher first, then cover with oil.

Electrical burns
- Asystole more common after high-frequency shock.
- Low voltage <1000V, high >1000V.
- Lightening—extremely high voltage, extensive deep muscle damage, may need fasciotomies, risk of rhabdomyolysis, myoglobinuria, acute renal failure, maintain high urine output >2mL/kg/hr.

Necrotizing fasciitis

Life-threatening condition. Call senior if any suspicion.

Think about

- Patients more at risk—diabetic, on steroids, recent surgery, trauma, chemotherapy, immunosuppressants.
- Usually a combination of bacteria including *Staphylococcus aureus*, group A streptococci and anaerobes.

Ask about

- What was the first sign/symptom noticed?—usually a small patch of erythema followed by pain and swelling.
- How rapidly has it progressed?—usually rapid over hours/days.
- If associated with penetrating injury, details and timing of this.
- Any treatment so far—antibiotics, surgery.
- Past medical history, drug history, allergies.
- More common in alcoholics and diabetics.
- Any culture results so far.
- When last ate and drank.

Look for

- Erythema, swelling, induration, crepitus, putrid discharge, extreme pain out of keeping with signs.
- Overlying skin may appear normal then dusky/purple as the infection progresses.
- Mark out extent of tissue affected and record time.
- Necrosis undermines between the skin and subcutaneous layer, leaving the skin loose over the area.
- Patient may lose sensation over the area affected.
- Muscle may be involved.
- Patient may look well or systemically toxic.

Investigations

- Pulse, RR, Sats, BP, BM.
- Baseline bloods—FBC, U&Es, CRP, clotting, G&S, cultures.
- ABG.
- Swab any pus/discharge.
- X-ray—look for gas in subcutaneous fascial planes.
- ECG,
- Chest X-ray if indicated for GA.

Management

- Resuscitate patient as necessary, IV access, fluids, oxygen.
- Prepare for theatre—will need extensive debridement and IV antibiotics (IVABs).
- At a later date wounds created may need cover with split skin grafts.

Postoperative problems

Breast

- Reduction—postop. risk of haematoma, nipple necrosis.
- Augmentation—postop. risk of haematoma, infection, rupture.

Flaps

Call senior immediately if any concerns re flap.

Pedicled

Flap left attached to supplying vessels, pedicle, swung on pedicle to different position:

- Latissimus dorsi for breast reconstruction, lower limb trauma.
- TRAM—transverse rectus abdominis muscle for breast reconstruction, sternal wound dehiscence.
- Gastrocnemius from calf for lower limb/knee soft tissue defects.

Free

- TRAM—transverse rectus abdominis myocutaneous. Associated skin paddle can include the ipsilateral or contralateral rectus. Anastomosed to either internal mammary or thoracodorsal vessels.
- DIEP—deep inferior epigastric perforator flap. Same skin flap taken but rectus muscle left intact.
- Gracilis—muscle from inner thigh. Used to cover soft tissue defects of the lower limb, often associated with fractures.

Postoperative monitoring

- Colour, temperature, capillary return, bleeding on pinprick, Doppler.
- Hb and haematocrit (Hct) 4–6hr postop—Hb should be 10–12g/dL; Hct 25–35%, give blood if <25, give colloid if >35.
- Keep warm with Bair Hugger®.
- UO >0.5mL/kg/hr.
- Systolic BP >100mmHg.
- Do not give diuretics or inotropes to a patient who has recently had a flap without discussing it with a senior.

Cleft palate repair

Call senior if any concerns.

- Try to calm down child and parents.
- Bleeding—avoid suction unless absolutely necessary.
- Airway obstruction—oxygen, nebulizers.
- May need nasopharyngeal airway—do not insert unless emergency without discussing with senior first.
- Pyrexia—septic screen, start antibiotics, usually Augmentin®. Check results of preop. nose/throat swabs.

Craniofacial

Usually have paediatrician on call immediately postop.

Call senior if any concerns: temperature, vomiting, headache, wound discharge (blood/CSF), altered/fluctuating behaviour/level of consciousness, distress.

Compartment syndrome

Any operation/injury to a limb is at risk of compartment syndrome. See 📖 Chapter 3.

ⓘ Pressure sores

Think about

- Paraplegia, quadriplegia, spina bifida, immobilization, multiple sclerosis.
- Consider malignant change.

Ask about

- Onset, duration of ulcer.
- Previous, concurrent ulcers.
- Prior medical, surgical treatment.
- Previous, current wound care.
- Mattress.
- Systemic symptoms—fevers, weight loss, loss of appetite.
- Diabetes.
- Steroid use.
- Malignancy, liver disease, any chronic disease.

Look for

- Barczak staging system:
  - Stage 1—Skin intact but reddened for >1hr after relief of pressure.
  - Stage 2—Blister or break in dermis ± infection.
  - Stage 3—Subcutaneous tissue involved.
  - Stage 4—Through deep fascia, involving muscle, bone or joint.

- Character of wound base, granulation/necrotic tissue.
- Size, shape, depth of wound.
- Edge—heaped, undermining, sloping, punched out.
- Position, usually over bony prominences—ischium, sacrum, trochanter, heels, occiput, scapula.
- Connection with underlying joint/urethra via sinus.
- Continence.
- Skin quality.
- Oedema.
- Evidence of infection.

Investigation

- Bloods—FBC, U&Es, LFTs, Bone, CRP, ESR.
- X-ray if osteomyelitis suspected.
- Wound swabs.

Management

- Stages 1 and 2 can be usually treated conservatively.
- Stages 3 and 4 may need excision and flap reconstruction.
- Debride necrotic ulcers.
- Antibiotics if infection.
- Pressure-relieving mattress and regular turning every 2hr.
- Improve nutrition, dietician review.
- Good control of diabetes.
- Appropriate dressings—discuss with plastic surgery sister, tissue viability nurse.

Chapter 11

Breast surgery

Rachell Bright-Thomas

Introduction

When describing breast pathology to a senior colleague it is important to state:

- The *side* (left or right breast).
- The *site* of the problem, in terms of quadrants of the breast (Fig. 11.1) and/or its position relative to the nipple (distance in cm from the nipple and position on the clock face of the breast).
- The *size* of any swelling and its consistency (hard, fixed to muscle or skin, fluctuant).
- A description of the overlying *skin* (oedematous, erythematous, necrotic, dimpled, tethered).
- The patient's *general state* (comfortable, in pain) and *vital signs* (pulse, blood pressure (BP) and temperature).
- What you are concerned about, *why you are ringing* or why you think the patient needs admission or to be seen urgently.

In a postoperative patient all of the above need to be noted along with:

- Details of the *operation* she has had performed.
- The position of *scars* (looking closely for those in the periareola region, at the lateral aspect of the breast or in the inframammary fold (IMF) as these can be easily overlooked). Associated scars on the back or abdomen (in flap reconstructions).
- The quantity of fluid in the *drains* in the previous 24hr and its character (serous, haemoserous, frank blood, turbid).

For example: 'I would like to ask your advice about a breast patient. She is a 55-yr-old woman who had a left skin-sparing mastectomy and axillary clearance performed 10 days ago for a 2.5cm central breast cancer with associated ductal carcinoma in situ (DCIS). She had a simultaneous implant-only subpectoral reconstruction and her only scars are a central purse-string suture and a short vertical axillary scar just behind the anterior axillary fold. She was discharged 5 days ago after both drains were removed. She is now feeling generally unwell, with night sweats and fevers, and she is currently flushed with a temperature of 38°C. Her pulse is 100bpm and her BP is 120/85. The left reconstructed breast looks swollen and the skin is generally erythematous and hot to touch. There appears to be a seroma extending under the skin into the axilla and I am concerned because I think she has a significant infection following her surgery. I wanted to discuss her case with you prior to her admission to decide on the best course of action with regards to drainage of the seroma and antibiotics.'

The problem should now be clear to the specialist registrar (SpR) or consultant, and they can give appropriate advice and decide whether or not they need to come to see the patient.

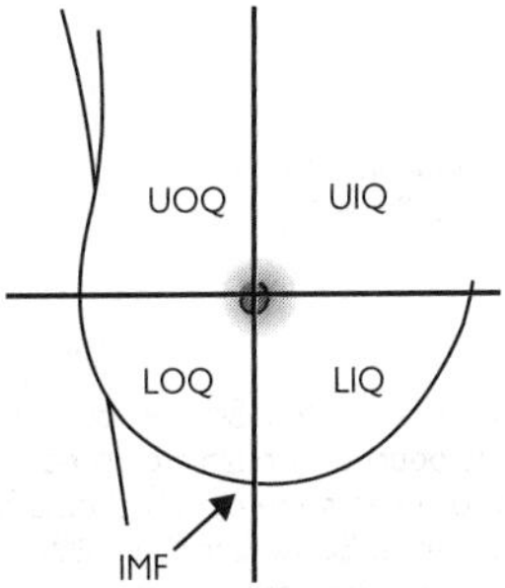

UOQ	Upper outer quadrant
UIQ	Upper inner quadrant
LOQ	Lower outer quadrant
LIQ	Lower inner quadrant
IMF	Inframammary crease

Fig. 11.1 Breast quadrants of the right breast.

Breast sepsis

- Alert senior if there is skin necrosis or an implant in situ.
- Admit if the patient is systemically unwell.

Think about

Breast sepsis can be:

- *Lactational*—mastitis or abscess. Generally due to a Staphylococcus aureus infection in engorged ducts, introduced through a cracked nipple. Continued breast-feeding and/or expression of milk should be encouraged despite lactational breast sepsis. Bacteria in the milk do not harm the baby and feeding helps to decompress engorged ducts.
- *Non-lactational*—generally periductal sepsis with or without abscess formation. Breast abscesses in this group usually arise in smokers, diabetics or those taking immunosuppressive drugs. They are associated with a mixed bacterial spectrum. Simple infected sebaceous cysts can also occur.
- *Postoperative*—a simple wound infection or an infected seroma, both of which are often staphylococcal although other organisms including pseudomonas and mycobacteria have been seen, particularly in association with breast implants.

But . . . beware the missed inflammatory cancer or acute post-radiotherapy changes that may mimic breast sepsis. Any 'mastitis' in postmenopausal or non-lactating patients have to be treated as suspicious and requires follow-up in the next breast clinic.

Ask about

- Recent breast or axillary surgery.
- Breast-feeding.
- Smoking and drug history.

Look for

- Signs suggestive of mastitis:
  - Generalized breast erythema and swelling.
- Signs suggestive of an abscess:
  - A fluctuant area with overlying erythematous shiny skin.
  - Skin necrosis (purple discoloration, thinning, desquamation, lack of blanching on compression).
  - A swinging pyrexia (as occasionally abscesses in the retromammary space may not be palpable but will lead to systemic upset).

Table 11.1 Antibiotics of choice

Nature of sepsis	Antibiotic of choice	If penicillin allergic
Lactational	Flucloxacillin 500mg QDS	Erythromycin 500mg BD
Non-lactational	Co-amoxiclav 375mg TDS	Erythromycin 500mg BD + metronidazole 200mg TDS
Postoperative	Co-amoxiclav 375mg TDS	Erythromycin 500mg BD + metronidazole 200mg TDS

Management

Mastitis or simple postoperative wound infection

Antibiotics as outlined in Table 11.1.

Abscess

- Requires *adequate* drainage. Delay may lead to breast tissue and skin loss, a poor cosmetic result and may also impede breast-feeding.
- The majority can be managed by simple aspiration in the A&E or outpatient setting. Only a small number require formal incision and drainage.
- After drainage, consider admission and intravenous antibiotics in systemically unwell ♀, particularly those on chemotherapy or other immunosuppressive drugs, or those with extensive cellulitis.

After complete aspiration or drainage the patient can be discharged but should return to the breast clinic within 48hr for review as many abscesses needing repeat aspiration and/or further evaluation to exclude underlying breast cancer.

If the skin is intact

- Treat with simple aspiration under antibiotic cover.
- Apply Emla® cream to the skin. Going through non-indurated skin is less painful.
- Using a 19G needle, aspirate the abscess, ideally under ultrasound guidance if an ultrasound machine or friendly radiologist is available.
- The needle should be inserted parallel to the chest wall to avoid the small chance of a pneumothorax.
- An appropriate volume of 1% lidocaine or similar local anaesthetic can be infiltrated into the abscess, and the abscess aspirated with a 'washing' in and out of the local anaesthetic.
- Send a sample of the pus to microbiology.
- Commence appropriate antibiotics, as outlined in Table 11.1.

Do not insert a needle blindly into a breast with an implant. If you think there is an abscess here, it is possible that the implant will need to be removed to eradicate the infection. Discuss with a senior first.

If the overlying skin is necrotic

This will need formal incision and drainage. However, remember that drainage will be gravitational so that when the patient sits or stands up you need to have the drainage point of a large abscess at the most dependant point of the abscess. This may mean drainage out through the IMF.

- Inform the surgical SpR, as it may need to be performed under general anaesthetic (GA) in the theatre.

If it is a small abscess and you are advised to continue with drainage in casualty:

- Clean the skin with povidone–iodine or chlorhexidine.
- Infiltrate local anaesthetic (1% lidocaine) circumferentially around the affected skin or apply Emla®. Remember, truly necrotic skin is insensate.
- The necrotic skin should be removed with a blade or scissors and a good pair of forceps. The cavity should be washed out with local anaesthetic and saline.
- Send a sample of pus to microbiology.
- The wound can be left open (not sutured) to improve drainage.
- Packing can be minimal (a small wick of Kaltostat®) to reduce discomfort.
- Commence appropriate antibiotics.

Post-surgical infected seroma

- Swab the wound with a Steret®.
- The wound is anaesthetic and can be opened with a blade just enough to allow the admission of a fine sterile suction catheter (10ch) and suction applied. Alternatively a 19G needle on a 20mL syringe can be introduced into the lower end of the wound under aseptic technique.
- Aspirate the infected collection.
- Send a sample of pus to microbiology.
- A single suture (absorbable or non-absorbable size 2/0 or 3/0 cutting suture) tied over the wound can be used to close any gap in the wound. Wound glue is a good alternative.
- Commence antibiotics if the patient has associated cellulitis, is systemically unwell, or is immunocompromised or continuing with adjuvant treatment for breast cancer other than simple hormonal manipulation.

ⓘ Postoperative seroma with no evidence of infection or overlying skin impairment

These are common, not an emergency, and the patient can be referred to the next breast clinic. If extremely tense and uncomfortable, the seroma can be aspirated through the most dependant point of the scar under aseptic technique.

Threatened flap

- Alert senior if flap appears compromised.
- The patient may need to return to theatre, as there may only be a short window of opportunity to save a flap before it is lost for good.

Think about

An increasing amount of breast surgery involves breast reduction techniques to excise a cancer (a therapeutic mammoplasty), or skin-sparing mastectomy combined with pedicled or free flaps (as described at the end of the chapter, p446) to recreate a 'breast'. The viability of the skin flaps, the nipple and the transposed flaps in this complex surgery can all be threatened by pressure on the flap, venous congestion, hypotension or arterial insufficiency.

Ask about

- Details of recent surgery.
- Is she a smoker or has other medical problems?
- What is her temperature and BP?

Look for

Any evidence of a bleed putting pressure on the flap:
- Pale, cold or cyanosed skin of the mastectomy flaps and/or of any transposed flap.
- Lengthened capillary return.
- Pallor or cyanosis of the nipple–areola complex (NAC).

Management

- Ensure good oxygenation.
- Keep the patient comfortable.
- Keep the patient warm, Gamgee on the flap, a warming blanket on the patient.
- Obtain IV access and keep well perfused with good urine output (50mL/hr).
- Consider the need to return to theatre and keep nil by mouth until reviewed.
- A congested NAC may need some sutures removed or leeches applied. Discuss with a senior first.

Differential diagnosis

- Generalized poor perfusion.
- Discoloration of breast skin with blue dye after sentinel lymph node biopsy.
- Bruising.

General points

- Free flaps are less robust than a pedicled latissimus dorsi flap.
- Smokers, the obese, diabetics and ♀ with prior radiotherapy are at greater risk of postoperative complications.

Postoperative bleeding/haematoma

Alert senior if bleeding is causing haemodynamic compromise or a haematoma is present.

Excessive bleeding must be taken seriously and seen rapidly.

Think about

Bleeding within 24hr of surgery is ongoing from the operation (due to a slipped clip or suture) or reactive when BP rises after surgery.

Ask about

- Details of recent surgery.
- Anticoagulation use and known coagulopathies.
- Systemic disorders including hypertension (treated or untreated) and liver disease.

Look for

- Vital signs (collapse is sometimes the first sign of excessive postoperative bleeding).
- Marked bruising/discoloration of the overlying skin.
- Excessive discomfort/pain due to tension on the flaps.
- A tense swelling (mastectomy wounds should be flat).
- ↑ purple discoloration of the nipple after a breast reduction or reconstruction (as ↑ pressure may impede nipple blood flow).

Management

- Think airway, breathing, circulation (ABC).
- Initiate resuscitation and inform a senior colleague.
- Regular, well documented observations.
- Check FBC, U&Es, clotting and group & save.
- Likely to need to return to theatre to evacuate haematoma and identify the bleeding point.

General points

- Excessive bleeding is often associated with minimal blood in the drains (as the drains clot off).
- Mastectomy flaps can hide large volumes of blood (litres).
- Haematomas are common after ♂ mastectomy or surgery for gynaecomastia.

ⓘ Nipple necrosis and postoperative wound breakdown

Think about

Small areas of wound breakdown or nipple necrosis are frequently seen several days or weeks after complex breast surgery. 'The angle of sorrow' (the 'T' junction of scars in the IMF produced after some breast reduction operations) is a common place for wound problems; see below.

Ask about

- Details of recent surgery.
- Is there an implant in situ?—this can be at risk if the wound breaks down.

Look for

- Evidence of skin necrosis or sepsis.

Management

A small area of simple wound breakdown can be cleaned up and sutured and the patient can be referred on to the next breast clinic.

- Clean the skin with povidone–iodine or chlorhexidine.
- Remove small necrotic areas of skin with a blade. They will be anaesthetic so do not generally require local anaesthetic.
- Insert a few simple sutures (absorbable or non-absorbable 2/0 or 3/0 cutting sutures). Wound glue may suffice in a small defect not under tension.
- Give covering antibiotics (as described previously) if there is any evidence of postoperative infection.

ⓘ New breast lump and nipple discharge

New breast lumps (even if fungating) and nipple discharge (even if bloody) are not emergencies. As long as the patient is otherwise well, she can be discharged and seen in the next breast clinic.

Malodorous ulcerating cancers may have an anaerobic infection and benefit from topical application of metronidazole gel.

Surgery for breast cancer

Mastectomy

There are many eponymous names for various types of mastectomy but a simple mastectomy combined with an axillary staging procedure is now the treatment of choice for large cancers, central cancers, widespread DCIS or multifocal disease. The breast tissue and overlying skin, including the NAC, is excised leaving the pectoralis muscles intact. The scar can be transverse, hockey-stick shaped or even vertical, but is flat to the chest with at least 1 drain in situ.

Locally advanced breast cancers can present specific surgical problems:

- Extensive skin resection may lead to difficulty with wound closure so the mastectomy may need to be combined with a skin graft or a flap to avoid closing wounds under tension.
- Local resection of the pectoralis muscle is required for tumours fixed to the chest wall.

Skin-sparing mastectomy

Skin-sparing mastectomy is increasingly being used to preserve the skin envelope of the breast in patients undergoing ablative surgery with immediate reconstruction. It can be done through a circumareolar incision if the NAC is to be removed, or occasionally from a lateral approach if the nipple is to be retained.

If a skin-sparing mastectomy is combined with a myocutaneous flap reconstruction (see below), a paddle of skin from the flap can be inserted into the defect left by the NAC. This is a useful guide to the 'health' of the flap and should not be covered up with dressings but checked regularly for warmth, colour and capillary return. If an implant-only reconstruction is used, the circumareolar incision can be closed as a short transverse scar or with a purse-string. The latter method can appear 'bunched up' initially but it settles with time to give a good cosmetic result.

Conservative breast surgery

Wide local excision (WLE) of the breast

This is excision of the breast cancer with a 1cm margin in all directions. The tumour is excised in a cylindrical way, taking the tissue from the skin anteriorly to the pectoral fascia posteriorly. Wider undermining of the skin and breast parenchyma can be performed to re-cone the breast at the same time. This re-coning can increase the degree of bruising and swelling after a simple WLE. The use of drains is variable. The position of scars is highly variable (to improve cosmesis) and not always over the resection site.

Quadrantectomy (segmental excision of the breast)
This is a larger procedure removing a pyramid of breast tissue pointing towards the NAC. There should be a large (2cm) margin of normal tissue around the tumour. This sort of surgery leaves a very poor cosmetic result and is usually performed as part of an oncoplastic procedure to re-shape the breast.

Axillary surgery

The arguments for and against axillary dissection have been extensively covered elsewhere. Suffice it to say that axillary surgery can vary from a sentinel lymph node biopsy (where the aim is to remove the first node draining the cancer) to full axillary clearance. All of these operations provide important prognostic information to aid in the choice of adjuvant treatment. Axillary clearance is also of therapeutic value.

The axillary incision for a sentinel lymph node biopsy alone should be small and a drain is not generally required. The patient may have an area of blue dye on the breast skin or develop a transient generalized bluish skin tone or even blue tears, urine and vomit. The complications from this procedure (in terms of arm pain and swelling) are less than for a standard axillary dissection, although there is a very small documented risk of anaphylactic reaction to the dye.

A traditional axillary dissection can be performed through a vertical or transverse axillary scar, or via a mastectomy incision. The common complications of this surgery are given on page 448.

Surgery for benign breast disease

Excision of gynaecomastia

Techniques vary from simple liposuction to the use of a vacuum-assisted biopsy device (Mammotome®) to a more traditional surgical approach with the incision placed around the areola margin, in the IMF or at the lateral aspect of the breast. This surgery is associated with a high incidence of postoperative haematoma, so many patients return to the ward with drains in situ or a compression garment is applied and they are observed overnight.

Microdochectomy

This is the removal of a single duct from the breast, usually performed for single-duct bloody discharge. There is only a small scar around the areola margin, no drains are required and the patient is normally discharged on the same day. Complications are unusual.

Total duct excision

All the major ducts under the areola are removed but it is approached through a similar scar to a microdochectomy. The use of postoperative drains is variable. There is ↑ risk of partial nipple necrosis. This normally develops over time rather than being apparent in the first 24hr. Once again the patient is frequently discharged on the same day.

Cosmetic breast surgery

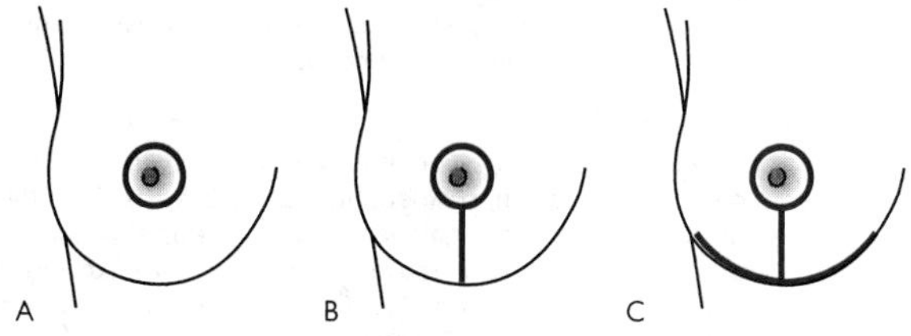

Fig. 11.2 (a) Circumareolar or Bennelli type scar for small reductions or lifts. (b) Single or vertical scar. (c) Wise pattern (with anchor-shaped scar).

Reduction mammoplasty/mastopexy techniques

There is a variety of breast reduction techniques, which are described in terms of the retained blood supply to the nipple (the pedicle) and the type of skin excision used. *Mastopexy* is an operation to lift the ptotic breast and raise the nipple height without a reduction in breast volume. The techniques used are very similar to those of *breast reduction*. The commonest scars for both operations are shown in Fig. 11.2.

The commonest nipple pedicles are inferior, superior and supero-medial, although this can be adjusted endlessly. The skin pattern does not necessarily tell you what type of pedicle has been used, although the operation note should. Most patients will have at least 1 drain in situ after surgery. The potential complications are given below. The risk of vascular insufficiency of the pedicle and skin flaps is ↑ in smokers, the obese and patients who have had radiotherapy.

Breast augmentation

This is the insertion of a silicone or saline implant to increase breast size. The implant can be inserted under the breast parenchyma or under the pectoral muscle. It can be achieved through a 5cm incision in the IMF, under the NAC, or at the lateral aspect of the breast. The use of drains is variable. Some patients with subpectoral implants complain of feeling pressure on the chest wall initially after surgery, but this settles with time.

Oncoplastic breast surgery

This is a fusion of aesthetic surgical and ablative/oncological surgical techniques to remove and stage breast cancer adequately whilst retaining or restoring a natural breast shape and symmetry.

Therapeutic mammoplasty

A breast cancer is removed using a breast reduction technique. In this way larger tumours or those in cosmetically sensitive areas (e.g. the medial aspect of the breast) can be removed without leaving a misshapen breast. The scars, drains and postoperative complications are like those seen after breast reduction. This procedure is often combined with a contralateral breast reduction to retain symmetry.

Breast reconstruction

Reconstruction begins with an assessment of 'what is missing' and 'what is available' to replace it. Traditional mastectomy leads to a deficiency in skin and volume. The skin can be replaced by tissue expansion or it can be recruited from another part of the body. Volume can be replaced with a subpectoral implant/expander, a myocutaneous flap or a combination of the two.

Flap surgery itself is undergoing a revolution and can vary from a pedicled flap to a free flap. The most common pedicled flap is the latissimus dorsi (LD) flap, swinging the LD muscle with its overlying fat and skin round from the back through the axilla to lie in the breast. This procedure is generally well tolerated and the flap is robust. Occasionally a pedicled transverse rectus abdominis flap (TRAM) is brought up from the abdomen, but this has a risk of later abdominal herniation where the rectus muscle is removed and the blood supply is less reliable.

All flaps containing muscle will leave a functional deficit at the donor site and will atrophy and decrease in volume with time. The free deep inferior epigastric perforator (DIEP) flap, where the abdominal pannus is harvested on a perforator vessel without sacrificing the rectus muscle, addresses both of these problems, but is a highly specialized technique performed only by plastic surgeons with microvascular expertise.

All patients having flap surgery should be kept warm and well perfused with good analgesia after surgery to ensure good flap perfusion. LD reconstructions are generally nursed on a ripple mattress to avoid prolonged pressure on the back. Alternatively regular turning is important. Patients having TRAM/DIEP reconstructions are nursed with the hips and knees flexed for 48hr postoperatively (to avoid undue tension on the abdominal closure). The complications of flap surgery are described below.

All reconstructions should be viewed as a journey for the patient. They generally require a series of operations with minor adjustments and contralateral procedures to achieve symmetry. Immediate reconstruction is increasingly being offered. This is efficient in terms of overall operating time and it allows skin-sparing mastectomy techniques that give an excellent cosmetic result.

Nipple reconstruction

There is a variety of techniques available for nipple reconstruction, which can be performed as a day-case procedure under local anaesthetic or combined with other minor adjustments under GA. Early complications are rare.

Complications of breast surgery

Breast and axillary surgery are remarkably well tolerated. If well counselled about what to expect, many ♀ having a straightforward mastectomy or WLE, experience little pain and are comfortable with oral analgesia (regular co-dydramol 2 tablets QDS and/or diclofenac 50mg TDS). Other units routinely supply patient-controlled analgesia (PCA) for the first 24hr after surgery. Perioperative intercostal nerve blocks can also be of benefit. These latter measures are more commonly used following complex reconstructive procedures, where pain can be troublesome.

Early specific complications of surgery seen on the wards include:

- Anaesthesia of the armpit and/or paraesthesia of the inner aspect of the upper arm after axillary surgery, resulting from damage to the intercostobrachial nerve. This is extremely common after an axillary dissection (up to 80% of ♀). It may improve gradually over 2yr.
- Haematoma (discussed above).
- Nipple congestion/discoloration after the use of reduction techniques (discussed above).
- Skin flap necrosis after skin-sparing mastectomy or reduction techniques (discussed above).
- Possible myocutaneous flap failure (discussed above).
- Sloughing of abdominal wounds or umbilical necrosis after TRAM/DIEP, to extensive tissue undermining and tension on wound closure. May need debridement and re-suturing. Associated sepsis may need antibiotic treatment.

The risks of deep vein thrombosis and pulmonary embolism are also to be remembered in ♀ with malignancy, especially those having long reconstructive operations. The risk is ↑ in ♀ on tamoxifen and those who have recently had chemotherapy. Thus all ♀ with no contraindication should receive prophylactic Clexane®.

Later complications that the GP may ring up concerned about include:

- Seroma (particularly common after axillary surgery, 50% after axillary clearance). This does not need draining if it is not too tense or uncomfortable, as aspiration carries a small risk of introducing infection.
- Stiff or frozen shoulder after axillary surgery. This benefits from exercise and physiotherapy.
- Necrosis or breakdown of wound edges (discussed above).
- Lymphoedema (swelling of the arm after axillary surgery) should be referred to the breast or lymphoedema clinic. It is not an emergency.
- Wound infection (discussed above).

Chapter 12

Urology

Alex Chapman

Introduction

Urology is a specialty that is often greeted with some trepidation by junior doctors, in part because of a lack of familiarity with its common pathologies. This is unfortunate as these common presentations are interesting and varied, and often easily managed by the junior doctor on-call which as a result can make it very rewarding. This chapter aims to guide the user through many urological presentations from both the emergency department and the ward in a simple and logical manner.

Abbreviations

AAA	abdominal aortic aneurysm
BPH	benign prostatic hyperplasia
CRP	C-reactive protein
CT	computed tomography
DMSA	dimercaptosuccinic acid
ESWL	extracorporeal *shock* wave lithotripsy
FBC	full blood count
GA	general anaesthetic
G&S	group and save
KUB	kidney, ureter and bladder
IVU	intravenous urogram
MC&S	microscopy, culture and sensitivity
MSU	midstream urine
NSAIDs	non-steroidal anti-inflammatory drugs
PSA	prostate-specific antigen
TURP	transurethral resection of prostate
U&Es	urea and electrolytes
USS	ultrasound scan
UTI	urinary tract infection

Caution in using IV contrast (e.g. for IVUs)

- Contains iodine. Check for allergies.
- Do not use in renal failure and with patients taking metformin.
- Caution with use in diabetics, dehydrated patients and those at risk of renal failure.
- Caution in asthmatics and patients with shellfish allergies (often due to iodine).
- Minor reactions include flushing, nausea and vomiting, and itching.
- Anaphylaxis may occur—patients who have had a severe reaction should not be exposed to it again.
- Ensure patient is adequately hydrated prior to receiving contrast, i.e. bolus 1 litre of normal saline IV.

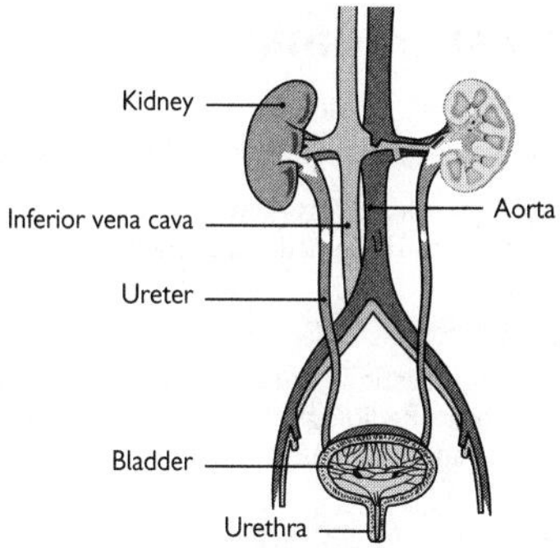

Fig. 12.1 Anatomical diagram of the urinary system.

Urological trauma

Inform on-call urologist.

Approximately 10% of trauma cases involve the genitourinary system; 90% of this is blunt trauma. These patients should be assessed and managed by the trauma team.

Renal trauma

There are various classifications to enhance communications between healthcare professionals. Radiological staging deems grade 1 and 2 as minor, and grades 3, 4 and 5 as major.

Renal Trauma

- Grade 1 —contusion to the kidney without a minor laceration.
- Grade 2 —non-expanding perirenal haematoma or cortical lesion <1cm deep without extravasation of urine.
- Grade 3 —parenchymal laceration >1cm without extravasation of rine.
- Grade 4 —parenchymal laceration extending into the collecting system.
- Grade 5 —shattered kidney or an injury to the renal pedicle.

Think about

- Children's kidneys are at greater risk from trauma as they are relatively larger than an adults, more mobile and less protected.
- Deceleration injuries.
- Compression injuries.

Look for

- Evidence of flank trauma.
- Rib fracture or overlying bruising.
- Frank or microscopic haematuria.
- Documented evidence of hypotension.
- Penetrating injuries.
- Flank tenderness.
- Tachycardia.
- Pallor/shock.

Investigations

- MSU/dipstick—haematuria (frank/microscopic).
- FBC—anaemia.
- U&Es—raised urea and creatinine.
- G&S/cross-match.
- Most patients with blunt renal trauma and all penetrating renal trauma require radiological investigation.
- An IVU can be performed once resuscitation has commenced. This can demonstrate the renal cortical borders, presence and position of both kidneys and the collecting systems and ureters. It may also demonstrate extravasation of contrast (beware of contraindications).

- CT remains the 'gold standard' investigation for staging renal trauma. It clearly defines parenchymal lesions, haematoma and extravasations of urine. In addition it provides information on other organs.
- Ultrasound has a role in minor blunt trauma and arteriography may be used additionally where there is a suspicion of a vascular injury or in cases where embolization may be beneficial.

Management

- Resuscitate—advanced trauma life support (ATLS) protocol (📖 p88–90).
- Overall mortality rate from renal trauma is 0.8–4%, usually from haemorrhage/sepsis.
- Blunt trauma—90% of cases are minor and do not require surgery. Bleeding normally settles with bed-rest and rehydration.
- If displaying ongoing retroperitoneal haemorrhage, urinary extravasation and evidence of non-viable parenchyma—may require surgery.
- Penetrating trauma—these injuries need formal surgical exploration.
- Some renal trauma is only found in the operating theatre, in which case an on-table IVU is essential.
- Extravasation/calyceal disruption/non-function—require exploration. Expanding or pulsatile haematoma also needs exploration after vascular control has been gained.

Injury resolution may be monitored with USS or DMSA scan instead of CT. Follow-up blood pressure (BP) monitoring is essential for 6 months and an IVU at 3 months will ensure that any perinephric scarring has not caused hydronephrosis or vascular compromise.

Ureteric trauma

- These make up <1% of all genitourinary trauma.
- Haematuria may be present in an few as 50%.
- IVU is usually diagnostic, but definitive diagnosis may require retrograde urography. Many are discovered intraoperatively.
- Repair requires debridement, tension-free anastomosis and stenting with insertion of a retroperitoneal drain.

Bladder trauma

- Occur in up to 25% of patients with pelvic fractures.
- Mortality rate can be up to 30% due to co-existing injuries.
- Bladder trauma can also occur with penetrating injuries or be iatrogenic in origin.
- Frank haematuria is almost always present; a retrograde cystogram is diagnostic and can usually demonstrate the three types of bladder injury:
  - Bladder contusion.
  - Intraperitoneal rupture.
  - Extraperitoneal rupture.

Intraperitoneal rupture is treated with surgical repair, whereas extraperitoneal rupture is usually treated with catheterization for at least 2 weeks.

Urethral trauma

- Most commonly caused by straddle-type injuries or direct blows to the perineum with bruising/swelling or local tenderness.
- Injuries can be divided into anterior and posterior.
- Posterior injuries are commonly associated with pelvic fractures due to the shearing forces of fractured bone against the relatively fixed membranous urethra. They occur in 3–4% of pelvic fractures; 90% of these have blood at the urethral meatus and many will have a high-riding prostate on digital rectal examination. **Do not pass a urethral catheter if urethral trauma is suspected.**
- Place a 12Fr urethral catheter at the urethral meatus and place 2–3mL into the balloon to keep it in place. Inject 30mL water-soluble contrast and look for evidence of extravasation on X-ray (Fig. 12.2).
- Urethral disruption may be complete or incomplete.
- Treatment is usually insertion of a suprapubic catheter and delayed repair at ~ 6 months.

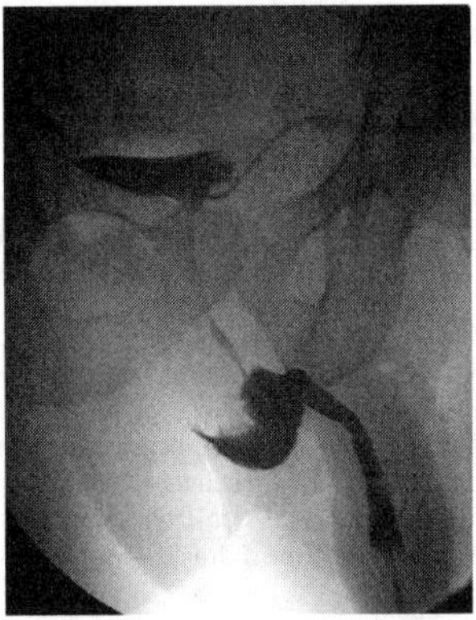

Fig. 12.2 Retrograde urethrogram with ruptured urethra.

Genital trauma

- Injuries are associated with bruising, pain and swelling.
- Scrotal injuries are well characterized by USS and can determine whether the underlying testis is merely traumatized or ruptured, requiring surgical repair.
- Penile injuries are often caused by excessively vigorous sex or masturbation, and are uncommon. The term 'fracture' is reference to rupture of the tunica albuginea or the corpora, and is treated surgically. Refer to registrar.

Urinary retention

- The inability to pass urine.

Think about

- Transient causes:
  - Medication, e.g. anticholinergic/antidepressants.
  - Alcohol or drugs, e.g. opiates.
  - Constipation.
  - Urinary tract infection (UTI).
  - General/regional anaesthesia.
- Permanent causes:
  - Benign prostatic hyperplasia (BPH).
  - Bladder neck obstruction.
  - Prostate cancer.
  - Acute prostatitis.
  - Bladder/urethral calculi.
  - Urethral strictures.
  - Neurological disease.
  - Posterior urethral valves (only in children).
  - Pelvic masses.
  - Idiopathic urinary retention in ♀ (Fowler's syndrome).

Ask about

- Painful retention—usually describe history of lower urinary tract symptoms (LUTS):
  - Obstructive (voiding)—poor stream, hesitancy, post-micturition dribbling.
  - Irritative (storage)—urgency, frequency, dysuria, nocturia, urge incontinence.
  - Transient causes (as above), but most commonly BPH in ♂.
- Painless retention—usually neurological or gradual in onset. Often have a history of LUTS and some associated with overflow incontinence.
- Spinal cord injury.

Look for

- Painful retention—pain, palpable/percussable bladder:
  - Digital rectal examination—assess prostate size and consistency.
  - Pelvic and neurological examination (particularly important in ♀). Consider spinal pathology.
- Painless retention—enlarged, painless, palpable, percussable bladder.

Investigations

- Urine analysis—to identify infection (microscopic/macroscopic haematuria is common in patients with retention of urine).
- U&Es—a proportion of patients will have acute or chronic renal impairment due to upper tract obstruction and hydronephrosis.

- USS will display such upper tract dilatation and bladder scanning will confirm volume of urine in bladder prior to catheterization.
- PSA should not be checked as retention causes ↑ level and thus should only be done by a urologist or someone with the knowledge to explain the significance of a raised result. The need for biopsy and further treatment, if appropriate, may arise and should be handled by someone with appropriate experience.

Management

- Immediate drainage by insertion of a urethral catheter. If this is not appropriate or possible, a suprapubic catheter should be used. Be sure to note the residual volume clearly in the notes. Decompression of a distended bladder may cause some haematuria. This can be avoided by slow decompression (keeping the catheter bag above the bladder).
- A post-obstructive diuresis may occur, especially in painless retention and with abnormal U&Es. After recording the residual bladder volume post-catheterization, if the patient passes >200mL/hr urine for 2 consecutive hours then intravenous fluids should be given to match input to output. 20mL/hr may be added for insensible losses and an accurate fluid input/output chart recorded. Monitor K^+ and check weight daily.
- Patients with severe renal failure may need referral to renal physicians for consideration of dialysis. If appropriate, do so early.
- α-blockers have been shown to be beneficial in patients presenting with acute retention of urine when removing the catheter, and may be started at diagnosis and continued for at least 48hr before attempts at catheter removal.
- Otherwise treatment is targeted at any of the permanent causes as listed above. Many of these options are surgical including:
  - Urethral dilatation/urethrotomy.
  - TURP.
  - Bladder neck incision.
  - Resection of posterior valves.
- Treat any underlying treatable cause.

ⓘ Haematuria

Haematuria is the presence of blood in the urine and can be frank (visible) or microscopic. The difference between these is quantitative and really only represents a degree of pathology rather than separating them.

Think about

- It is essential to confirm haematuria. Other causes of red urine include:
  - Dietary intake (beetroot/rhubarb).
  - Drugs (rifampicin/phenothiazines).
  - Myoglobinuria/haemolysis.
  - Vaginal bleeding.
- Causes outside the urogenital tract:
  - Blood dyscrasias.
  - Thromboembolic events affecting the kidneys.
  - Drugs.
  - Extra-urogenital inflammatory/malignant causes in direct contact.
- Causes within the urogenital tract:
  - Tumours (bladder, renal, prostatic, urethral).
  - Infection/inflammation (pyelonephritis, cystitis).
  - Calculi (renal, ureteric, bladder).
  - BPH.
  - Trauma.

Ask about

- If frank haematuria, where in stream:
  - Beginning—usually from penile/bulbous urethra.
  - Entire—usually from above the bladder neck.
  - Terminal—usually prostatic or from bladder neck.
- Pain:
  - Renal angle—tumour, infection, calculus In kidney.
  - Loin to groin—commonly associated with ureteric calculi.
  - Voiding—infection/inflammation of bladder or urethra.
- Painless—suspicious for tumours, commonly bladder, BPH.
- Associated symptoms:
  - Fevers, rigors, malaise, nausea, vomiting—pyelonephritis.
  - Weight loss—tumour.
- Risk factors for malignancy—smoking, aniline dyes, aromatic compounds, family history, schistosomiasis, chronic UTI, stasis of urine.

Look for

- Systemic signs—cachexia, pyrexia, rigors, pallor, tachycardia, hypotension.
- Renal mass (kidneys are not usually palpable).
- Renal angle tenderness—obstructed kidney, pyelonephritis.
- Suprapubic tenderness—cystitis, clot retention.
- Digital rectal examination—BPH, prostate cancer.
- Palpate urethra and corpora—urethral cancer, diverticulum with calculus.

Investigations

- Blood—FBC, clotting screen, U&Es, G&S, cross-match.
- Urine—dipstick, cytology, microscopy, culture.
- Radiological—not always necessary acutely:
  - Renal tract USS—good views of kidneys.
  - IVU—good for pelvi-calyceal system and ureters.
  - CT—KUB for stones (non-contrast); later for staging malignancies.
- Cystoscopy:
  - Usually flexible cystoscopy under local anaesthetic.
  - Occasionally under GA for patient preference, young patients, ongoing bleeding.
  - Allows biopsies for histological diagnosis.
- Patients with asymptomatic microscopic haematuria, i.e. on suspicion or incidental discovery, should be investigated as up to 20% will have highly significant lesions. MSU and urine cytology are essential. USS and flexible cystoscopy should be performed on an urgent outpatient (<2 weeks) basis. and clinical judgement will guide further investigations such as an IVU/retrograde studies.

Management

- Of the underlying condition, e.g. infection, blood dyscrasias.
- If ongoing frank haematuria and clots—insertion of three-way irrigation catheter and bladder irrigation. Initial bladder washout with normal saline under strict aseptic technique until urine clot-free. Irrigation should start immediately thereafter and be continuous until urine is clear.
- If ongoing frank haematuria without clots—can be managed without catheterization if only 'rose' coloured, if patient can maintain a good oral intake. May require catheterization and irrigation if clots appear or urine becomes more heavily blood-stained.
- Persistent haematuria, especially requiring ongoing transfusion should be managed with a GA cystoscopy and washout ± diathermy.
- In the presence of uncontrollable life-threatening haematuria, bladder instillations (e.g. prostaglandins), embolization or ligation of the internal iliac arteries may be considered. In long-standing cases, urinary diversion or cystectomy should be considered.

Renal and ureteric calculi

Up to 5% of the population will at some point be affected by urolithiasis (♂:♀ 4:1).

Think about

- 75% calcium oxalate stones but many also contain calcium phosphate and some contain uric acid.
- Stone formation requires supersaturated urine.
- Predisposing factors:
  - Impaired urinary drainage—where urine stagnates (e.g. bladder diverticulum, hydronephrosis).
  - Excess urinary solutes—low urine volume (e.g. dehydration, low fluid intake):
    - ↑ excretion of calcium (e.g. hyperparathyroidism)
    - ↑ excretion of uric acid (e.g. gout, chemotherapy)
    - ↑ excretion of oxalate (high intake of leafy vegetables, rhubarb, tea).
  - Abnormal constituents present:
    - Infection: epithelial sloughs allow calculi to form (especially with obstruction)
    - Foreign bodies: stents, catheter fragments
    - Cystinuria (inborn error of metabolism).

Ask about

- Previous urinary tract calculi.
- Severe lower abdominal/flank/loin to groin pain. Classically colicky but commonly constant.
- Nausea and vomiting.
- Lower urinary tract symptoms (especially when calculus at lower ureter)—frequency, urgency, genital pain.
- Fevers/rigors—significant risk of infection in an obstructed system, needs to be looked for and treated promptly and effectively.
- Haematuria.

Look for

- Pyrexia, sweating, restless patient unable to lie comfortably.
- Loin/flank tenderness.
- Occasional peritonism as the posterior peritoneum overlies the ureter.

Investigations

- Urinanalysis—microscopic haematuria (commonly but not always present), MSU.
- Blood: FBC, U&Es, Ca, Phosphate, urate.
- Radiological:
  - Plain abdominal X-ray; specifically KUB shows 90% of calculi.
  - IVU for renal anatomy, e.g. hydronephrosis, site of obstruction.
- A completely obstructed kidney may show no contrast.
- CT (gold standard)—replacing IVU; highly sensitive for calculi and can diagnose other conditions, e.g. AAA.

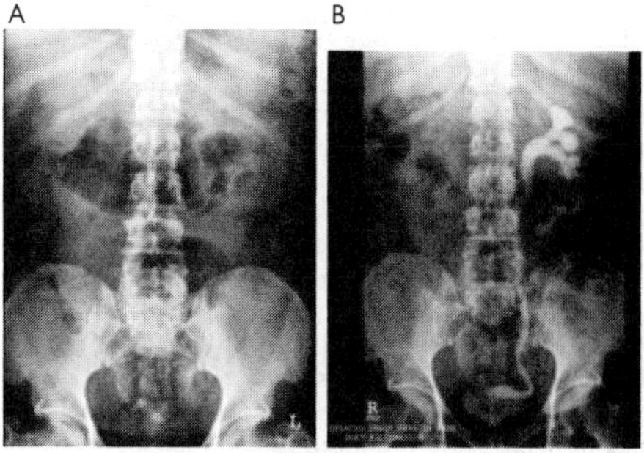

Fig. 12.3 Left renal tract obstruction. (A) Calcific density in the pelvis just to the left of the midline. This is shown on the delayed post-micturition film (B) to be causing obstruction, with a standing column of contrast to this level and no emptying of the pelvi-calyceal system on the left. The calculus is shown to be within a ureterocele (abnormal congenital implantation of the ureter into the bladder), and can be seen with a 'cobra's head' appearance. Of note the standing column delineates the course of the normal ureter and is the line that should be checked on any control image to look for calculi.

A limited IVU (control, 15min film post contrast, and post-micturition film) should be performed if there is a clinical suspicion of calculous obstruction. Some centres now perform CT urography routinely. Bear in mind that this requires a significant contrast load, and a history of allergy, metformin use and renal failure should be taken.

Treatment

- Analgesia—diclofenac 50–100mg PR/PO/IM ± pethidine + antiemetic.
- Hydration—patient should be adequately hydrated with oral or, if necessary, IV fluids (2.5L/day); excessive IV hydration may exacerbate pain.
- Stones tend to lodge at three sites:
  - Pelvi-ureteric junction.
  - Pelvic brim.
  - Vesico-ureteric junction.
- Further treatment as an outpatient is possible if:
  - Pain is controlled with oral analgesia.
  - Renal function tests are normal (U&Es, renogram).
  - Only mild to moderate obstruction of the affected side.
  - Patient is well enough to maintain an adequate PO fluid intake.
  - Patient is apyrexial with no features suggestive of concurrent infection.
  - An appropriate system is in place for review in outpatient clinic within 4 weeks.
- Ureteric calculi are best treated by allowing spontaneous passage, which occurs in up to 90% of patients with calculi <5mm in diameter.

- Calculi up to 1cm in diameter can pass spontaneously, although many do not. Follow-up is best by KUB X-ray with radio-opaque calculi; otherwise by USS, IVU or CT.
- It is justifiable to wait for weeks/months for spontaneous passage of a stone unless:
  - There is a high-grade obstruction behind which renal damage may occur.
  - There is evidence of impaired renal function.
  - There is infection in an obstructed system which is very serious and potentially life threatening.
  - Pain is not controlled with moderate oral analgesia.
- Infection in an obstructed system is a *urological emergency* requiring IV antibiotics and urgent decompression either by placement of a percutaneous nephrostomy tube (usually by radiologist) or with retrograde JJ stent insertion under anaesthetic. **Must be discussed urgently with on-call urologist**:
  - Look for renal angle tenderness, pyrexia, obstructed renal tract on IVU or CT.
- If calculus does not pass spontaneously, other interventions are possible:
  - ESWL—upper ureteric and renal calculi.
  - Ureteroscopy—lower ureteric and after failed ESWL: stone retrieval, electrohydraulic lithotripsy, laser disintegration.
  - Open or laparoscopic surgery.

Differential diagnosis

- AAA.
- Biliary colic.
- Diverticular disease.

Urinary tract infection and pyelonephritis

Urinary tract infection

Defined as the presence of a pure growth of >10^5 colony-forming units/mL urine, infections that occur in the bladder are the most common and known as cystitis. They may develop into pyelonephritis. ♂ can develop prostatitis or epididymo-orchitis.

Urinary tract infections may be termed complicated if they occur:

- In ♂.
- With abnormal renal tract anatomy.
- With abnormal renal function.
- In immunocompromised patients.
- With virulent organisms.

Think about

- Previous UTI.
- Catheterization/sexual intercourse.
- More common in ♀.
- Common in elderly due to urinary obstruction (especially in men).
- Atrophic vaginitis.
- Cystocele.
- Recent instrumentation of urinary tract.
- Foreign body/calculus of renal tract.
- Organisms:
  - *Escherichia coli*—80% of community-acquired and 50% of hospital-acquired infections.
  - *Proteus*, *Klebsiella*, *Enterococcus*, *Pseudomonas* and *Staphylococcus saprophyticus* are other likely pathogens.

Ask about

- Dysuria, frequency, urgency, suprapubic discomfort.
- Haematuria in as many as 10% of UTIs in healthy ♀ (haemorrhagic cystitis).
- Fever, rigors, loin pain and vomiting occur in pyelonephritis.
- Back pain, malaise and a tender prostate occur in prostatitis.

Look for

- Pyrexia, tachycardia and hypotension.
- Suprapubic discomfort.
- Palpable bladder.
- Loin pain (pyelonephritis).
- Swollen tender prostate (prostatitis).

Investigations
- Urinalysis (if contains leucocytes and nitrates: 70% chance of UTI) and MSU for microscopy, culture and sensitivities.
- FBC, U&Es, CRP—if unwell. Blood cultures if pyrexial.
- KUB X-ray if calculous disease is suspected.
- USS (can often be done as an outpatient) should be performed in most cases, especially in complicated UTIs and in the presence of haematuria. IVU may be considered.

Management
- Plenty of oral fluids, frequent urination, voiding after intercourse.
- Treat any underlying cause.
- Consider admission if complicated UTI, elderly, frank haematuria or unwell.
- Cystitis—trimethoprim 200mg BD for 3–5 days (first-line); cefalexin 500mg TDS for 5–7 days.
- Prostatitis—ciprofloxacin 500mg BD for 28 days (doxycycline can be used as second line).
- Patients with complicated/recurrent UTIs should be referred to the urology outpatient department.

Pyelonephritis

Mild/moderate cases
- Home with 14 days oral antibiotics (cefalexin/ciprofloxacin).
- Urology outpatients follow-up.
- Advise patient to return if they deteriorate.

Severe cases unwell, septic
- Admit.
- IV rehydration.
- IV antibiotics—cefuroxime 750mg TDS (± gentamicin 5–7mg/kg if renal function normal). Adjust antibiotics according to cultures.
- Needs ultrasound the following day and consider KUB/IVU if not settling, to exclude obstruction of urine.

An obstructed, infected kidney needs urgent decompression by percutaneous nephrostomy (or retrograde stenting in centres with no out-of-hours interventional radiology). Inform on-call urologist immediately.

☠ Testicular torsion

Inform on-call urologist immediately.

Twisting of the spermatic cord causes the blood supply to the testis to be compromised.

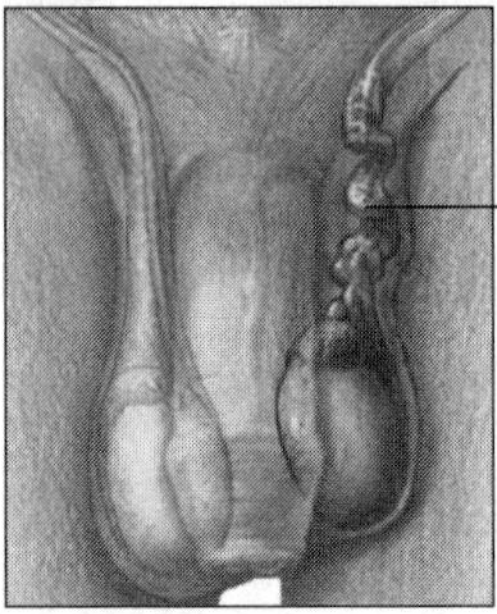

Fig. 12.4 Torsion of testicle.

Think about

- Usually occurs in patients under 30yr, common in children.
- Abnormal investment of testis by tunica vaginalis.
- Long mesorchium.
- Previous episode of testicular torsion.
- Prompt surgery (<6hr after onset) saves the testis.
- May occur with minimal swelling.

Ask about

- Sudden onset of unilateral pain.
- Pain radiating to the abdomen.
- Nausea and vomiting are common.
- Pain worse on walking.
- Absence of urinary tract symptoms and usually afebrile.
- Beware of intermittent pain, which rarely occurs but may represent intermittent torsion.

Look for
- Tender swollen testis, hot.
- Transverse lie.
- High-riding testis on affected side.
- Tender thickened cord.

Investigations
- Doppler USS may have a role in distinguishing differential diagnoses but this *must* not delay surgical intervention. It remains a clinical diagnosis.

Management
- Urgent scrotal exploration <6hr after first onset of symptoms.
- Alert urologist on-call, anaesthetist and theatres.
- Nil by mouth, when did they last eat or drink?
- Consent for possible orchidectomy ± bilateral orchidopexy.
- At operation expose and untwist the testis. If it is viable it must be fixed ± fixation of contralateral testis.

Differential diagnosis
- Epididymitis/orchitis.
- Torsion of the cyst of Morgagni (remnant of the Mullerian ducts).
- Testicular trauma.
- Acute hydrocele.
- Tumour.
- Strangulated inguinoscrotal hernia.

⚠ Acute epididymitis and orchitis

Inflammation of the epididymis or testis. Usually unilateral but may be bilateral. Rare before puberty. Important to *differentiate* from testicular torsion (above).

Think about

- Commonly caused by sexually transmitted pathogens—*Chlamydia trachomatis* and *Neisseria gonorrhoeae*, particularly in younger ♂.
- In ♂ >35yr, commonly caused by urinary pathogens, e.g. *E. coli*.
- Viral orchitis—recent ↑ incidence of mumps orchitis.
- Occasionally may be tuberculous.

Ask about

- Recent UTI, dysuria and other lower urinary tract symptoms.
- Urinary tract instrumentation.
- Unprotected sex (especially with new partner).
- Urethral discharge.
- Fevers and malaise.
- Pain and swelling of scrotum.

Look for

- Pyrexia.
- Scrotal swelling, erythema, tenderness.
- 2° hydrocele.
- Urethral discharge.

Investigations

- Urine MC&S.
- Raised WCC and CRP.
- Urethral swabs.
- Blood cultures if systemically unwell.
- Scrotal USS—if abscess suspected and to exclude underlying tumour.

Management

- Bed-rest.
- Scrotal support.
- NSAIDs.
- PO ofloxacin 200–400mg BD for 2–4 weeks in patients <35yrs (as has good *Chlamydia* cover); PO ciprofloxacin 500mg BD may be used in older patients. Change antibiotics according to cultures.
- If an abscess is identified (on USS) it may need urgent drainage.
- Occasionally admission may be required for IV antibiotics and analgesia.
- Advise sexual partners to have STI check, where indicated.
- Urology outpatients in 4–6 weeks.

Fournier's gangrene

Inform on-call urologist immediately.

Infection of the scrotal skin → gangrene, usually with multiple pathogens and carrying a significant mortality. Often presents with an unwell, septic or confused patient.

Think about
- More common in the elderly.
- Underlying immunocompromise, especially diabetes mellitus.
- Occurs following perianal sepsis and scrotal abscess.

Ask about
- Fevers and malaise.
- Scrotal/perineal pain.
- Immunocompromise.

Look for
- Signs of sepsis.
- Scrotal oedema, erythema, tenderness, gangrene and necrosis.
- Expanding affected area, often within a few hours.

Investigations
- Swabs for MC&S.
- FBC, U&Es, CRP.
- Blood cultures.

Management
- IV fluid resuscitation.
- Nil by mouth.
- Broad-spectrum IV antibiotics, e.g. metronidazole 500mg TDS, gentamicin 5–7mg/kg OD (reduce with impaired renal function), amoxicillin 500mg TDS.
- Urgent radical surgical debridement with second look in 12–24hr.
- Early involvement of plastic surgeons.

Priapism

Inform on-call urologist.

A painful, prolonged erection, occurring in the absence of sexual stimulation and not relieved by orgasm.

Think about

- The erection involves the cavernosal bodies but not the corpus spongiosum or glans penis.
- Classification:
  - High flow:
    - Rare
    - Caused by penile or perineal trauma which results in an arteriovenous fistula within the corpus cavernosum
    - Bright red, well oxygenated blood.
  - Low flow:
    - Most common
    - Often no known aetiology
    - Caused by haematological conditions, e.g. leukaemia, sickle cell anaemia
    - Caused by drugs, such as α-blockers, phosphodiesterase 5 inhibitors and other erectile dysfunction medication (e.g. prostaglandin E1)
    - Dark deoxygenated blood.

Ask about

- Previous episodes.
- Medication and underlying haematological problems.
- Trauma.
- Medical or non-medical drug use (e.g. cocaine, Viagra®).

Look for

- Soft glans penis and corpus spongiosum.
- Rigid corpora cavernosa.

Investigations

- FBC to look for underlying cause ± sickle cell screen.
- Blood gas analysis of cavernosal blood may be helpful in classification.

Management

Low flow

- Ask patient to run up and down stairs.
- Firm manual compression.
- Aspirate blood from corpora with butterfly needle inserted into the lateral aspect of shaft to avoid urethral trauma.
- Once corpora aspirate is bright red and if priapism persists, irrigation of the corpora can be performed with an α-agonist (10mg phenylephrine in 500mL normal saline). This can be repeated after 10–15min (use of phenylephrine is contraindicated in high-flow priapism and continuous BP monitoring is required due to risk of severe hypertension).
- Surgery—creation of a shunt between the erect corporal body and the corpus spongiosum/glans penis/saphenous vein as a last resort.

High flow

- Pudendal artery embolization/open ligation of abnormal vessels may be required.

All patients with priapism should be warned of impotence (8% if resolves within 24hr) and those with unknown aetiology should be warned of chance of recurrence of up to 40%.

Paraphimosis

This is when the retracted foreskin cannot be reduced to its normal position. As the foreskin is maintained in its retracted position, at the coronal sulcus, the ensuing oedema of the glans makes reduction more difficult.

Think about
- If untreated, vascular insufficiency of the glans penis may occur.
- Usually due to a tight foreskin retracted during intercourse or during catheterization.

Ask about
- Previous difficulty retracting foreskin.
- Pain in glans penis or foreskin.

Look for
- Swelling and tenderness of glans penis and foreskin.
- Retracted foreskin.

Management
- Manual compression of glans and foreskin.
- Use of topical 2% lidocaine gel for lubrication and analgesia.
- Place thumbs on to glans and, using the index and middle fingers of both hands, attempt to pull the foreskin forward. Wet gauze may be needed to maintain grip.
- If unsuccessful, try covering the glans in 50% dextrose solution for 0.5–1hr and then repeating as above.
- This may be uncomfortable for the patient, in which case strong analgesia should be given ± sedation.
- If unsuccessful, inform urologist on-call as a dorsal slit may be needed under GA/LA.
- This is likely to recur, so patient should be advised to have an elective circumcision at 6–8 weeks.

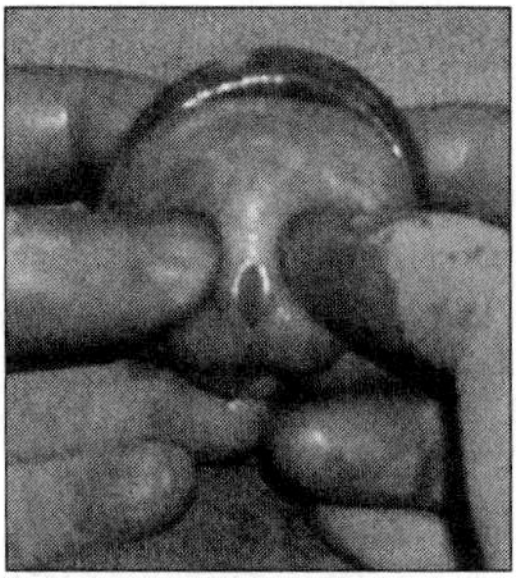

Fig. 12.5 Reduction of paraphimosis.

Procedures

Catheters

- Size, in French gauge:
  - 12Fr—small.
  - 16Fr—medium.
  - >16Fr—large.
- Latex is soft and for short-term use.
- Simplastic®/silicone catheters are firmer and may be used long term (up to 3 months).

Urethral catheterization

- Contraindicated in urethral injuries and acute prostatitis (usually).
- Male doctors should always have a female chaperone when catheterizing ♀ (although this is normally carried out by nurses).
- Gain verbal consent from the patient if possible.
- Lie patient supine in a well lit area (♀ with knees flexed and hips abducted with their heels together).
- Under strict aseptic technique with sterile gloves and the catheter pack opened and prepared on a trolley at the bedside with an appropriately sized catheter.
- In ♂, retract the foreskin with one hand (dirty hand) and clean the glans with gauze soaked in cleaning fluid (e.g. chlorhexidine). The dirty hand should not be used to touch the catheter.
- Use a sterile drape to keep the cleaned area away from the scrotum.
- In ♀, again use a 'dirty' hand to separate the labia and 'prep' the urethral meatus (wipe from pubis to anus). The 'dirty' hand should not touch the catheter.
- In ♀, put sterile lidocaine gel (2%) on the catheter tip and ~5mL into the urethra, then advance the catheter with gentle pressure. Insert to the hilt until urine is draining freely, then inflate the balloon with 10mL water and retract the catheter gently until you feel the balloon rest at the bladder neck.
- In ♂, put 10mL lidocaine gel (2%) into the urethra and massage it down by stroking the urethra on the ventral surface of the penis. Allow 2–3min for the anaesthetic to work.
- Holding the penis with the 'dirty' hand upwards, pointing towards the ceiling (with some traction to eliminate any urethral folds and reduce the chance of creating a false passage), insert the catheter with gentle pressure.
- When the tip reaches the prostate gland, whilst maintaining traction on the penis, tilt it downwards pointing to the feet (this eases its passage through the prostate). Again, insert to the hilt until urine is draining freely and then inflate the balloon with 10mL water.
- Gently pull the catheter so the balloon rests at the bladder tip, and reduce the foreskin.
- Connect to a catheter bag.
- If significant resistance is encountered during insertion, stop, withdraw and reinsert.

(A)

(B)

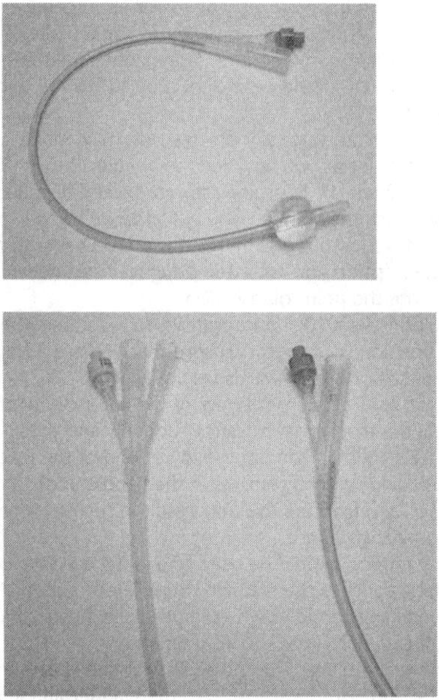

Fig. 12.6 Urethral catheters.

Tips for difficult ♂ catheterization

- Use 20mL 2% lidocaine gel.
- If resistance is encountered, try using a larger catheter as this is less likely to create a false passage.
- Maintenance of longitudinal traction, first upwards and then pointing to the feet, is essential when negotiating a difficult prostatic urethra.
- Never force a catheter as, once a false passage has been created, urethral catheterization may become impossible.
- If you have used these guidelines and failed—DO NOT PERSIST:
  - Suprapubic catheterization.
  - Call the on-call urologist.

Suprapubic catheter insertion

- Confirm the patient has a palpable/percussable bladder. Confirm volume with bladder scan.
- Obtain verbal/written consent.
- Ideally perform with flexible cystoscopy to guide placement (although this is seldom possible in the emergency setting).
- Have an assistant available and do not attempt this procedure without prior, adequately supervised experience.
- Lie the patient supine.

- Under sterile conditions, 'prep' the lower abdomen.
- Prepare the suprapubic pack and catheter on a trolley at the bedside.
- Using 1% lidocaine ± epinephrine (adrenaline), infiltrate at the point of insertion, which should be 2–3cm superior to the pubic symphysis in the midline.
- Ensure you infiltrate vertically downwards, maintaining a midline position, aspirating as you advance the needle.
- Infiltrate ~10–20mL 1% lidocaine (do not exceed 0.3mL/kg 1% lidocaine). When you reach the bladder, you will aspirate urine in the syringe.
- Never insert a suprapubic catheter if you are unable to aspirate urine in the position you are attempting to insert it.
- Carefully note the point of insertion.
- At this point make a 10–15mm transverse incision in the skin.
- Into this, position your trocar. Ensure that you are advancing it in the midline and straight downwards vertically.
- Beware that, as the different layers of the anterior abdominal wall are passed, the trocar may advance suddenly and thus it is essential to place the stabilizing hand at the lower end of the trocar (whilst the force-providing hand remains at the handle end) to control it in the event of this. Ignoring this may result in severe damage to intra-abdominal structures.
- A screwing motion should be used to avoid excessive force.
- As the trocar reaches the bladder you will feel a 'give'. At this point, maintaining gentle downward pressure, retract the trocar from the sheath and urine should drain out.
- Now remove the trocar altogether, leaving the sheath in place; pass the catheter through the sheath into the bladder and inflate the balloon. The sheath can then be removed by tearing down the side of it using the tag.
- Ensure haemostasis at the entry point and if necessary use a suture, being careful not to damage the catheter.
- Ensure that urine is still draining from the catheter freely and attach a catheter bag and dry dressing.

Patients may complain of bladder spasm when catheterized, as the tip and balloon irritate the bladder. This will normally settle in time, but anti cholinergics may be used to alleviate this in the short term (e.g. oxybutinin 2.5mg TDS).

On urine dipstick, patients with a catheter often appear to have an infection. It is not normally necessary to treat these unless the patient is systemically unwell.

Dorsal slit

- Perform under penile block or GA.
- Sterile conditions.
- Using a scalpel, incise the dorsal surface of the entire foreskin.
- Ensure good haemostasis.
- This will then allow the foreskin to be reduced.
- Ultimately the patient will need a formal circumcision, but this is best performed several days later once the oedema has settled, and in an elective setting.

Blocked catheters and nephrostomy tubes

Blocked catheters

- Some 40–50% of patients with long-term catheters have blockages.
- Patients presenting to the emergency room with a blocked catheter usually require the catheters to be changed.
- **NOTE:** Was there recent urological surgery? Do not change the catheter of patients who have had a recent urethral anastomosis (e.g. after radical prostatectomy, radical cystoprostatectomy) without discussing with the urologist on call, as the anastomosis may be disrupted. In addition, avoid changing catheters in patients who have had recent *TURP* or *urethral surgery* (e.g. after stricture surgery).
- Blockage of catheters due to blood clots requires a bladder washout and bladder irrigation to be continued until the urine is clear.

Bladder washout

- Under strict aseptic technique.
- Use a 50mL bladder syringe and sterile water.
- Insert a syringe-full with firm pressure and then aspirate the same volume back.
- Continue this with fresh water until the aspirate is clot free.
- If it is difficult to aspirate back, deflate the balloon fully, manipulate the position of the catheter, and then reinflate the balloon.
- Always restart bladder irrigation immediately after a washout in order to stop clots reforming in the bladder. Ensure nursing staff change irrigation bottles promptly and do not allow irrigation to stop.

Blocked nephrostomy tube

- Look for other causes of low urine output.
- Consider whether the urine could be passing internally via the ureter.
- If blocked—may be flushed gently with 10mL normal saline under strict aseptic technique.
- If unsuccessful, discuss with on-call urologist.

TUR syndrome

An uncommon complication of transurethral surgery (normally occurs only after TURP), caused by absorption of irrigation fluid.

Think about

- Occurs in 1–2% of patients who undergo TURP.
- ~10–30mL irrigation fluid is absorbed systemically per min of resection, → fluid overload and acute hyponatraemia.
- Glycine is a constituent of irrigation fluid and an inhibitory neurotransmitter. Glycine toxicity causes reduced consciousness and visual disturbances.

Look for

- Confusion.
- Bradycardia.
- Nausea and vomiting.
- Collapse.
- Fluid overload.
- Pulmonary oedema.
- Reduced level of consciousness—cerebral oedema.

Investigations

- U&Es—hyponatraemia <120mmol/L is usually symptomatic.
- ECG—hyponatraemic changes include widening of QRS complex, ST elevation and T-wave inversion.
- Hyperammonaemia—byproduct of glycine metabolism.
- Low serum osmolarity.
- High anion gap.

Management

- Stop irrigation immediately.
- Consider use of diuretics (furosemide 40mg IV).
- Discuss with on-call urologist/anaesthetist.
- Fluid restriction <800mL/24hr may ↑ serum levels at 1.5mmol/24hr.
- If hyponatraemic encephalopathy evident, patient should be monitored in an ITU setting. Hypernatraemic fluids (e.g. × 2 normal saline) may be given when correcting serum sodium. Raise serum sodium by a maximum of 1mmol/L per hr or 20mmol/L per 48hr to prevent cerebral oedema.

TUR syndrome

Chapter 13

Gynaecology

Rufus Cartwright

The gynaecological history

A full gynaecological history includes sensitive personal issues. Particularly in the very young, in the very old, and in the distressed patient you may find it difficult to broach these topics. Use discretion, but do not underestimate the importance of these areas. In ♀ of reproductive age, at least three questions should always be asked:

- Date of last menstrual period (LMP).
- Current contraception.
- Last smear test date and result.

These simple questions should help you avoid common medicolegal pitfalls and provide pointers for the full history.

Menstrual history

- Age of menarche.
- Regularity and length of cycle.
- Time between periods.
- Usual number of days of bleeding. It is conventional to express this as:

  k = 5 (number of days bleeding)/28 (length of cycle)

- Character of last period—heaviness or pain.
- Presence of post-coital bleeding.
- Presence of intermenstrual bleeding.
- Presence of post-menopausal bleeding (if appropriate).
- Relation of other symptoms (e.g. pain) to bleeding.

Other gynaecological history

- Urinary history (as for urology).
- Pre-menstrual syndrome (PMS).
- Sensation of prolapse ('bulge down below').
- Presence or character of any discharge:
  - Itching.
  - Offensive odour.
  - Colour.
  - Relation to menstrual cycle.

Obstetric history

- Total number of pregnancies (gravida or G).
- Total number of deliveries over 24 weeks (parity or P).
- Outcome of each pregnancy:
  - Miscarriage (ask about reasons and gestation).
  - Termination (ask about gestation and method).
  - Stillbirth.
  - Spontaneous vaginal delivery.
  - Caesarean (elective or emergency).
  - Instrumental delivery (forceps or ventouse).
- Gestation and birthweight of each baby.
- Previous pregnancy complications.

Sexual history

- Currently, or ever, sexually active.
- Sexuality.
- Method of contraception or intention to become pregnant.
- History of sexually transmitted diseases including pelvic inflammatory disease (PID).
- Dyspareunia—superficial or deep.

If appropriate to the presenting complaint, enquire about number of partners, types of sexual activity, coitarche (age of first sexual intercourse), libido, etc.

Vaginal examination

Many ♀ are extremely apprehensive about vaginal examination, particularly if you are ♂. Regardless of your sex, always have a chaperone present and ask them to sign in the notes. Explain carefully to the patient what you intend to do and seek her verbal consent. Try to ensure some privacy; if possible avoid the curtained bays in A&E or on the ward.

Speculum examination

Cuscoe's speculum is much the most useful kind of speculum for general purposes. It has two hinged blades that can be locked open in a range of positions. To insert a Cuscoe's speculum, first warm it slightly if possible, and lubricate the blades with jelly. Ask the patient to lie on her back with her hips flexed and moderately abducted. Gently part the labia and, with the blades rotated 90° to one side, insert the speculum a small distance down and back. Rotate the speculum so the handles are again upwards, and then insert it as far as it will comfortably reach. Partly open the blades with pressure on the handles, and if necessary apply the lock. Angle the speculum to get a view of the cervix. If this is impossible consider whether the uterus is in an unusual retroverted, or overly anteverted, position, or whether you need a larger or smaller speculum.

To remove the speculum, unlock the blades and, without closing them entirely, slowly withdraw it, attempting to visualize the vaginal walls. Be careful not to trap the cervix or tissue from the vaginal side walls between the blades.

Bimanual examination

Particularly in a thin patient, bimanual examination can be very informative. The patient lies on her back, in the same position as for Cuscoe's speculum examination. If possible the patient should have an empty bladder. Stand at the right side of the bed if you are right handed. Lubricate the gloved index and middle fingers of your right hand only. Gently insert both fingers until they reach the posterior fornix. Place the left hand suprapubically and try to palpate the organs that lie between your two hands. You should be able to elicit the following information:

- Uterus—size, shape, consistency, mobility, anteversion or retroversion, and tenderness.
- Cervix—patency of the os (nulliparous, multiparous, or open), consistency, presence of cervical excitation.
- Adnexae—presence, size and consistency of any mass, and associated tenderness.

Cervical excitation is also known as cervical motion tenderness. Gently brushing the cervix to one side stretches the fallopian tube, causing immediate pronounced pain—characteristic of PID or ectopic pregnancy.

Vigorous palpation of an ectopic pregnancy, or an ovarian cyst may rarely cause it to rupture. Although it is usually necessary to perform bimanual examination, in order not to miss physical signs, you should seek senior advice first.

Glossary of gynaecological acronyms

Gynaecological notes are littered with jargon and acronyms. Although some specialist terminology is necessary, where possible you should try to avoid using obscure acronyms. If anything, the situation is worse in obstetrics.

AFP:	A-fetoprotein—a tumour marker also employed in fetal screening.
BV:	bacterial vaginosis.
CA125, CA199 and CEA:	Commonly employed markers from ovarian tumours.
CIN:	cervical intraepithelial neoplasia, graded from 1 to 3.
CS:	caesarean section, sometimes elCS for elective caesarean, and emCS for emergency caesarean.
CVS:	chorionic villus sampling.
DCDA:	dichorionic diamniotic twins, the commonest sort of twinning.
DO:	detrusor overactivity.
EDD:	estimated date of delivery.
G_xP_y:	a confusing and frequently argued notation for previous pregnancies and deliveries. Gravidity refers to the total number of pregnancies, including any current pregnancy. Parity is the number of babies delivered after 24 weeks' gestation, whether alive or stillborn.
GIFT:	gamete intra-fallopian transfer.
HCG:	human chorionic gonadotropin.
ICSI:	intracytoplasmic sperm injection.
IMB:	intermenstrual bleeding.
IUI:	intrauterine insemination.
IUCD or IUD:	intrauterine contraceptive device—confusingly in obstetrics IUD can also be used for intrauterine death.
IUP:	intrauterine pregnancy.
IVF:	in vitro fertilization.
LLETZ:	large loop excision of the transformation zone, an excision biopsy. performed at colposcopy
LMP:	the first day of the last menstrual period.
NT:	nuchal translucency—an ultrasound marker, measured at 13 weeks' gestation, to estimate risk of trisomy 21.
OAB(S):	overactive bladder (syndrome).
OHSS:	ovarian hyperstimulation syndrome.

PCB:	post-coital bleeding.
PID:	pelvic inflammatory disease.
PMB:	post-menopausal bleeding.
RU486:	mifepristone, an anti-progestogen used to terminate pregnancy up to 9 weeks.
STOP:	suction termination of pregnancy.
SVD:	spontaneous vaginal delivery.
TCRE:	trans-cervical resection of the endometrium.
TOP:	termination of pregnancy.
TOT:	trans-obturator tape, inserted for stress incontinence.
TVS:	trans-vaginal scan.
TVT:	tension-free vaginal tape; also for stress incontinence.
USI:	urodynamic stress incontinence (formerly genuine stress incontinence).
VIN:	vulval intraepithelial neoplasia.
ZIFT:	zygote intra-fallopian transfer.

Bleeding in the first trimester

Think about

Some bleeding occurs in the first trimester in up to half of all pregnancies. Although it is always a negative prognosticator, only about half of these pregnancies are not viable. The diagnosis will often be made some time after presentation, using ultrasound and serial β-HCG. This does not, however, diminish the importance of history and examination.

Ask about

LMP

It is important to establish the date of the LMP. The gestation of a pregnancy is dated from the LMP, not from the time of conception. However, this must be adjusted, depending on the length of a woman's menstrual cycle. Ovulation typically occurs 14 days before the onset of menstruation. A ♀ with a regular 35-day cycle should have conceived ~21 days after her last period. A ♀ with a regular 21-day cycle should have conceived ~7 days after her last period. Applying common sense, re-date the pregnancy as:

- Time elapsed from probable date of conception + 2 weeks.

Character and duration of bleeding

Most ♀ will recognize a 'normal period' as bleeding lasting from 3 to 7 days, with heavier bleeding on the first few days. Check that the apparent last period fits with a woman's normal pattern of bleeding.

Heavy bleeding with a positive pregnancy test is suggestive of incomplete miscarriage. An ectopic pregnancy is typically associated with a small amount of dark red blood or brown discharge, although this is by no means reliable.

Equally though, a history of passing tissue is suggestive but not diagnostic of complete or incomplete miscarriage. Blood clots or mucus are easily mistaken as tissue, unless sent for histology.

Pain and coincident symptoms

Pain associated with a miscarriage is similar in character to dysmenorrhoea or period pains, but may be worse. It is usually felt as a low central crampy pain. An ectopic pregnancy causes unilateral pain but the pattern of pain, like bleeding is very unreliable as to the diagnosis. Significant intra-abdominal bleeding from an ectopic may cause the classic referred shoulder tip pain.

The passage of large clots through the cervix may be associated with severe pain and even cervical shock. However, a history of fainting or dizziness must suggest ectopic pregnancy.

The triad of early pregnancy symptoms are nausea, urinary frequency and breast tenderness. After fetal death, ♀ may notice a remission in these symptoms even before the onset of bleeding.

Risk factors

The principal risk factors for miscarriage are multiple previous miscarriages and advanced maternal age. It is more important to consider the risk factors for ectopic pregnancy:

- History of PID.
- Current use of progestogen-only pill (POP), Depo-Provera® or IUCD.
- Previous tubal surgery, including sterilization.
- Previous ectopic pregnancy.
- Emergency contraception.
- Assisted conception.

Look for

Emergency

If a patient has intra-abdominal or heavy vaginal bleeding she may become shocked. As for any surgical emergency, assess airway, breathing and circulation (ABC) when resuscitating. Large clots or tissue passing through the cervix may cause severe pain or bradycardia. Perform a speculum examination and check for products visible at the cervical os. These can be removed with sponge holding forceps. This simple action can rapidly reduce pain and bleeding, and improve haemodynamic status.

Incomplete miscarriage and ectopic pregnancy are both conditions that may need early transfer to theatre, so do not delay in involving senior help.

Non-emergency

Assess gynaecological patients just as for other surgical patients. Look for signs of anaemia and circulatory compromise, and consider whether these are consistent with the history of bleeding. Abdominal examination should assess the site and character of the tenderness. Unilateral tenderness suggests an ectopic pregnancy. Peritonism, distension or ileus suggests a haemoperitoneum, associated with a ruptured ectopic.

Vaginal and pelvic examination should not be repeated unnecessarily. However, in many cases they may make the diagnosis (Table 13.1).

Table 13.1 Bleeding in the first trimester

	Bleeding	Cervical os	Uterine size	Adnexae
Threatened miscarriage	Scanty	Closed	Consistent with date of LMP	Normal
Inevitable miscarriage	Heavy fresh blood	Open	Consistent with date of LMP	Normal
Incomplete miscarriage	Heavy fresh blood ± tissue	Open or closed	Variable	Normal
Complete miscarriage	Nil or minimal	Closed	Normal	Normal
Ectopic pregnancy	Dark brown blood	Cervical excitation and closed os	Slightly enlarged	Unilateral tenderness ± mass

Investigations

- FBC.
- Group and save—even if bleeding is very slight you must establish whether the ♀ requires anti-D.
- β-HCG is often helpful when the diagnosis is unclear, particularly when ectopic pregnancy is suspected.
- Progesterone is also employed in some units as a prognostic factor for a failing pregnancy.
- High vaginal swab (HVS), although PID is rare during pregnancy.
- Send any tissue obtained for histology, but see note below about handling of fetal tissue.

Management

Whom to admit?

Management will often depend on the local availability of scanning. Patients with heavy bleeding or haemodynamic compromise will obviously require admission for resuscitation and immediate investigation. Any suspicion of ectopic pregnancy should also usually prompt admission, unless local protocols dictate otherwise. This may require diagnostic laparoscopy if scanning is not available immediately.

Women with a threatened miscarriage can often be allowed home, with an outpatient scan arranged as soon as possible to confirm fetal viability. Women with a complete miscarriage can also be allowed home, and may benefit from a scan to confirm that the uterus is empty.

Women with incomplete or inevitable miscarriage should be admitted. With heavy bleeding they may require urgent evacuation of retained products of conception. Otherwise they should be stabilized and await a scan to confirm the clinical findings. Further management will depend on gestation, clinical condition and patient's wishes.

Sensitive handling of fetal tissue

The handling of fetal tissue has increasingly complex regulations. Your unit will undoubtedly have a policy covering this area, and may have a specialist bereavement midwife, who can guide you. The difficulties occur because there is a wide variation in attitudes to a pregnancy loss, partly depending on the gestation, the circumstances, and the ♀ herself.

The disposal options available include incineration with clinical waste, formal cremation (privately or through the NHS Trust) and burial (usually privately arranged).

No clear rules can be given for dealing with this. The Royal College of Obstetricians and Gynaecologists (RCOG) has provided some general guidance[1]:

'Any personal, religious or cultural needs relating to the disposal of the fetal tissue should be met wherever possible and should be documented in the woman's medical notes.

Some women or couples may not wish to receive information about, or take part in, the disposal of the fetal tissue. Provided that the woman or couple has been made aware that the information is available, these wishes should be respected. It should be clearly documented in the woman's medical notes whether information has been requested or not and, if so, whether it has been given.'

When to give anti-D

Use of anti-D immunoglobulin in early pregnancy protects the current and subsequent pregnancies from Rhesus disease of the newborn. 250iu anti-D should be given as soon as possible after a 'sensitizing event' to all Rh-negative ♀. Sensitizing events are all circumstances in which significant quantities of fetal blood may enter the maternal circulation leading to alloimmunization:

- Ectopic pregnancy.
- Termination (medical or surgical).
- Evacuation of retained products of conception (ERPC).
- Threatened miscarriage or spontaneous fetal loss after 12 weeks.

There are certain exceptions. Anti-D should not be given to ♀ who are already known to be sensitized. It does not need to be given within 6 weeks of a previous dose. If a large fetomaternal haemorrhage is suspected, send a Kleihauer test (same vacutainer as G&S, to haematology lab), and giving 500iu anti-D. 500iu should always be given for terminations after 20 weeks.

1 RCOG (2005). Disposal Following Pregnancy Loss Before 24 Weeks of Gestation. London: RCOG.

Ectopic pregnancy

Think about

Ectopic pregnancy occurs in ~2% of all pregnancies and 10% of 1st trimester ♀ presenting to the emergency room with pelvic pain or vaginal bleeding. The rate is rising in concert with the increasing incidence of chlamydia. It remains a significant cause of maternal death. An ectopic pregnancy is one in which the fertilized ovum implants outside the uterus. In 97% of cases this will be in the fallopian tubes, but rarely it can be on the cervix, ovary or peritoneum.

Typically ectopic pregnancies present after 6–8 weeks of amenorrhoea, but they can present at any stage during pregnancy. In an acute presentation the diagnosis should always be made clinically.

Ask about

80% of patients are now diagnosed on the basis of an early pregnancy scan. However, the classical history is of unilateral iliac fossa pain accompanied by brown discharge, eventually leading to collapse with severe peritonitic pain. None of these features is invariably present. 25% of patients will not even have a history of amenorrhoea. A high index of suspicion is required.

- Establish likely gestation from LMP.
- Even if there are no missed periods, ask about symptoms of early pregnancy.
- Assess character, onset and site of the pain.
- Ask about risk factors for ectopic pregnancy:
  - Previous ectopic pregnancy.
  - Previous pelvic surgery, especially tubal.
  - Previous PID, or chlamydia.
  - Use of POP, emergency contraception or IUCD.

Look for

- Check vital signs, and for postural hypotension.
- Perform a full abdominal examination, eliciting the site of tenderness, presence of rigidity or guarding, and presence of bowel sounds.
- Perform a gentle pelvic examination after seeking senior advice. Cervical excitation, adnexal tenderness, an adnexal mass and bogginess in the posterior fornix are all compatible with a diagnosis of ectopic pregnancy.

Investigations

- FBC.
- G&S. If signs of hypovolaemia, cross-match according to local protocol.
- Rh type.
- Serum β-HCG.
- Progesterone (some units).
- Trans-vaginal ultrasound.
- Diagnostic laparoscopy—if unwell, or after confirmation of diagnosis.

Management

- Patients can rapidly decompensate. Acquire large IV access, as may need rapid fluid resuscitation.
- If Rh negative, patient should be given Rh immunoglobulin.

Management is determined by local protocol and clinical condition. Historically ectopic pregnancy was always treated with laparotomy and salpingectomy. Gradually this has ceded to laparoscopy and salpingectomy or salpingostomy. Recent years have also seen the emergence of conservative methods of management, including the administration of methotrexate. As a cross-covering doctor you cannot be expected to make management decisions at this level. However, remember that even a stable patient may deteriorate suddenly following admission if the tube ruptures. Always consider the possibility that an urgent laparoscopy may be required.

Hyperemesis gravidarum

Think about

Most ♀ experience nausea and possibly vomiting in early pregnancy. By definition, hyperemesis presents before 20 weeks' gestation. It consists of persistent, severe vomiting leading to dehydration, weight loss, ketosis and electrolyte imbalance. A combination of physiological, psychological and sociological factors is implicated. Sequelae include Mallory–Weiss tears, low birth-weight infants and, rarely, Wernicke's encephalopathy or even death. Although genuine hyperemesis occurs in only 0.1% of pregnancies, vomiting in early pregnancy is a common cause of admission for rehydration and anti-emetics.

Differential diagnosis

- Normal physiological 'morning sickness'.
- Pyelonephritis.
- Gastroenteritis.
- Pancreatitis.
- Appendicitis.
- Hepatitis, including acute fatty liver of pregnancy.
- Ovarian torsion.
- Degenerating fibroid.
- Diabetic ketoacidosis.
- Addison's disease.
- Hyperthyroidism—hyperemesis is often associated with deranged thyroid function test results.
- Molar pregnancy (hyperemesis is associated with raised β-HCG).
- Raised intracranial pressure.
- Migraine—hyperemesis is epidemiologically associated with migraine.
- Psychological factors.

Ask about

- Date the pregnancy based on LMP or early pregnancy scans.
- Assess the onset and severity of the vomiting, including ability to tolerate food or fluids.
- A personal or family history of hyperemesis can be helpful.
- Try to exclude other diagnoses.
- Especially when the history is disproportionate with the physical findings, take a careful social history and make an assessment of mental state.
- Always remember that a confused or amnesic patient may be developing Wernicke's encephalopathy.

Look for

A thorough examination of all systems is required. There are no signs specific to hyperemesis, but an assessment of dehydration must be made, and other signs may clarify the differential diagnosis.

Investigations

- Dipstick + MSU to exclude urinary tract infection (UTI) and ketosis.
- U&Es to guide rehydration.
- FBC, LFTs to exclude other causes.
- Amylase.
- Thyroid function tests (TFTs) are frequently deranged but may suggest 1° thyroid disease.
- Severely dehydrated patients should be placed on an input/output chart.
- A transvaginal scan should be arranged to exclude molar pregnancy.

Management

If ♀ are neither dehydrated nor ketotic, and are managing to drink fluids, they should be allowed home with anti-emetics and dietary advice. Metoclopramide (10mg TDS PO) or prochlorperazine (25mg PR max BD) are appropriate first-line choices. The patient should be encouraged to eat frequent light meals, and be prescribed a multivitamin in addition.

Women who are clinically dehydrated, with ketosis or electrolyte disturbance, should be admitted for IV fluids and IV anti-emetics. Typically metoclopramide 10mg IV TDS is used first line, but cyclizine and prochlorperazine may also be employed. If the patient fails to respond to a combination of two anti-emetics, ondansetron or prednisolone may be of benefit. It is essential to give thiamine 100mg PO OD to avoid Wernicke's encephalopathy. Women with dehydration during pregnancy are at high risk of deep vein thrombosis (DVT), so consider thromboprophylaxis.

Interpretation of ultrasound findings in early pregnancy

As a cross-covering doctor, you may be asked to review out-of-hours scans with patients. Most scan departments will produce excellent reports that state not just the diagnosis, but the preferred course of management. When you are required to make the interpretation, remember these simple rules:

An ectopic pregnancy can never be excluded on the basis of a scan.

Ectopic pregnancies may be very difficult to visualize on scan (Fig. 13.1). Even with a viable intrauterine pregnancy, a co-existing ectopic pregnancy can occur. Although the quoted rate is 1 in 40 000, this rises to 1 in 100 in association with assisted conception techniques. With a positive pregnancy test, an empty uterus and pain, the default diagnosis remains an ectopic pregnancy until proven otherwise.

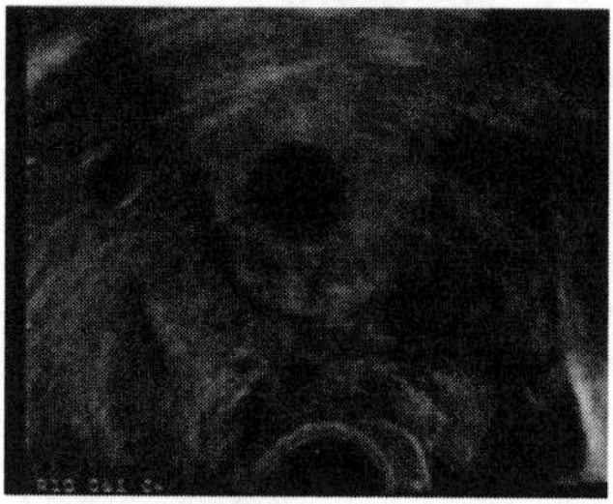

Fig. 13.1 Ectopic pregnancy.

A viable pregnancy cannot be confirmed until the β-HCG is over 1000. If the β-HCG is >1000IU/L you should see scan evidence of an intrauterine pregnancy, if it is present. If not, consider ectopic pregnancy.

A pregnancy can now be visualized (Fig. 13.2) from the middle of the 4th week of gestation. This corresponds to a β-HCG of at least 1000. If the uterus appears to be empty, but the β-HCG level is low, the scan is inconclusive. A definitive diagnosis will be made by repeating the scan when the β-HCG is over 1000.

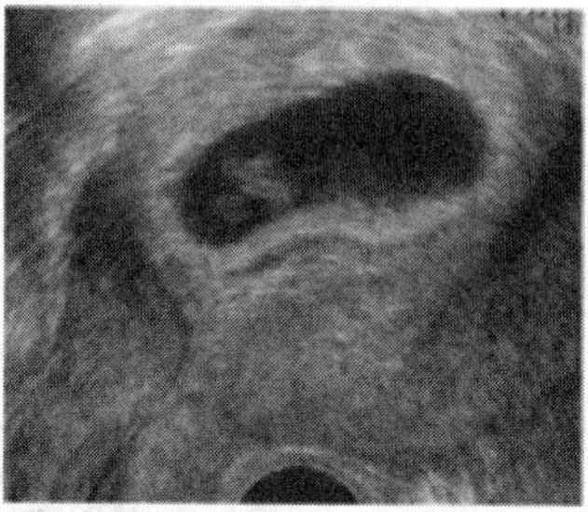

Fig. 13.2 Viable intrauterine pregnancy.

In the second trimester, retained products should usually be evacuated surgically.

Conservative management of inevitable or missed miscarriages is acceptable to many ♀. However, retained products following a miscarriage at gestations beyond 12 weeks are unlikely to pass spontaneously. In the first trimester, ERPC may be indicated when there are large retained products (Fig. 13.3) or the ♀ is symptomatic.

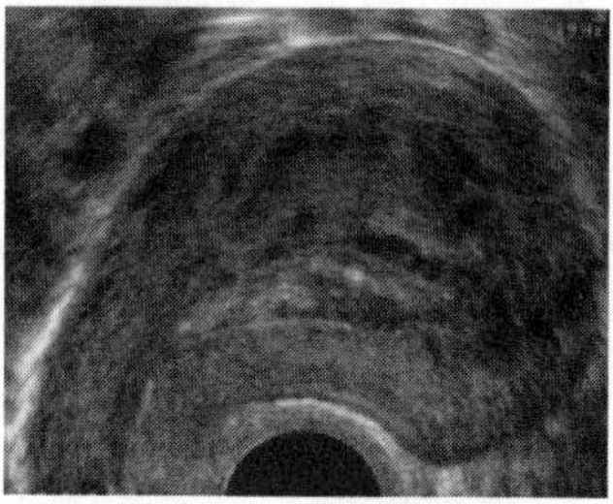

Fig. 13.3 Retained products of conception.

Table 13.2 The five indications for termination of pregnancy (Abortion Act 1991, Certificate A)

A.	The continuation of the pregnancy would involve risk to the life of the mother greater than if the pregnancy were terminated.
B.	The termination is necessary to prevent grave permanent injury to the physical or mental health of the pregnant ♀.
C.	The pregnancy has not exceeded its 24th week and that the continuance of the pregnancy would involve risk, greater than if the pregnancy were terminated, of injury to the physical or mental health of the pregnant ♀.
D.	The pregnancy has not exceeded its 24th week and that the continuance of the pregnancy would involve risk, greater than if the pregnancy were terminated, of injury to the physical or mental health of any existing child(ren) of the family of the pregnant ♀.
E.	There is a substantial risk that if the child were born it would suffer from such physical or mental abnormalities as to be seriously handicapped.

Termination of pregnancy

One in three of all ongoing pregnancies in the UK ends in termination. Even if you do not approve on ethical or religious grounds, it is important to treat ♀ having an abortion with the same kindness and respect you would extend to other patients.

Most terminations in the UK are performed for essentially social reasons, justified as protecting the 'mental health' of the mother or her existing children. These terminations are allowed up to 24 weeks' gestation. The limits of viability have steadily reduced with advances in neonatal care. It is now commonplace for babies born in the 23rd week of gestation to survive. The 24-week cut-off is thus increasingly anachronistic.

Beyond 24 weeks, termination can be performed only if the pregnancy will result in grave permanent injury or death of the mother, or if there is a substantial risk that the baby would be born with severe disability.

As a junior doctor you are unlikely be asked to participate in routine terminations, but might become involved in emergency situations. Even if you hold a conscientious objection, you have a legal duty to provide care if the long-term health or life of the mother is at risk.

Medical terminations

Early medical termination can be offered up to 9 weeks' gestation. Patients need the same preparation as for a surgical termination:

- Hb.
- G&S.
- Scan to confirm gestation.

There are many different protocols for early medical termination in use. Commonly in the UK, the patient takes 200mg mifepristone (RU486) orally, followed 48hr later by 800mcg misoprostol inserted vaginally, either at hospital or self-administered at home. Although medical termination before 9 weeks is safer than surgical termination, complications include:

- Nausea, diarrhoea and hot flushes associated with misoprostol.
- Severe dysmenorrhoea-like pains.
- Incomplete termination requiring subsequent ERPC.
- Failed termination (~3%).
- Endometritis.

Mid-trimester medical terminations are performed in almost the same way, at gestation beyond 14 weeks. However, multiple doses of misoprostol are usually required. This should be done only on an inpatient basis.

Surgical termination

See section on Common gynaecological operations (📖 page 514).

☉ Pelvic pain

Think about

With a negative urine pregnancy test, the list of causes of acute pelvic pain unique to ♀ is relatively short:

- Ectopic pregnancy—must be excluded with serum β-HCG estimation.
- PID.
- Endometrioma.
- Dysmenorrhoea.
- Ovarian or adnexal torsion.
- Ovarian cyst rupture or haemorrhage.
- Degeneration of fibroid.
- Ovarian hyperstimulation.
- Mittelschmerz.

Even in ♀ of reproductive age, non-gynaecological causes of pelvic pain must of course be considered.

Initial assessment

As in any cause of abdominal pain, resuscitation and analgesia may need to come before full history and examination.

Ask about

Take a normal history but focus on the full gynaecological history. Dyspareunia, menstrual irregularities and discharge may all point towards a gynaecological cause. Although urinary symptoms, bowel symptoms, or nausea and vomiting may suggest a surgical cause, they may equally be present with a gynaecological condition. Nausea and vomiting in particular are seen in 66% of ♀ with ovarian torsion.

Look for

- Examine the abdomen to help localize the tenderness and define its character.
- Listen for bowel sounds.
- Perform a speculum examination and take high vaginal and cervical swabs.
- If you suspect ectopic pregnancy or ovarian hyperstimulation, proceed with bimanual examination *only after taking senior advice*—rupturing ovarian cysts or a distended fallopian tube will cause a bad situation to become immediately worse.
- Bimanual examination should otherwise further confirm the site of tenderness—uterine, unilateral adnexal or bilateral adnexal.
- Check for cervical excitation—subtle signs on vaginal examination include bogginess in the pouch of Douglas, suggestive of haemoperitoneum or free fluid.

Table 13.3 gives the likely examination findings for the common gynaecological causes of pain, but remember that common surgical conditions, such as appendicitis, can also cause adnexal tenderness.

Table 13.3 Gynaecological differentiation of pelvic pain

Diagnosis	Examination findings
Ectopic pregnancy	Unilateral adnexal tenderness Possible adnexal mass Possible brown vaginal bleeding Cervical excitation
PID	Bilateral adnexal tenderness Heavy vaginal discharge Cervical excitation Possible fever Possible adnexal mass
Ovarian cyst accident	Unilateral adnexal tenderness Possible adnexal mass Possible low-grade fever
Ovarian hyperstimulation	Abdominal distension Bilateral abdominal tenderness Omit bimanual examination!
Degenerating fibroid	Hard fibroid uterus Single tender fibroid

Investigation

For all of the conditions in Table 13.3 consider:

- FBC, CRP, G&S, serum β-HCG, vaginal and cervical swabs, MSU.
- Ovarian hyperstimulation requires U&E and LFTs in addition.
- Any patient with a high fever should have blood cultures sent.

Further investigation will be determined by clinical condition, clinical suspicions and availability of ultrasound.

Management

Ectopic pregnancy

See section on Ectopic pregnancy (📖 page 492).

PID

Strict criteria exist for the diagnosis of PID, because it has important sequelae (infertility and subsequent ectopic pregnancy) and requires contact tracing. However, many doctors advocate a low threshold for starting antibiotics. 'Triple antibiotics' are usually given, although the exact treatment regimen depends on local protocol:

- Aim to cover the common organisms: chlamydia, gonorrhoea and vaginal anaerobes.
- Treatment should be continued for 2 weeks.
- Patients with an adnexal mass, peritonism/severe pain, or fever should be admitted for analgesia, IV antibiotics and IV fluids.

- Rarely patients require laparoscopy. Even if patients are allowed home, arrange a pelvic ultrasound to exclude other causes of pain. Advice about barrier contraception, contract tracing and future risk of ectopic pregnancy is appropriate once the diagnosis has been confirmed.

Ovarian cyst accident

Most patients can be admitted for analgesia and IV fluids while awaiting a pelvic scan. Judgement as to when to intervene early with laparoscopy will require senior review. Worsening pain, or the onset of nausea and vomiting, are both indications for considering laparoscopy before confirming the diagnosis on scan.

Ovarian hyperstimulation

Management of ovarian hyperstimulation varies widely. Most assisted conception unit have their own protocol. Analgesia and careful fluid management are always appropriate though.

Degenerating fibroids

These can usually be managed conservatively with analgesia.

Bartholin's abscess

Bartholin's abscess

Think about

Bartholin's gland lies beneath the labia minora, between the superficial and deep layers of the urogenital diaphragm (Fig. 13.4). Its normal function is to provide lubricating secretions during sexual arousal. The duct opens within the vagina, just exterior to the hymenal ring. Ordinarily the gland is impalpable. However, if the duct becomes blocked the gland may swell to form a cyst, or become infected forming an abscess. The presentation is similar to that of a perianal abscess, sometimes causing confusion.

Ask about

The history is often of a recurrent painful swelling or a previously treated Bartholin's abscess. The swelling may have ↑ and then ↓ in size as the abscess discharges pus. Try to elucidate any risk factors, including diabetes, and take a full sexual history, as Bartholin's abscess can sometimes be due to gonococcal infection.

Look for

On examination a tender fluctuant swelling is felt deep in the vaginal wall. A small abscess will be palpable ~3cm anterolateral to the posterior fourchette, but as the abscess grows it may track anteriorly or posteriorly. The duct may be seen within the vagina, and may sometimes be observed to discharge pus.

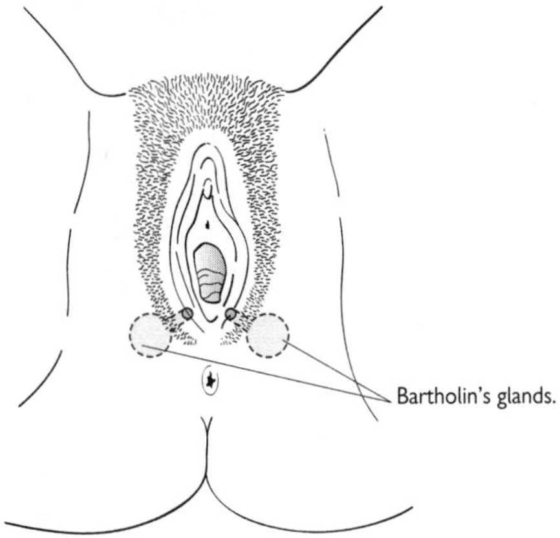

Fig. 13.4 Location of Bartholin's glands.

Investigations

- FBC.
- G&S.
- Low vaginal swab (LVS), HVS and cervical swabs.
- Swab any pus expressed.

Management

The abscess should be laid open or marsupialized under general anaesthetic to minimize the risk of recurrence. It is usual practice to cover the procedure with broad-spectrum IV antibiotics.

Sexual assault and vaginal trauma

Rape and sexual assault

Most ♀ who have been sexually assaulted never report it to the police or to a doctor. If they do present, they need specialist care. Many ♀ will be seen at dedicated units, offering security and privacy, ♀ staff, and the expert skills of a police surgeon in gathering the forensic evidence. If you are asked to see a patient who has been assaulted in A&E it may be because the ♀ is too unwell to be treated in a specialist unit. Your first priority must be assessment and resuscitation, although it is important to remember that your notes can be submitted to court and that you could be asked to write a statement. It is very important to ask a few simple questions: when, where, who, what happened. Always remember to time and date your notes and, as ever, make them legible.

Medical care

- Vaginal lacerations or haematomas may require exploration or suturing (see below).
- Arrange treatment for co-existent non-genital injuries.
- Hepatitis B vaccination should be offered to all victims of sexual assault if penetration has occurred.
- Antiretroviral treatment can also be offered. This is usually for 1 month in duration and needs to be started within 48hr. It is especially indicated for anal rape, multiple assailant rape, high-risk assailant rape (e.g. intravenous drug user, from endemic area), if there are genital injuries or if the assault resulted in loss of virginity.
- Consider the need for emergency contraception, morning-after pill or IUCD.
- Hepatitis A/tetanus vaccination if clinically indicated.
- Bacterial prophylaxis—azithromycin and cefixime as stat doses will treat existing infection but may not treat newly acquired infections.
- Mental health—many ♀ reporting sexual assaults are from vulnerable groups. Ask about any history of mental health problems and consider whether psychiatric assessment is needed.
- Arrange sexual health screening as part of follow-up.

Forensic issues

If the patient wants to report the assault to the police you can assist them by reporting it to the police in the area where the assault took place. The police will then arrange a forensic examination.

Forensic examination involves taking a history of the assault, documenting injuries and collecting samples. Both DNA and microbiological samples may be presented in court. The earlier examination is done after the assault the better—DNA can still be found up to a week later in a case of vaginal rape with no condom and ejaculation. For anal rape the cut-off is usually 2–3 days. Forensic medical examiners should usually carry out the examination. Advice can be sought from these doctors regarding the best management for a particular assault.

Vaginal trauma

Paradoxically most ♀ with vaginal laceration presenting to A&E will have sustained it during consensual intercourse. The other common mechanism of genital injury is the 'fall astride' leading to vulval laceration or haematoma.

Ask about

Assess the mechanism of injury, excluding any possibility of retained foreign bodies. Although most injuries will be related to consensual intercourse, have a low threshold for suspecting an assault (as for non-accidental injury).

Look for

- Perform a bimanual examination and try to palpate any laceration.
- Rarely the pouch of Douglas or the bladder may have been perforated.
- Gentle speculum examination should visualize any laceration.
- Vulval haematoma will be obvious from pain, discoloration and asymmetry.

Management

- Superficial lacerations may not require suturing at all.
- Conversely heavily bleeding lacerations may need to be packed to reduce haemorrhage while transfer to theatre is arranged.
- Small haematomas may respond to ice and compression. However, a large haematoma can lead to substantial haemorrhage and should be explored in theatre.

Complications of IUCDs

There are two types of intrauterine contraceptive device (IUCD or coil) in common use in the UK. Copper IUCDs contain a length of copper wire wound around a T-shaped plastic former. They act as a contraceptive through the spermicidal action of the copper. Copper coils tend to ↑ dysmenorrhoea and exacerbate menorrhagia.

The Mirena® IUCD is also T-shaped, but carries a 'cartridge' of progestogen on its stem. This progestogen is released over 5yr into the endometrium. It thins the endometrium → absent or much lighter periods and in addition thickens the cervical mucus preventing spermatozoa from entering the uterine cavity.

There are several common difficulties associated with both types of coil.

Removing a coil

An IUCD can cause severe dysmenorrhoea like pains after insertion, particularly in nulliparous ♀. The treatment for this ought to be analgesia, not removal. If you do need to remove it:

- Insert a Cuscoe's speculum to get a good view.
- Grasp the strings with sponge-holding forceps.
- Warn the patient to expect brief discomfort and then, with firm, constant traction, gently withdraw the coil.
- If you suspect infection send the coil for microbiological culture and sensitivities.
- If the patient has had unprotected sexual intercourse within the previous 5 days offer emergency contraception.

Pregnancy with coil in situ

The Mirena® IUCD is a more effective form of contraception than even sterilization. If patients do become pregnant with a IUCD in situ, always consider the possibility of an ectopic pregnancy. Check to see that the strings of the coil are still visible and then arrange an early transvaginal ultrasound. This should be able to confirm an intrauterine pregnancy, and demonstrate that the coil has not migrated (see below). If the pregnancy has implanted inside the uterus, and the strings are visible, the patient will need careful counselling. Leaving the coil in situ increases the risk of first-trimester miscarriage, and second- and third-trimester sepsis. Removing the coil may precipitate immediate miscarriage.

The lost coil

When IUCDs are inserted the strings are cut to about 1cm from the cervical os. Patients are usually advised to palpate the cervix intermittently to ensure the IUCD is still in situ. IUCDs can become 'lost' in one of three ways:

- They may fall out during a heavy period—surprisingly this is not always noticed by the patient.
- They may become rotated or malpositioned so that the strings are not visible.
- Through incorrect insertion or subsequent infection, they may migrate into the peritoneum, bowel or bladder.

If the patient is shocked or unwell, resuscitate and then check with a Cuscoe's speculum that the strings cannot be seen. Arrange an erect chest X-ray and a transvaginal ultrasound. If you suspect perforation into bowel, bladder or peritoneum, and the strings are visible, do not try to remove the coil.

If a scan demonstrates that the IUCD is in utero, but the strings are not visible, the IUCD can sometimes still be retrieved without resorting to hysteroscopy. Bearing in mind the possibility of precipitating cervical shock, very gently probe the external os with Spencer–Wells forceps and attempt to grasp any strings.

Infection in the presence of a coil

The presence of a IUCD acts as a focus for infection, increasing the risk of PID. No consensus exists as to whether it is best to remove the IUCD in this circumstance. Take high and low vaginal swabs, as well as cervical swabs, and seek senior advice.

Other emergency cases

ⓘ Foreign bodies

Condoms, diaphragms and other items may become lodged in the vagina. This is among the more embarrassing problems presenting to A&E, and requires the utmost tact and sensitivity. Passing a medium or large Cuscoe's speculum should enable you to retrieve the item using sponge-holding forceps. Some frequently misplaced items, such as the cap from a deodorant bottle, may require removal under anaesthesia.

Menorrhagia

- If the patient is shocked or unwell, commence resuscitation with oxygen and fluids.
- Send off an urgent haemoglobin and cross-match, but perform vaginal examination early to exclude cervical shock.

Most ♀ who present to A&E complaining of heavy vaginal bleeding will be well, with normal Hb levels. Send off a FBC to reassure you and her, and then offer simple medical management and a gynaecology outpatient appointment.

Ask about

The commonest causes of menorrhagia are anovulatory cycles and fibroid disease. However, the full differential diagnosis is long, including gynaecological cancers, PID, clotting disorders and thyroid disease. Take a full history. It is notoriously difficult to estimate the volume of vaginal bleeding from history. Some ♀ grossly overestimate their loss, whereas others may minimize potentially life-threatening loss. Try to quantify the loss with these questions:

- Number of pads/tampons used per day.
- Presence of large clots.
- Previous requirement for iron tablets
- Always ask about dizziness, chest pain and palpitations.

Look for

- Perform a general examination, as you would for any cause of anaemia.
- Look for signs of systemic illness, including polycystic ovary syndrome (PCOS) and thyroid disease.
- Remember that a young patient may compensate well for hypovolaemia.
- Check for postural hypotension, and ↑ pulse on standing.

As part of your full examination you must visualize the cervix and exclude the presence of a pelvic mass with a bimanual examination.

Investigations
- FBC.
- G&S.
- International normalized ratio (INR)/activated partial thromboplastin time (APTT).
- Thyroid function.
- HVS.

Management
Many patients respond well to tranexamic acid 1g TDS. When this is contraindicated, a 10-day course of norethisterone 10mg BD may be effective. Arrange a trans-vaginal ultrasound scan for all patients, and treat any anaemia.

Packs, catheters and other gynaecological paraphernalia

Catheters

After most vaginal operations patients are transferred to the ward with a catheter and vaginal pack in situ. Surgeons follow different protocols, but it is common to remove the catheter on the second postoperative day (48hr post-procedure).

Particularly if the patient has had a continence procedure (colposuspension, TVT, obturator tape, bladder neck bulking), she is at risk of voiding difficulties or retention. A bladder overdistension injury can easily be avoided by careful documentation of fluid balance.

After removal of the catheter the patient should try to void spontaneously. After each void the residual urinary volume should be measured, by either ultrasound or in–out catheterization. If the patient is unable to void after 6hr, an indwelling catheter should be re-inserted.

Patients with persistent residual urine volumes >100mL may need to learn clean intermittent self-catheterization.

Vaginal packs

Vaginal packs are traditionally inserted following vaginal hysterectomy or pelvic floor repair to minimize the possibility of vaginal haematoma. They may also occasionally be used for difficult cervical bleeding or vaginal trauma. They are extremely uncomfortable for the patient and require adequate analgesia. The pack is typically a 2-inch gauze roll soaked in proflavin antiseptic cream. It is usual to remove the pack on the first postoperative day (24hr post-procedure).

Instruments for assisting at gynaecological laparoscopy

You may be surprised to find that gynaecological instruments are often entirely different from those used in general surgery. Most of them are self-explanatory. However, if you are assisting at a laparoscopy you need to familiarize yourself with the use of a Sims speculum, the Spackman cannula and vulsellum forceps. They are used together to isolate and manipulate the cervix and uterus.

The *Sims speculum* is a curved retractor with two blades. When used in surgery, one blade lies along the posterior wall of the vagina and the other blade serves as a handle for retraction. The *vulsellum* is a locking toothed forceps that clamps on to the anterior lip of the cervix. The *Spackman* is a long metal cannula, with a widening ~2 inches from the tip, and with a movable clip to attach to the vulsellum. It is inserted into the cervical os and, once in place, can be angled to antevert or retrovert the uterus.

To use them correctly:

- Swab the vagina with a Betadine®-soaked sponge on a sponge-holding forceps.
- Perform an in–out catheterization.
- Bimanually palpate the uterus to assess its position and size.
- Pass the Sims speculum to visualize the cervix.
- Apply the vulsellum gently to the anterior lip of the cervix.

- Under direct vision, insert the tip of the Spackman into the os.
- Pass the hooks of the Spackman through the handles of the vulsellum, and lock them under tension.
- Moving the Spackman posteriorly will now cause anteversion of the uterus, and vice versa.
- At the end of the procedure carefully remove the Spackman and vulsellum, and check that the cervix is not bleeding.

Common gynaecological operations

Hysterectomy

Hysterectomy is one of the commonest major operations performed in the UK. The three main indications are fibroid disease, dysfunctional uterine bleeding and uterovaginal prolapse. Other indications include endometriosis, and benign or malignant disease of the ovaries or endometrium. Since the advent of cervical screening, very few Wertheim's hysterectomies are now performed for cervical malignancy.

There are several possible routes available:

- *Abdominal hysterectomy* is performed through a transverse or vertical abdominal incision. This may be total, including the uterus and cervix, or subtotal, leaving the cervical stump behind. It is often combined with salpingo-oophorectomy (removal of tubes and ovaries), particularly in post-menopausal ♀.
- *Vaginal hysterectomy* is performed entirely through a vaginal incision. It is associated with less pain and a shorter postoperative stay. It is technically difficult if there is no degree of prolapse, or if the uterus is enlarged. It does not allow easy access for salpingo-oophorectomy. It is a convenient approach when simultaneous pelvic floor repair is required. Patients will return to the ward with a urethral catheter and vaginal pack in situ.
- *Laparoscopic hysterectomy* and laparoscopically assisted vaginal hysterectomy are gaining in popularity. In common with other minimal-access procedures, they are associated with ↓ postoperative stay but ↑ operating time.

Preoperative preparation

Patients need to be medically optimized where possible. Unless there are special considerations, most patients require only routine preop. blood work-up, and not a cross-match. Some surgeons give bowel preparation.

Postoperative complications

Immediate

- Bleeding (intra-abdominal or vaginal).
- Wound infection and dehiscence.
- Pelvic haematoma or abscess.
- Injuries to ureter or bladder, and formation of fistulae.
- Chest and urinary tract infection.
- DVT and pulmonary embolism (PE).

Delayed

- Even when the ovaries are not removed, menopause is advanced by a mean of 18 months.
- ~30% of ♀ will have recurrent prolapse.

Abdominal myomectomy

Abdominal myomectomy is indicated in ♀ with subfertility and intramural or subserous fibroids. It may also be performed for ♀ with menorrhagia and fibroids who wish to preserve their uterus. The procedure is associated with greater haemorrhage than abdominal hysterectomy. Most surgeons quote a risk of 1–2% of conversion to hysterectomy in the event that haemorrhage cannot be controlled.

Preoperative preparation

Some surgeons request a 2-unit cross-match. This will depend on local blood ordering schedules.

Postoperative complications

Immediate

Abdominal myomectomy is associated with the same immediate complications as abdominal hysterectomy. In addition, ~ one-third of patients experience a fever during the first 48hr; this is not necessarily associated with sepsis.

Delayed

Fibroids may recur.

Laparoscopy

As per general surgery, but note that there are differences in technique. As gynaecological patients are less likely to have acute infection, or bowel adhesions, most gynaecologists use a Veress needle for insufflation, followed by blind trocar entry. Diagnostic laparoscopies are usually performed as day-case procedures, although patients having operative laparoscopy may require overnight admission for observation and analgesia.

Hysteroscopy

Hysteroscopy is the commonest procedure performed by most gynaecologists. The main indications are the investigation of menorrhagia, dysfunctional uterine bleeding and post-menopausal bleeding. Hysteroscopy is commonly combined with endometrial sampling (curettage). Other hysteroscopic procedures include resection of the endometrium, resection of submucous fibroids, and thermal or microwave endometrial ablation.

Preoperative preparation

Routine bloods.

Postoperative complications

Immediate:

- Vaginal bleeding.
- Uterine perforation.
- Fluid overload—rare with modern infusion pumps.
- Endometritis.

Suction termination of pregnancy (STOP)

The indications are discussed in the section on termination (📖 p498). The procedure is the conventional method of termination between 7 and 12 weeks' gestation, but can also be performed outside that range. The cervix is usually primed with vaginal prostaglandins 4hr before the procedure. The cervix is dilated to allow a suction curette into the endometrial cavity. Once the products of conception have been passed, IV syntocinon is given to reduce haemorrhage.

Preoperative preparation

Most terminations are arranged via dedicated clinics and separate operating lists. No practitioner is under any duty to participate in an abortion procedure if they have a conscientious objection, provided that this does not involve risk of grave permanent injury or death to the patient.

- All patients require Hb and blood group.
- Rh-negative ♀ require anti-D after surgery.
- Ideally all ♀ should have ultrasonography to confirm gestation, viability and site of pregnancy.
- If there is no policy of giving routine intraoperative antibiotics, you should screen for chlamydia.
- It is appropriate to discuss future plans for contraception; Depo-Provera® can be given during surgery if desired.

Postoperative complications

Immediate

- Vaginal bleeding.
- Uterine perforation.
- Further retained products of conception.
- Endometritis.

Delayed

- Subfertility, associated with postoperative pelvic infection.

Evacuation of retained products of conception (ERPC)

This procedure is indicated for management of incomplete miscarriages as well as missed or inevitable miscarriages depending on clinical condition and the patient's wishes. The cervix is dilated to allow passage of either a rigid curette or a suction curette. Once the uterus is felt to be empty, IV syntocinon may be given.

Preoperative preparation

Hb and blood group are required for all ♀. In Rh-negative ♀ anti-D may already have been given at the onset of bleeding. If not, it will be required after surgery. Current RCOG guidelines suggest that 250iu should be given within 72hr.

When there is suspicion of a molar pregnancy or heavy bleeding before surgery, a cross-match should be ordered.

Postoperative complications

As for suction termination of pregnancy; see above.

Continence procedures

Colposuspension is the 'gold standard' operation for stress incontinence. It is usually performed as an open abdominal procedure, but in some centres can be performed laparoscopically. The retropubic space is dissected and sutures are placed on either side of the bladder neck, anchored to the iliopectineal ligament. This provides support for the bladder neck and treats anterior wall vaginal prolapse.

The use of colpo-suspension is gradually being superseded by a range of less invasive vaginal procedures that aim to suspend the urethra with a hammock of synthetic material. The commonest of these performed in the UK is the TVT. This can be performed either under general or local anaesthesia. In some centres it may be done as a day case. A Prolene® mesh is inserted vaginally either side of the urethra. It is passed on two trocars through the retropubic space, emerging in the anterior abdominal wall. The tape is then tightened to support the mid-urethra.

Preoperative preparation

- The RCOG recommends that all patients should have had urodynamics performed before surgical intervention for stress incontinence.
- Routine bloods.

Postoperative complications

Immediate

- Bleeding (intra-abdominal or vaginal).
- Wound infection.
- Pelvic haematoma or abscess.
- Injuries to bladder.
- Chest and urinary tract infection.
- DVT and PE.
- Voiding difficulties and retention.

Delayed

- New-onset urgency and frequency.

Chapter 14

Paediatric surgery

A. Kate Khoo

Vital signs

Think about

Children have the same nursing observations performed as adults do, but the normal range varies with age. The following should help you assess your patient.

Table 14.1 Normal paediatric observations

Age (yr)	Respiratory rate (breaths/min)	Pulse (bpm)	Systolic BP (mmHg)
<1	30–40	110–160	70–90
1–2	25–35	100–150	80–95
2–5	25–30	95–140	80–100
5–12	20–25	80–120	90–110
>12	15–20	60–100	100–120

Remember that a drop in blood pressure (BP) is a very late sign and indicates imminent arrest (📖 p530).

Recognizing the sick child

In differentiating between a 'normal' well child and an unwell child, it is not only the vital signs that are useful. A child's behaviour, coupled with information from the nursing staff, can help you to form a rapid impression of how well he or she is.

Think about

Is this child unwell?

Look for

In addition to checking the vital signs, the following points indicate general status:

Table 14.2 General assessment of the child

	Well	**Unwell**	**Severely unwell**
Demeanour	Smiling	Miserable	Irritable/ unconscious
Feeding	Feeding and drinking normally	Irregular feeding and drinking/ reduced intake	Unable to feed
Interaction	Interacting, playing	Uninterested in surroundings	Unresponsive
Observations	No cardio-respiratory compromise	Early changes in basic observations	Severe cardiorespiratory compromise

If the child is unwell, proceed to ABC assessment (📖 p526) and call for help.

Recognizing the sick infant

An infant's normal behaviour is age dependent, and this must be taken into account when assessing the severity of illness. The parents are a good source of information as to whether the infant's behaviour is 'normal'.

Think about

Is the infant unwell?

Look for

Table 14.3 Recognition of a sick infant

	Well	Unwell	Severely unwell
Demeanour	Smiling (>6 weeks), Making eye contact, (>2 months)	Miserable (any age)	Irritable/ unconscious (any age)
Feeding	Feeding/drinking normally (any age)	Irregular feeding and drinking/reduced intake (any age)	Unable to feed (any age)
Nappies	More than 4 wet nappies a day	Fewer than 4 wet nappies (any age)	No wet nappies a day (any age)
Posture	Sits unsupported (>7 months)	Unable to sit unsupported (>7 months)	Floppy (any age)
Interaction	Fixes and follows (>2 months), Recognizes parents/ main carers (>7 months), Vocalizing sounds (>3 months)	Uninterested in surroundings (>2 months)	Unresponsive (any age)
Observations	No cardio-respiratory compromise (any age)	Early changes in basic observation (any age)	Severe cardio-respiratory compromise (any age)

If the child is unwell, proceed to ABC assessment (📖 p526) and call for help.

Weight

Centile charts can be used to plot weight (as well as height and head circumference) against age to ensure it is appropriate. They should be available on your ward and in the patient's notes, to chart their progress. Most children are weighed on admission to hospital. However, in an emergency, an estimate can be made for children aged over 1yr:

Weight in kg = (2 x Age in yrs) + 8

- Weight of a term neonate is around 3–4kg.
- Average weight of a 6-month baby is around 8kg.

Blood results

Be aware that not all biochemistry and haematology normal ranges are the same in children as in adults. Your local haematology and biochemistry lab should provide their own paediatric reference ranges.

As a guide, haemoglobin values are higher in newborns. Your local haematology lab will be able to provide their normal ranges, but for a guide see Table 14.4.

Table 14.4 Average haemoglobin ranges in children

Age	Average Hb (g/dL)
Day 1 of life	13–22
2 weeks	14–20
3 months	10
2yr	11
3–5yr	12
5–10yr	13
>10yr	14

ABC assessment

Early identification and prioritization of the sick child is of the utmost importance when cross-covering paediatric surgery. The unwell child requires rapid assessment and treatment following the ABC approach that is used for unwell adults. (See also 🕮 p520 for more on vital signs and recognition of an unwell child.)

The ABC assessment gives a structure for rapid evaluation of the unwell patient.

Think about

- Airway.
- Breathing.
- Circulation.
- Disability
- Exposure and
    - Don't
    - Ever
    - Forget
    - Glucose
- Is this a respiratory or circulatory problem?
- Is the child compensated or decompensated?
- Do I have enough skilled help? If not, who else should I call?

Management

Airway

- Is the airway patent?
- Is there evidence of obstruction?—mucus, history of foreign body, vomit, snoring.
- Is the airway patent? If not, open it by placing the head in neutral (1yr or less) or extension (>1yr). Check the position. As children have relatively large heads and short necks, they are prone to neck flexion when recumbent (which closes the airway). However, over-extension can also cause obstruction if a large tongue flops back or a malleable infant trachea collapses.
- Remember to check the nose—infants under 6 months are obligated nasal breathers, so mucous crusting can cause difficulty breathing. Suction if necessary.

- Call for help—you may need senior surgical help, anaesthetic help or the paediatric crash team,
- Open the airway with a chin lift/jaw thrust.
- Consider airway adjuncts (e.g. a Guedel) and/or suction.
- The airway may need securing by endotracheal intubation. Get anaesthetic help.

Breathing

- Is the effort of breathing increased? This is an indicator of the severity of respiratory disease and helps you identify patients at risk of potential respiratory failure.
- Observe the child with the chest exposed if possible. Signs of ↑ effort of breathing include tachypnoea (see 📖 p520 for a guide to respiratory rate with age), intercostal, subcostal or sternal recession, use of accessory muscles and grunting.
- Alar flaring and head bobbing (caused by sternomastoid use) may be seen in infants.
- Remember that a slow respiratory rate may indicate fatigue, and be a pre-terminal state.
- Gasping is a sign of profound acidosis and is extremely worrying.
- How effective is the child's breathing? Look at the chest expansion (or abdominal excursion in infants) as an indicator of the amount of air being inspired and expired.
- Auscultate the chest, listening for reduced, asymmetrical or bronchial breath sounds. Inspiratory noise (stridor) indicates laryngeal or tracheal obstruction, expiratory noise (wheeze) indicates lower airway narrowing. A silent chest is an ominous sign.
- Pulse oximetry is useful, but remember that it is inaccurate at saturations <70%, in cases of shock, when the oximeter is placed on a cold periphery and in the presence of carboxyhaemoglobin. A child's saturation reading in air can gives an indication of the efficacy of breathing but do not be falsely reassured by good sats in a patient on supplementary oxygen.
- Other indicators of respiratory inadequacy include agitation or drowsiness.
- Central cyanosis and unresponsiveness are pre-terminal signs.

- Call for help.
- Give high-flow oxygen through a non-rebreathing mask with a reservoir bag.
- If the breathing is inadequate, commence bag mask until the airway can be secured.
- Call for anaesthetic help immediately.

Circulation

- Check the pulse—the carotid is usually most accessible, except in infants with short fat necks, when the brachial or femoral can be used instead.
- Note tachycardia—may be present in shock or pain (heart rate may be extremely high, up to 220bpm, in small infants).
- Bradycardia or a rapidly falling heart rate is a pre-terminal sign. (For heart rates by age see 📖 p520).
- Assess perfusion—is the skin mottled, pale or cool?

- Check capillary refill by pressing on the sternum for 5sec (in children with pigmented skin, the nail-beds are useful, and the sole of the foot may be used in small babies), It should refill within 2–3sec.
- BP measurements may be useful, but do not be falsely reassured by a normal BP.
- Hypotension in children is a late, pre-terminal sign of circulatory failure—if present, get help immediately.
- Urine output charts may be available—a urine output <1mL/kg/hr in children (or <2mL/kg/hr in infants) indicates inadequate renal perfusion.

- Call for help.
- Ensure that high-flow oxygen is being given.
- Obtain IV access (or intraosseous access) and give a fluid bolus of 20mL/kg crystalloid (normal saline) if the child is in shock.
- Take urgent blood samples.

Disability

Determine AVPU category:

A alert
V responds to voice
P responds to pain
U unresponsive.

This gives a rapid idea of the level of consciousness of a patient. If the patient is unresponsive to voice, give a painful central stimulus by applying pressure to the supraorbital ridge or sternum. A score of 'P' corresponds to a Glasgow Coma Score ≤8. Note also any reduced tone (seriously ill children are often floppy), abnormal posture, and pupil size and reactivity.

- Call for help.
- A patient with a GCS <8 is unable to protect their airway, and endotracheal intubation must be considered.

Don't Ever Forget...Glucose

Hypoglycaemia can resemble shock, especially in neonates.

- Check BM (blood sugar level) and that a lab glucose has been sent.
- If hypoglycaemia (BM <2.6) give 5mL/kg 10% dextrose IV bolus.

Table 14.5 Children's Glasgow Coma Score

	Score
Eye opening (max 4)	
Spontaneous	4
To verbal stimuli	3
To pain	2
No response to pain	1
Best verbal response (max 5)	
Alert, babbles, coos, uses words to usual ability	5
Reduced verbal ability, spontaneous irritable cry	4
Cries only to pain	3
Moans to pain	2
No response to pain	1
Best motor response (max 6)	
Obeys verbal commands/spontaneous movement	6
Localizes to pain/withdraws from touch	5
Withdraws from pain	4
Abnormal flexion to pain (decorticate)	3
Abnormal extension to pain (decerebrate)	2
No response to pain	1

Exposure

Expose the patient and examine for other signs of illness (e.g. rash).

Once the 1° assessment has taken place and treatment of any threat to life has commenced, you may take a medical history, perform a fuller clinical examination and arrange any specific investigations.

In the event of cardiac or respiratory arrest, call for the paediatric crash team and commence CPR. The paediatric ALS algorithm is shown in Fig. 14.1.

If you are working with children, do consider attending the resuscitation council's paediatric resuscitation courses (NLS, newborn life support; EPLS, European paediatric life support; APLS, advanced paediatric life support) for valuable training.

Paediatric advanced life support algorithm

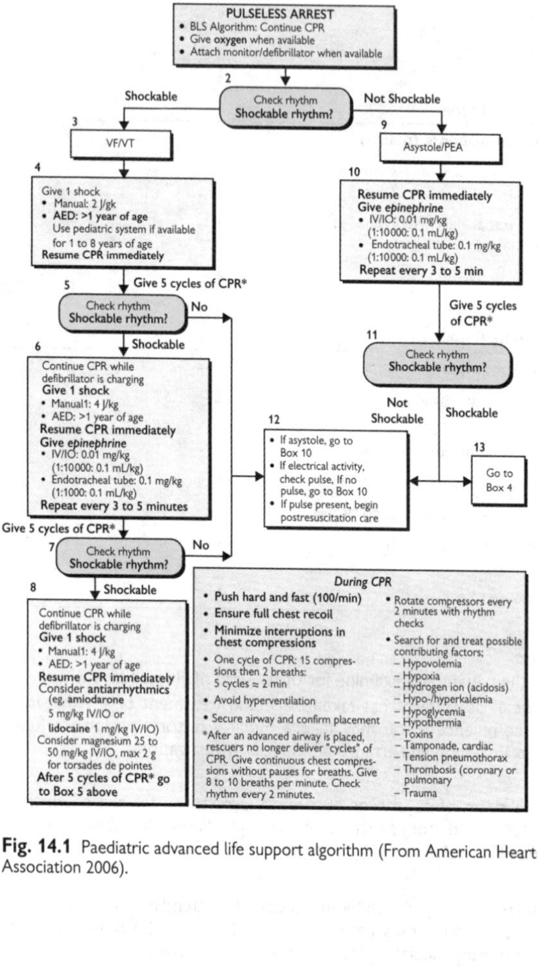

Fig. 14.1 Paediatric advanced life support algorithm (From American Heart Association 2006).

Taking blood

This can be a lot trickier in children than adults, not only because of their size, but also because they are less likely to be able to cooperate.

Think about

What is the indication for this blood test? Avoiding unnecessary venepuncture not only saves time and money, but also spares patient anxiety and discomfort. Some well children undergoing simple elective surgery will not require routine preop. investigation. Don't overlook simpler options—if the child has, for example, a working Hickman line, use that for sample collection instead (remember to use aseptic technique).

Analgesia

- Topical anaesthetic reduces discomfort and makes the child more cooperative.
- Place 4% amethocaine gel (Ametop™) on venepuncture sites and cover with a transparent occlusive dressing. In children >2yr the antecubital fossa can usually be used, but for children <2yr hands and feet are easier. It is wise to prepare more than one site, just in case. It takes 45min for the local anaesthetic to take effect. If you really can't wait, cooling the area with ethylchloride spray (Cryogesic®) can diminish the sensation a little but the effect lasts for only a few seconds.

Method

- Can I realistically find a vein in this child for venepuncture (preferable), or must I revert to a heel-prick collection (newborns only)?
- Will this child need IV access too? If so, insert a line and take blood via this to prevent unnecessary repetition (see technique below).

Blood bottles

- Children's blood bottles are different colours to those of adults!
- Check your hospital practice to ensure that you send the right samples, but, as a rough guide, commonly used tubes are listed in Table 14.6.
- Note the volume of blood required for each test before proceeding, to ensure that you take an adequate amount of blood and don't need to repeat the test—this is often marked on the side of the tube.

Environment

- Make use of the ward treatment rooms or draw the bedside curtains to prevent spreading distress to the other patients.
- Explain to the child and parents what you are about to do and why.
- Use play specialists (if available) and parents to help distract and reassure the child.
- In addition, have a nurse with you to help keep the child still and to act as a tourniquet, squeezing the limb.

Table 14.6 Commonly used blood tubes (check hospital lab protocol)

Tube colour	Chemical agent	Tests for
Orange	Lithium–heparin	Most routine biochemistry, B12, folate, ferritin, microbiology assays
Green	Sodium citrate	Clotting and thrombotic screening
Red	EDTA	Haematology, molecular genetics, PTH, ACTH, ciclosporin levels Transfusion (may have a separate colour EDTA/larger tube for blood bank)
White	Serum tube	α-fetoprotein
Brown	Serum gel	Immunology, virology, microbiology antibody tests
Yellow	Sodium fluoride	Glucose, lactate

EDTA, ethylene diamine tetra-acetic acid; PTH, parathyroid hormone; ACTH, adrenocorticotropic hormone.

Equipment

- Alcohol wipe.
- Gauze swabs or cotton-wool.
- Tape.
- Syringe—2.5 or 5mL is usually sufficient.
- Appropriate blood bottles.
- Butterfly needle (conventional blood taking) or heel-prick device (Tenderfoot™)/green needle + petroleum jelly (heel prick).

Conventional blood-taking

- Remove Ametop™, prepare skin with alcohol wipe and insert butterfly needle into vein as for adults.
- Draw up blood into syringe.
- When enough blood has been drawn, tell the assistant to stop squeezing, withdraw the needle and place cotton-wool/gauze over the puncture site.
- Reassure the child that the procedure is over and praise their good behaviour.

The heel prick (Fig. 14.2)

- Prepare venepuncture site with alcohol wipe.
- You may have a specialized heel-prick device (Tenderfoot™) available—if so, snap off the safety catch of the device and place firmly on to the child's heel, with the arrow pointing at the intended puncture site on the heel (Fig. 14.3).

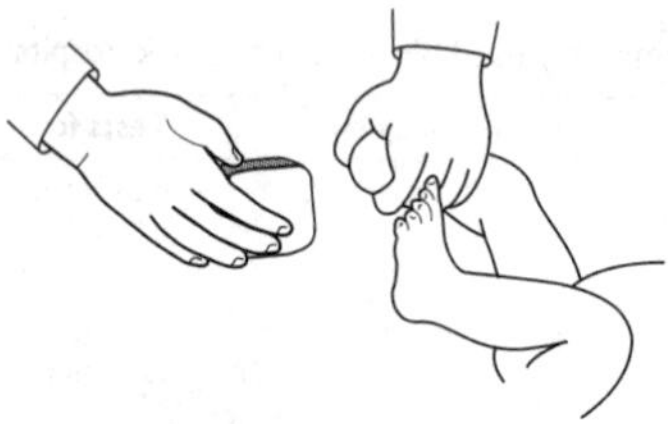

Fig. 14.2 Performing a heel prick with a Tenderfoot™ device. Grasp the baby's heel firmly. (Adapted from Capehorn DMW, Swain AH, Goldsworthy LL, eds (1998). Handbook of Paediatric Accident and Emergency Medicine. Harcout Brace, London).

- Have a blob of petroleum jelly waiting on your nearby tray and your blood bottles open, ready at hand. Line them up in the correct order—you will need to fill lithium–heparin tubes (U&E) before EDTA tubes (FBC), as EDTA can contaminate the other tubes and make results unreadable.
- Hold the heel securely. Warn the patient and assistant. Push the button, which will fire the spring-loaded puncture device, then put the Tenderfoot™ aside.
- Quickly smear a light coating of petroleum jelly over the heel—this makes the drops of blood easier to collect.
- Squeeze the heel and collect the blood droplets in the bottle, tapping it on a hard surface from time to time to send the blood to the bottom of the tube. Remember, U&Es first. Do make sure that you have enough blood in the bottle to process—it may take some time to collect enough.
- When the tubes are full, clean off the petroleum jelly and place a small dressing over the puncture site.

If you do not have a Tenderfoot™ device, make your puncture with a 20G needle, then proceed as above.

Note: The technique of breaking the hub off a 20G needle and leaving it in situ during a heel prick to channel the drops of blood into a blood bottle tube is now deeply discouraged on grounds of patient safety—do not do this.

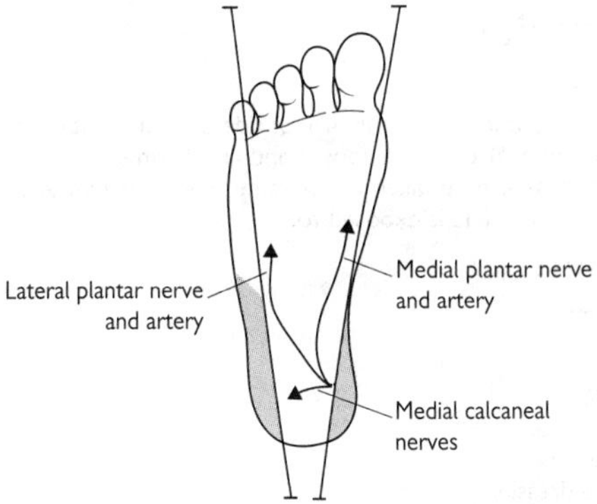

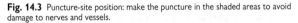

Fig. 14.3 Puncture-site position: make the puncture in the shaded areas to avoid damage to nerves and vessels.

Cannulation

Think about

Check the indication for the cannula, decide upon a suitable environment and method of analgesia (see above) and check whether blood tests are needed, as these can be taken at the same time to minimize the number of procedures the child is exposed to.

Management

Environment

See above.

Equipment

- Alcohol wipe.
- Gauze swabs.
- Adhesive dressing.
- Splint and bandage for younger children.
- Appropriate cannulas—24G (yellow 'neoflon') in neonates, 22G (blue) in infants, 20G (pink) or 18G (green) may be appropriate in older children requiring faster infusions.
- Syringe.
- 5mL normal saline for flush.

Method (Fig. 14.4)

- Apply local anaesthetic cream and wait for it to take effect—ensure a suitable environment and assistant, as described above.
- Clean off the cream, identify a vein, prepare the skin with an alcohol swab and insert a 22G (blue) or 24G (neoflon) cannula using the same technique as in an adult. Secure the cannula with an adhesive dressing.
- If you need to take blood, attach a syringe to the 22G cannula and withdraw. For smaller cannulas, either allow the blood to drip from the end of the cannula straight into the bottle or use a 2mL syringe with a 25G (orange) needle attached to draw blood up slowly from the end of the cannula.
- Cap off the cannula end and flush with normal saline to ensure patency.
- Secure with adhesive dressing. Cannula sites are usually bandaged and splinted in order to protect them from little fingers. Don't let go of the limb until you are sure that the cannula has been patient-proofed—or your good work will be in vain.
- Reassure the patient that the procedure is over and praise their good behaviour.

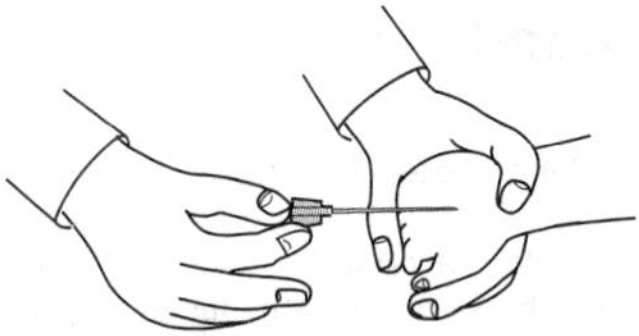

Fig. 14.4 Inserting a cannula into an infant—you may need to use your index finger to secure the baby's wrist.

Difficult access

- Call for help.
- If you are unable to cannulate a patient successfully after a maximum of three attempts, do not continue blindly but call a more experienced colleague for assistance—don't forget that members of the nursing staff may be experienced in paediatric cannulation. Other members of the surgical team, paediatricians and anaesthetists may also be able to offer help.
- In cases of extreme difficulty, alternative access may be needed. Call senior. Central lines and PICC (peripherally inserted central catheter) lines are inserted under general anaesthesia in children. In an emergency, intraosseous access may be used. Venous cut-downs, femoral lines and, in the neonate, umbilical venous catheterization are other alternatives.

Capillary blood gases

Think about

In children, arterial blood gases are rarely performed without arterial access in situ. Instead, venous blood gases and capillary blood gases are used. These are collected in capillary tubes and usually processed on portable machines on the ward—ask the nurses to prepare the analyser before you take the sample.

Method

Venous samples

- From a newly inserted cannula—place the capillary tube in the open end of the cannula before capping/flushing and blood will move up into the tube by capillary action.
- From a venous blood sample—having taken blood with a needle and syringe, insert the capillary tube into the mouth of the syringe and the blood will move into up into the tube by capillary action.

Capillary samples

- Perform a heel prick, as above. Place the capillary tube on the skin and the sample will move up into the tube.
- Having filled the tube, occlude the ends using gloved fingers to prevent the blood from spilling out, and load the sample into the gas analyser.

Extravasation injury

Think about

Extravasation is the leakage of a substance into the subcutaneous tissue from a vascular access device. Symptoms include swelling, oedema or erythema around a line site. It can result in skin necrosis, tendon exposure, 2° infection, abscess formation, amputation of digits and contracture of affected limbs. It is a clinical emergency—you must see these patients promptly and take steps to minimize the injury.

Management

- Ensure that the injection or infusion has been stopped.
- Ensure that the residual drug or fluid has been aspirated from the device.
- Remove affected cannulas to prevent further use, and refrain from using long lines and central access lines for further drug administration.
- If a limb is affected, elevate it.
- Assess the extent of the injury, taking account of the volume of fluid extravasated, the substance extravasated and the site of extravasation. Look for colour (erythema), sensitivity and swelling. Irritant drugs (e.g. doxorubicin) and hypertonic solutions (e.g. total parenteral nutrition [TPN]) are most likely to cause harm. Use universal indicator paper to determine the pH of the substance if in doubt.
- Alert the plastic surgery team and request urgent review. They may proceed to saline and/or hyaluronidase flush-out of the site, if indicated—hyaluronidase is an enzymic spreading factor that helps to disperse the fluid.
- Ensure the patient has alternative venous access if IV drugs/fluid/TPN are required.

Differential diagnosis

- Local allergic reaction ('flare').
- Vein irritation due to administration of irritant substance.

Calculating fluid requirements

If you are not used to working with children, a simple task like this can seem daunting. However, as children vary so much in size and requirements, it is vital that you take a moment to calculate appropriate individual fluid regimens. Never guess: the sequelae of hyponatraemia from erroneous fluid prescription can be devastating. The scheme below should help.

Think about

- How much does the child weigh? What do I ∴ calculate the child's daily maintenance water requirement to be?
- Is the child in the first 3 days of life, premature, or recently had surgery? If so, this maintenance volume may need increasing or decreasing.
- What type of fluid would be most appropriate?
- Are there any other fluid losses that need replacing? If so, what type of fluid should be used?

Management

Calculate maintenance

- For the first 10kg, give 100mL/kg/day = 4mL/kg/hr.
- For the next 10kg, give 50mL/kg/day = 2mLl/kg/hr.
- Above 20kg give, give 25mL/kg/day = 1mL/kg/hr.

Adjust for circumstances

Needs less fluid: scale down maintenance.

After surgery

- Day 1 postop—give 60% of calculated maintenance.
- Day 2 postop—give 70% of calculated maintenance.
- Day 3 postop—give 80% of calculated maintenance.
- Day 4 postop—give 100% of calculated maintenance.

After birth

- Day 1 of life—give 60% of calculated maintenance (60mL/kg).
- Day 2 of life—give 80% of calculated maintenance (80mL/kg).
- Day 3 of life—give 100% of calculated maintenance (100mL/kg).

Needs more fluid: scale up maintenance.

After birth (see also above)

- Day 4 of life—give 120% of calculated maintenance (120mL/kg).
- Day 5 of life—give 150% of calculated maintenance (150mL/kg).
- Thereafter throughout neonatal period—give 150% of calculated maintenance (150mL/kg).
- Prematurity—may need more fluid. Consult with neonatal intensive care unit (NICU).

Note: It is not expected that you will be cross covering special care or NICU patients. They are outside the scope of this book—seek advice from your unit neonatologists.

Which maintenance fluid?

Children require 2–4mmol sodium/kg/day, 2–4 mmol potassium/kg/day, 1 mmol calcium/kg/day and 0.5 mmol magnesium/kg/day.

For children with normal U&Es

- Newborn—give dextrosaline mixture of 10% glucose and 0.18% saline, with 10mmol potassium chloride in each 500mL bag.
- Older child—give dextrosaline mixture of 5% glucose and 0.45% saline, with 10mmol potassium chloride in each 500mL bag.

Potassium

- 10mmol potassium chloride is usually added to every 500mL maintenance bag. However, do not give potassium within 48hr of surgery or to patients in whom you do not know the serum potassium level.

Abnormal sodium

- Hyponatraemia—give 0.45% saline and 5% glucose solution and recheck Na in 6hr.
- Hypernatraemia—give 0.45% saline and 5% glucose solution, but give the fluids at two-thirds the normal rate (66% maintenance) until the Na <150mmol/L. This prevents fits from a sudden fall in Na.

Other losses

Add in replacement fluid to maintenance regimen according to measured losses:

Nasogastric (NG) losses/diarrhoea.

- Replace mL for mL with normal saline + 10mmol KCl per 500mL bag.

Ileostomy

- Replace half of lost volume with normal saline + 10mmol KCl per 500mL bag.

Write it up

- Write out the fluid and concentration in full to avoid any confusion (e.g. N/S could be read as normal saline, or 1/5th normal saline).
- Prescriptions are usually made for 500mL of the appropriate fluid, to run at the appropriate rate. So, for a 10kg child, you might write:
  - 500mL of 0.18% saline/4% glucose IV, to run at 40mL/hr.

Fluids for the acutely unwell child

Think about
Is this child dehydrated?

Management

- Acutely dehydrated—give maintenance + deficit.
- Percentage dehydration is the percentage of body-weight lost (not of body water). It is assessed on vital signs and clinical examination. If known, weight loss can also give an indication of level of dehydration. (see worked example below).

Table 14.7 Clinical signs of dehydration

Mild dehydration	0–5%	Dry mucous membranes, thirsty
Moderate dehydration	5–10%	Sunken fontanelle and eyes, ↓ skin turgor, weight loss, may be lethargic, dry mucous membranes, oliguria
Severe dehydration (unusual)	>10%	Drowsy, cardiovascular instability, tachypnoeic, mottled skin, anuric

- Fluid deficit = (percentage dehydration x weight in kg x 10).
- Give this volume in addition to the maintenance volume over 24hr.

Example
Kemal is a 6-yr-old boy admitted via A&E for incision and drainage of an abscess on the emergency list later in the day. His mother says that he has been miserable, refusing all food and most drinks the previous day, and when he is weighed on the ward he is found to be 19kg. When he was seen at the health centre last week, he weighed 20kg. On examination he has dry mucous membranes and admits to being thirsty.

What to prescribe
The patient is nil by mouth and also show clinical signs of around 5% acute dehydration, which is supported by a known 5% weight loss. He ∴ needs a maintenance fluid regimen plus rehydration.

- Calculate maintenance—remember to use Kemal's normal weight (not current dehydrated weight):
  - First 10kg—4mL/kg/hr = 40mL/hr.
  - Second 10kg—2mL/kg/hr = 20mL/hr.
  - Total weight 20kg—rate = 60mL/hr.
- No adjustment for circumstances necessary.
- Which maintenance fluid?
  - He's not an infant, so use dextrosaline with 5% glucose and 0.45% saline.
  - He has not had any blood tests so his K^+ is unknown—omit for now.
- Other losses?
  - No history of vomiting/diarrhoea, but Kemal is water-depleted.
- Rehydration:
  - Fluid deficit = percentage dehydration x weight in kg x 10 = 5 x 20 x 10 = 1000mL.
  - Give this over 24hr = 41.6mL/hr.
- Write it up:
  - 500mL 0.45% saline/5% glucose IV, to run at 102mL/hr' (rounded up).

Note: The regimen for correcting a 5% fluid deficit is just under double maintenance—a good way to check that your calculation looks correct.

- Don't forget to adjust the fluid regimen once the fluid deficit has been corrected.
- Don't forget to adjust the chosen fluid once the U&Es are known.
- Never just copy the previous prescription—calculate each fluid prescription individually.

Prescribing fluids in shock

Fluid boluses

- Call registrar.

If a child is shocked, fluid boluses form part of resuscitation:

- Give 20mL/kg colloid or normal saline as a bolus and reassess.
- Further boluses may be required if no response.

Haemorrhagic shock

- Call registrar.

Although fluids can be used to restore some circulating volume, if there is significant ongoing bleeding urgent blood transfusion is called for. In the emergency situation when there is no time to wait for a full cross-match, 'flying squad' (O Rhesus negative) blood and occasionally group-specific (partially cross-matched) blood is used:

- Give 10mL/kg blood as a bolus and reassess. If there is no response, give further boluses.

Table 14.8 Estimation of blood loss

	Blood volume lost			
	10–15%	**20–25%**	**30–35%**	**>40%**
Urine output (mL/kg/hr)	1–3	0.5–1	<0.5	None
Pulse*	Mild tachy cardia	Tachycardia	Tachycardia	Tachycardia
Respiratory rate	↔	↑	Tachypnoeic	Tachypnoeic/ apnoeic
Systolic BP	↔	↓	↓	Severely ↓
Mentation	↔	Anxious	Confusion	Unconscious

* Remember that absolute pulse rate will vary with age (📖 p520). See also ABC assessment (📖 p526).

Prescribing for children

As children vary greatly in age and size, individual medication doses are always given per kg. Never try to guess what a drug dose might be for a child: check in the British National Formulary (BNF) for Children or the Royal College of Paediatrics and Child Health's formulary 'Medicines for Children' and calculate the dose properly. Most paediatric wards will have a copy. The child's weight is often recorded on the front of their drug chart.

Analgesia

Think about

In the past, analgesia in children was frequently under-prescribed. This was due to a mistaken perception that children did not experience pain to the same extent as adults, and clinicians' fears of the side-effects of potent analgesics. However, good analgesia is important not only to reduce a child's distress but also to allow patients to relax, making accurate diagnosis and management easier. Some hospitals use visual analogue scores to help children communicate their pain level (e.g. smiley and frowning faces). However, talking to the child, their parents and nurses can help you to gauge whether a patient's pain is well controlled. For good pain control:

- Give simple analgesia regularly rather than PRN.
- Give multiple drugs to take advantage of synergistic action.

Management

- Mild pain:
  - Paracetamol or a non-steroidal anti-inflammatory drug (NSAID).
  - Paracetamol + NSAID.
- Moderate pain:
  - Paracetamol + NSAID + codeine.
- Severe pain:
  - Morphine + paracetamol ± NSAID.

Routes

Oral

Elixirs are the usual formulation for younger children. Prescribe in mg, not mL, to avoid confusion. Don't forget that opiates can be given orally too.

Rectal

Some patients who have recently undergone anorectal surgery will need to avoid this route. Check the operation note before prescribing if in doubt.

IM

This route can be painful—avoid if possible. Poor control over rate of release mean that side-effects may be unpredictable. Never use in the hypovolaemic patient.

IV

Some hospitals now stock IV paracetamol for patients in whom other routes are contraindicated—check your local policy. IV injections may be titrated to response. Postoperative systems such as patient-controlled analgesia (PCA) or nurse-operated nurse-controlled analgesia (NCA) deliver boluses on demand. These are usually supervised by the anaesthetic/pain control team, who should be contacted if the dose or device needs reviewing.

IN
Intranasal diamorphine utilizes mucosal absorption to exert its effects and is used for acute pain in some hospitals—check your local policy.

Inhaled agents
A 50:50 mixture of oxygen and nitrous oxide (Entonox®) may be used in the acute setting for short-term analgesia during procedures. It is contra-indicated in bowel obstruction or suspected pneumothorax as it rapidly diffuses into enclosed gaseous spaces, worsening matters.

Doses and formulations
Paracetamol
- Good antipyretic,
- Maximum single dose 1g.
- Slow PR absorption (2–4hr).

Table 14.9 Paracetamol

	Dose (mg/kg)	Maximum in 24hr (mg/kg)	Frequency
Neonate			
PO	Loading dose: 20		One-off
	Then: 10–15	60	Every 6hr
If jaundiced	5	20	Every 6hr
PR	Loading dose: 30		One-off
	Then: 20	60	Every 8hr
>1 month			
PO	Loading dose: 20		One-off
	Then: 15	60	Every 6hr
PR	Loading dose: 30		One-off
	Then: 20	60	Every 8hr
>3 months			
PO	Loading dose: 20		One-off
	Then: 15	60	Every 6hr
PR	Loading dose: 40		One off
	Then: 15	90	Every 6hr

NSAIDs: ibuprofen

- Antipyretic.
- Use with caution in asthma, renal failure, liver failure, low platelets and risk of major haemorrhage.
- Risk of gastric irritation with prolonged use.
- Maximum single dose 400mg.

Table 14.10 Ibuprofen

	Dose (mg/kg)	**Maximum in 24hr (mg/kg)**	**Frequency**
>3 months			
PO	10	30	Every 8hr
PR	Not available		

NSAIDs: diclofenac

- Well absorbed PR—onset within 1hr.
- Elixir is very bitter—consider ibuprofen instead.

Table 14.11 Diclofenac

	Dose (mg/kg)	**Maximum in 24hr**	**Frequency**
>6 months			
PO	0.3–1	3mg/kg	Every 8hr
>6yr			
PO	0.3–1	150mg total	Every 8hr
PR	1–2	150mg total	Every 8hr

Codeine phosphate

- Note maximum daily doses.
- Codeine can be given IM/SC, but try to avoid injections unless absolutely necessary. Never give IV.

Table 14.12 Codeine phosphate

	Dose	**Maximum in 24hr**	**Frequency**
<12yr			
PO	0.5–1mg/kg	3mg/kg	Every 4–6hr
PR	0.5–1mg/kg	3mg/kg	Every 4–6hr
≥12yr			
PO	30–60mg per dose	240mg total	Every 4–6hr
PR	30–60mg per dose	240mg total	Every 4–6hr

Morphine

- IV boluses are used as acute rescue analgesia.
- If a child requires a regular infusion, contact anaesthetist for PCA/NCA.
- Sedation level and respiratory monitoring are essential.
- Also prescribe an antiemetic and PRN opiate antagonist (naloxone 4–10mcg/kg IV, repeat as necessary) for respiratory depression.
- Consider regular lactulose (0.5mL/kg BD to max 10mL).
- Note that in children aged 6 months to 5yr, morphine has a half-life <2 hr, as they metabolize it faster than adults. IM and SC are alternative delivery routes if absolutely necessary, but absorption is unpredictable.

Table 14.13 Morphine

	Dose (mcg/kg)	Maximum in 24hr	Frequency
Neonate			
Slow IV	40	Titrate dose to response	6 hourly
1–6 months			
PO (Oramorph®)	80		4 hourly
Slow IV	100–200	Titrate dose to response	6 hourly
6 months to 1yr			
PO (Oramorph®)	80		4 hourly
Slow IV	100–200	Titrate dose to response	4 hourly
1–2yr			
PO (Oramorph®)	200–400		4 hourly
Slow IV	100–200	Titrate dose to response	4 hourly
2–12yr			
PO (Oramorph®)	200–500		4 hourly
Slow IV	100–200	Titrate dose to response	4 hourly

Need more help?

Many hospitals have multidisciplinary acute/chronic paediatric pain teams who can offer advice and expertise. Your seniors/anaesthetists may also be able to help.

Parenteral nutrition

Think about

Surgical indications for parenteral nutrition include prematurity, necrotizing enterocolitis, intestinal failure (short gut, post-abdominal surgery, radiation/ cytotoxic therapy), hypercatabolic states (extensive burns, severe trauma, gastroschisis) and organ failure (acute renal or hepatic failure).

There are two components to parenteral nutrition: Vamin® (vitamins, amino acids, trace elements and carbohydrates) and lipids. These are made up in separate bags.

TPN can be administered as a cyclical or continuous regimen. In a cyclical regimen, TPN is stopped for 1–12hr a day. This is used when the child is on a stable regimen. Continuous TPN is a 24hr treatment during which Vamin® is given over 24hr and lipids over 20hr.

Management

To start a patient on TPN:

- Arrange access—this is usually central venous access (e.g. Hickman line or long line).
- Send baseline bloods—these are used to guide the PN prescription. Send U&Es, LFTs, Ca, Mg, phosphate, albumin, glucose, total protein and trace elements.
- Nutrition team review–follow the calculated PN regimen based on the patient's age, weight, baseline bloods and requirements.
- Write up prescription as advised by nutrition team. Initially lipids are given over 20hr and Vamin® over 24hr in a continuous regimen.

Whilst on TPN:

- Regular blood tests.
- Requires daily U&Es and regular BMs.
- Twice-weekly LFTs, Ca, Mg, phosphate, triglycerides.
- Monthly trace elements—selenium, copper, zinc, manganese.
- Adjust prescription as advised by nutrition team.

Preoperative preparation

Preoperative assessment

Think about

As in adults, a full history, examination, appropriate investigations and confirmation of the indication for surgery are required before an operation takes place. This may occur at the pre-admission visit or on admission to the ward. The management of specific co-morbidities is described later in the chapter (see Perioperative management of specific conditions, 📖 p554), as are the preoperative investigations, blood ordering schedules and bowel preparation schedules for specific operations (see Common operations, 📖 p598).

Preoperative fasting schedule

Think about

Check for local variation, but a typical preoperative fasting schedule for children would be:

- Children:
  - Last food—6hr preop.
  - Clear fluids—up to 3hr preop.
  - Nil by mouth—for 3hr preop.
- Babies:
  - Formula-fed—last milk feed 6hr preop.
  - Breast-fed—last feed 4hr preop.
  - Clear fluids—may be given up to 3hr preop.

Seeking consent for surgery in children

Think about

- Am I the appropriate person to seek consent for this surgical procedure?
- Who can give consent for this surgery?

Management

- Do not try to obtain consent for a procedure unless you are sufficiently experienced and informed.
- If you do not feel that you can comfortably discuss the aims, alternatives, risks and complications of a procedure, ask your senior to step in.

- Before you ask a child or their carer to sign a consent form for a procedure, check that they are able to give consent. People who can consent for surgery are:
  - Those with parental responsibility (guardianship)—mothers automatically have parental responsibility for their children; fathers also have parental responsibility if they were married to the mother when the child was conceived or born, or if they got married later or are registered on the birth certificate. If a child is in local authority care, you need to liaise with the child's social worker and obtain consent from the appropriately authorized person.
  - Patients >16yr.
  - Patients <16yr but have been judged to be competent to give consent. A child who is judged to have sufficient understanding and intelligence to enable them fully to understand the medical treatment that is proposed (thus considered 'Gillick competent') may consent to medical treatment. In cases where a competent child refuses treatment, in England the person with parental responsibility/court may give consent on their behalf for procedures that are in the child's best interest. However, in Scotland, a competent child's refusal of treatment may not be overruled in the child's best interest. If in doubt, seek legal advice.

Asthma

Think about

Before admission

- At pre-assessment clinic take a full history to determine the severity of the child's disease. This will include frequency of attacks, symptoms between attacks, date of last attack, treatment regimen (including steroid use and any recent changes to regimen), hospital admissions, ICU admissions and ventilatory support, current symptoms, current upper respiratory tract infection, triggers (especially NSAIDs) and associated atopy, and any recent pulmonary function tests and results (see Table 14.14).
- If there is evidence of an active viral upper respiratory tract infection (URTI), delay admission.
- If the child has had an acute attack in the last month, delay surgery.
- If there is wheeze on examination, or evidence from the history that the child is not optimized, delay surgery and refer to paediatrician for advice on management.
- Arrange a chest X-ray.
- If surgery is to proceed, advise the carer to continue regular medications until the operation.
- If in doubt, discuss the case with the anaesthetist.

Management

On admission

- Ensure normal medications are continued until time of surgery.
- Anaesthetic review—the patient may require further doses of inhalers immediately before going to theatre.

After surgery

- If child has atopy/NSAID-sensitive asthma, avoid NSAID analgesia.
- Exercise caution with opiates.

Table 14.14 Normal peak flow values

Height (cm)	Approx. age (yr)	Peak flow (mL)
110	5–6	150
120	6–7	200
130	7–8	250
140	8–10	300
150	10–12	350
160	12–14	400
170	>14	450

These values are reliable only in children >7yr.

Cystic fibrosis

Think about

Before admission

- Alert respiratory team to the planned surgical admission in good time as they will then be able to optimize the patient for surgery. It may be necessary to admit the child up to a week in advance for preoperative antibiotics. Seek advice about whether a PICU bed should be requested after surgery.
- Alert the anaesthetist in advance.
- Pulmonary function is often worse first thing in the morning. Do not schedule the patient first on the theatre list. Allow time for preoperative physiotherapy and clearing of secretions.

Management

On admission

- Follow respiratory team's advice; specific points to clarify are preoperative tests required, perioperative bronchodilator regimens, perioperative antibiotic regimens and whether parenteral vitamin K is required (if the patient is not on oral treatment).
- Ensure good hydration—if oral fluids are to be withheld for >3hr (i.e. operating time is uncertain), consider IV fluids before surgery.

After surgery

- Continuous pulse oximetry on ward. Oxygen as necessary.
- Regular chest physiotherapy.
- Continued involvement and advice of respiratory team.
- Opiates to be used with great caution—close monitoring required.

Diabetes

Think about

Before admission

- Put the patient first on the theatre list so starving times can be predicted accurately. Morning lists are less likely to be delayed than afternoon lists—let the admissions department know your preferences.
- Alert the anaesthetist and paediatric diabetes team to the planned admission.
- Admit the patient a day before surgery to allow time for preoperative reviews.

Management

The day before surgery

- Preoperative investigations should include U&Es, FBC, glucose (lab) and urine dipstick for ketones.
- Capillary blood glucose (BM) should be charted. Take pre-meal and pre-bedtime levels.
- Meals—normal supper.
- Insulin—normal SC insulin dose.
- Diabetes team to review before surgery.

On day of surgery

First on morning theatre list

- Meals—no breakfast, clear sweet drinks until 2hr before surgery.
- Insulin—omit morning dose. Insulin infusion may be commenced in anaesthetic room.
- Fluids—may be commenced in anaesthetic room once IV access has been obtained.
- Preop. BM and half-hourly measurement in theatre.

First on afternoon theatre list

- Meals—normal breakfast at least 6hr preop. (may need to wake up early).
- Insulin—give short-acting insulin before breakfast. The diabetes team will usually advise you on the dose, but as a rule this is half the patient's usual dose. If on M2® or Mixtard® (a mixture of long- and short-acting insulin), you will need to calculate the short-acting component (see Table 14.15). At noon, site a cannula and commence insulin infusion.
- Fluids—clear sweet fluids orally until 2hr preop.
- Preop. BM and half-hourly in theatre.

Table 14.15 Short acting insulin infusion according the BM results

BM (mmol/L)	Action
>28	Call doctor
18–28	Rate 0.1mL/kg/hr Call doctor
12–17	Rate 0.05mL/kg/hr
8–11	Rate 0.03mL/kg/hr
4–7	Stop infusion
<4	Call doctor

Insulin infusion

Many hospitals have their own guidelines for prescribing insulin infusions—if a local protocol exists, follow it. However, as a guide, an insulin infusion is prescribed as 50 units soluble insulin (Actrapid®) made up to 50mL with 0.9% saline (1 unit insulin/mL) and infused at a rate determined by hourly or 2-hrly BM results.

After surgery

- BM half-hourly for 2hr, hourly for 4hr, then 2 hourly until the next morning.
- Insulin and IV fluids—continue until taking full oral fluids and snacks.
- Suppertime—if eating and drinking well, and able to eat an evening meal, give normal dose of insulin before meal.

Latex allergy

Think about

Before admission

- Alert anaesthetist, theatres and ward of the planned surgery and admission.
- Familiarize yourself with your local latex protocol—most hospitals have local protocols for perioperative management of the latex-allergic patient.
- Book the patient first on the theatre list.
- Liaise with admissions to ensure the patient is admitted the night before surgery to allow time for pre-medication.

Management

On admission

- Ensure allergy is noted on patient's wristband/drug chart.
- Site cannula.
- Follow hospital latex allergy protocol if available. This may include:
  - IV steroids—1mg/kg methylprednisolone IV (to a maximum single dose of 50mg) 6hrly.
  - IV ranitidine—1mg/kg 6hrly, given over 2min.
  - IV antihistamine chlorpheniramine (Piriton®), given slowly:
    - 1 month to 1yr 250mcg/kg 6hrly.
    - 1–5yrs 2.5–5mg 6hrly.
    - 6–12yrs 5–10mg 6hrly.
  - If the patient is asthmatic, add salbutamol inhaler 6hrly.

These drugs are usually started 12hr before the procedure (2 doses).

After surgery

Continue medications for 24hr postoperatively.

Sickle cell anaemia

Think about

Before admission

Screening—patients from high-risk ethnic groups (western African, Central Indian, Afro-Caribbean, parts of the Middle East and Mediterranean) who do not know their sickle status should have preop. sickle cell screening. In children >6 months, you can perform an Hb solubility test at preadmission (Sickledex®, Sickleprep®). These are relatively quick to do, but do not differentiate sickle trait from sickle cell disease so, if the result is positive, it needs to be followed up with an Hb electrophoresis sample. Electrophoresis measures the proportion of HbS, thus differentiating sickle cell disease (70–90% HbS) from sickle cell trait (<50% HbS). In babies <6 months, Hb solubility tests are not reliable due to their high physiological HbF—send Hb electrophoresis from the start.

- Alert the anaesthetist and haematology team of the planned admission.
- Patients may require a preop. top-up or exchange transfusion, which will need to be arranged.
- FBC and group and save at preadmission, if possible—FBC result will help guide the haematologist's management. If the patient has had multiple previous transfusions, they may have atypical antibodies, which can make cross-matching take longer.
- Liaise with admissions to ensure that the patient is admitted the night before surgery.

Management

On admission

- Haematology review and follow specific advice.
- Ensure good hydration to avoid a sickle crisis. Insert a cannula and give IV maintenance (📖 P540) from midnight before the operation.

After surgery

- Continue IV fluids until drinking normally.
- Prophylactic antibiotics.
- Be alert for pulmonary/other complications and seek urgent haematology advice if concerned.

Postoperative pyrexia

Fevers in children are most frequently caused by viral illnesses, and are common in the community. However, they must always be taken seriously in the surgical population, and especially in children <6 months old. In this group the signs of serious infection can be few, so it is important to exercise caution.

Think about

- Is this patient seriously unwell? If so, I need to call for help and commence resuscitation.
- What is the cause of the pyrexia? What investigations are warranted?
- What management steps should I take?

Possible causes

- Infective—urinary tract infection (UTI), upper and lower respiratory tract infection (URTI and LRTI), gastroenteritis, central line infection, intra-abdominal sepsis, wound infection, otitis media, meningitis, other childhood infections.
- Non-infective—malignancy, drug/transfusion reaction (including anaesthesia), inflammatory, atelectasis, response to trauma/surgery, thromboembolism.

Management

- Assess ABC—if seriously unwell, call registrar and commence resuscitation.
- History—note any obvious focal signs such a cough or sites of pain. Note type of surgery and timing of surgery (respiratory/urinary infections may develop soon after surgery and anaesthesia, whilst wound infections take a few days to develop). Note age of lines and when they were last used—if source of bacteraemia is a central line, the spike may occur shortly after the device is used as bacteria are flushed through.
- Examination should include:
  - Respiratory examination.
  - Abdominal examination.
  - ENT examination.
  - Skin (rashes).
  - Wound site.
  - Line sites—central lines are potential sources.
  - Inspect contents of drains/urinary catheters
- Investigations—a partial septic screen consists of blood culture, FBC, throat swab, urine microscopy and culture, and chest X-ray. A full septic screen includes the above, plus a lumbar puncture. CRP, U&Es and, in the more unwell child, glucose and capillary blood gas may also be useful.

Pyrexia of unknown origin

- <6 months—full septic screen.
- >6 months:
  - Severely unwell—full septic screen.
  - Mildly unwell—partial septic screen.

Where focal signs exist, further specific investigations may be needed, e.g. suspected intra-abdominal collection, ultrasound or computed tomography scan.

- Give antipyretic—paracetamol + NSAID if no contraindications.
- Consider antibiotics.
- Clear focus of infection—commence appropriate treatment:
  - <6 months—call registrar; broad-spectrum antibiotics.
  - Severely unwell—call registrar; resuscitate (📖 p526); give broad-spectrum antibiotics (e.g. benzylpenicillin, amikacin, metronidazole).
  - Mildly unwell—may be appropriate to await investigation results before commencing treatment, unless deteriorates.
- If child has previously spiked fevers and is deteriorating despite antibiotics, review previous culture results and sensitivities, and seek microbiology advice.

Anaemia and blood loss

The most common cause of a low Hb in a surgical patient is bleeding. The average child has a blood volume of 80mL/kg, and a term infant has 90mL/kg. This means that the loss of even small volumes of blood during surgery can cause significant compromise to babies and young children.

Think about

- Is this patient's Hb normal for their age?
- Can I account for the low Hb? Is the patient known to have bled?
- Does the patient need a blood transfusion? If so, how much?

Management

- Check normal range of Hb values by age—see your local ranges, (📖 p524).
- First, consider the sample. Could it have been taken from an infusion site, thus diluted? Could it have clotted? If in doubt, repeat the sample urgently.

In the postoperative patient

- Check the operation note/anaesthetic charts for estimated blood loss, and note whether blood was given intraoperatively (in general, blood replacement at operation is considered if >15% of child's blood volume is lost).
- Also note preop. Hb, if available—are known losses consistent with the drop in Hb? If so, consider transfusion (see below). If not, examine the patient for cardiovascular compromise (📖 p520) for normal pulse rate by age) and find the source of ongoing blood loss—drains, urine, stools, vomit, wound dressings, haematomas, site of surgery and, importantly, examine abdomen for evidence of intra-abdominal bleeding.
- Alert registrar immediately (see 📖 p563 for haemorrhagic shock).

In the preoperative patient

- Review the history (including travel and diet) and examine the patient—specific features to look for are pallor, petechiae, hepatosplenomegaly and bony tenderness.
- Look at MCV, WCC and differential, and ESR/CRP. Consider possible causes:
  - Microcytic anaemia (MCV <70fl)—suspect iron deficiency/thalassaemia/sickle cell.
  - Macrocytic anaemia (MCV >100fl)—suspect folate deficiency (phenytoin/malabsorption), B12 deficiency (malabsorption/dietary, especially maternal deficiency in breast-fed infants), haemolysis.
  - Normocytic (MCV 81–97fl)—haemolysis, marrow failure, chronic disease.
  - Raised CRP/ESR may indicate chronic disease.
  - In patients with a history of travel to the tropics, eosinophilia with anaemia suggests hookworm rather than iron deficiency.

- Consider further investigations as appropriate—blood film, folate, B12, haemoglobinopathy screen, ferritin/transferrin, LFTs (billirubin/albumin), malaria screen, stool sample.
- Elective surgery may need to be postponed until investigations are complete. Discuss this with your registrar. Send a G+S to the laboratory as the child may require preop./postop. transfusion. If surgery is to proceed, ensure the anaesthetist is aware of the situation.
- Transfuse if patient is symptomatic or Hb <8.0g/dL.

Always discuss transfusion with the registrar. Certain specialties have different target Hb levels (e.g. orthopaedic surgeons may be more tolerant of a low Hb than plastic surgeons who have just sited a flap). Check the operation note for specific instructions.

Before prescribing a transfusion it is important to inform the patient and parents of the expected benefits and the potential risks of the procedure, and seek oral consent. Record your discussion in the notes.

Calculate transfusion volume

A transfusion of 4mL/kg packed cells raises the Hb by 1g/dL. Put another way, the transfusion volume can be calculated using the formula:

Volume required (in mL) = Weight (in kg) × 4 × Desired rise in Hb (in g/dL)

Haemorrhagic shock

- Call registrar.
- Blood may be required as part of resuscitation (📖 p526).
- If there is an obvious amenable source of bleeding, commence pressure and elevation.

Blood products

Platelets

- The transfusion volume is 10mL/kg.
- Discuss any platelet transfusion with the registrar.
- Consider giving a platelet transfusion in the following circumstances:
  - Platelet count $<10 \times 10^9$/L in a child.
  - Platelet count $<30 \times 10^9$/L in a neonate.
  - Platelet count $<50 \times 10^9$/L in a patient with mucosal bleeding.
  - Platelet count $<50 \times 10^9$/L in a patient about to have minor surgery (e.g. central line insertion).
  - Platelet count $<100 \times 10^9$/L in a patient about to have major surgery/surgery at a critical site.

You may be asked to prescribe other blood products:

FFP

The transfusion volume is 10mL/kg.

Cryoprecipitate

The transfusion volume is 10mL/kg.

Abdominal emergencies

Think about

- Most children presenting to A&E with abdominal symptoms have 'non-surgical' causes.
- As a rule, abdominal pain lasting >3–4hr should be considered to be evidence of an abdominal emergency until proven otherwise.

Overview

Causes of the surgical acute abdomen in the paediatric population

As paediatric surgical trainee the most common condition you will be called on to confirm or exclude is appendicitis (see Appendicitis, 📖 p586). However, it is important to bear in mind a range of possible surgical conditions causing abdominal symptoms, and can be useful to consider possible causes by age group (Table 14.16).

Table 14.16 Symptoms of acute surgical abdomen in children

	Predominant symptoms			
	Obstruction	**Pain**	**Bleeding**	**Mass**
Neonates (up to the first month of life)				
Meconium ileus	x	x		
Intestinal atresia or stenosis	x	x		
Hirschsprung's disease*	x	x		
Anorectal anomalies	x	x		
Malrotation and volvulus*	x	x		
Duplication abnormalities*	x	x	x	
Incarcerated inguinal hernia*	x	x	x	x
Necrotizing enterocolitis	x	x	x	
Infants (1 month to 2yrs)				
Intussusception	x	x	x	x
Pyloric stenosis	x			x
Children (≥2yrs)				
Appendicitis		x		x
Meckel's diverticulum	x		x	
Testicular torsion		x		x
Adhesions	x	x		

Note: This table gives the typical age group in which the conditions commonly occur. Conditions marked with an asterisk (*) may also present in infants and older children, and appendicitis and Meckel's diverticulum may be seen in younger children.

Table 14.17 Other causes of abdominal pain

Extra-abdominal	Intra-abdominal (medical)
Otitis media	Gastroenteritis
Lobar pneumonia	Mesenteric adenitis
Vertebral discitis	Constipation
Hip pain	Hepatitis
Diabetic ketoacidosis	Biliary colic
	Pancreatitis
	Peptic ulceration
	Crohn's disease
Gynaecological causes	Ulcerative colitis
Ectopic pregnancy	Urinary tract infection
Torsion of ovary	Renal calculus
Ruptured ovarian cyst	Pyelonephritis
	Sickle cell crisis
Pelvic inflammatory disease	Henoch–Schönlein purpura
	Recurrent abdominal pain of childhood
	Parasites

Other causes of abdominal pain in children

Table 14.17 shows some other causes of abdominal pain, which you should bear in mind as you assess the child. Remember that a full examination is necessary to exclude extra-abdominal causes of pain.

Neonatal bowel obstruction

Neonates presenting with bowel obstruction can be very sick, and require significant perioperative resuscitation. All require treatment at a specialist paediatric surgery centre, all require early senior surgical involvement, and many will need admission to the NICU for medical management by neonatologists. The day-to-day care of the critically ill neonate is beyond the scope of this handbook, but important surgical management points are highlighted below.

- Your surgical seniors will want to take the lead in the surgical management of these little patients.
- Management and investigation will include not only the steps described below, but also medical management and investigation by neonatal intensivists as befits the critically ill neonate.

Think about

The cardinal symptoms of neonatal bowel obstruction are:

- Bile-stained vomiting.
- Abdominal distension.
- Failure to pass meconium.

History and examination give an idea of the level at which bowel obstruction may be occurring. The obstruction may be due to mechanical factors or functional factors.

Mechanical causes of obstruction

- Upper GI obstruction:
  - Duodenal atresia/stenosis.
  - Malrotation with volvulus.
- Lower GI obstruction:
  - Meconium ileus.
  - Small bowel atresia.
  - Incarcerated inguinal hernia (see The groin, 📖 p589).
  - Anorectal malformation.

Functional causes of obstruction

- Hirschsprung's disease.
- Necrotizing enterocolitis.
- Sepsis (paralytic ileus).
- Postoperative ileus.

Duodenal atresia or stenosis

Abnormal duodenal development may result in either the complete absence of a segment of bowel, or a stenosis or membrane dividing a continuous duodenum (which may bulge distally inside the lumen as a 'windsock'). Duodenal atresia is associated with Down syndrome as well as renal and cardiac anomalies. There may also be other GI malformations (e.g. oesophageal atresia, anorectal anomalies).

Ask about

- Vomiting in the first few hours of life, usually bile stained (although if the obstruction is proximal to the ampulla of Vater it may not be). Note the frequency of vomits and duration of vomiting (may cause electrolyte disturbance). If the episodes are intermittent, this indicates partial obstruction, stenosis or malrotation.
- Meconium—may be passed even if obstructed.
- Abdominal distension—confined to the upper abdomen. The lower abdomen is scaphoid.
- Antenatal USS—may have been diagnosed prenatally with polyhydramnios and a dilated stomach and first part of the duodenum.

Look for

- An unwell child—basic examination and assessment (📖 p526).
- Specific features—upper abdominal distension with scaphoid (concave) lower abdomen. May be visible gastric peristalsis. If a nasogastric (NG) tube can be passed, aspirates will be high (>20mL) and usually bile stained.
- Associated conditions—assess the baby for dysmorphic features, e.g. Down's phenotype.

Investigation

- Send FBC, U&Es, LFTs, clotting, blood cultures (as sepsis is a differential diagnosis) and group and save.
- Check blood glucose.
- Consider capillary blood gas if unwell.
- Arrange plain abdominal X-ray. Immediately before the film is taken, inject 30mL air via the NG tube to provide contrast. A typical 'double bubble' appearance is seen in duodenal atresia.
- If partial obstruction is suspected, arrange an upper GI contrast study.
- Echo and renal USS should be performed to look for associated anomalies.
- Karyotype may be indicated if Down syndrome is suspected.

Management

- Urgent senior review and management.
- The patient should be treated in a specialist paediatric surgical centre.
- Neonatal intensive care may be needed.

- Admit patient.
- If shocked, attend to ABC. Call for help. Liaise with NICU if necessary.
- Keep nil by mouth.
- Insert NG tube.
- Obtain IV access. Send bloods (see above).
- Commence maintenance fluids/resuscitate as necessary (see IV fluids, p540).
- Give broad-spectrum antibiotics—there's a note on this with drugs.
- Liaise with theatres and anaesthetists.
- Proceed to laparotomy + duodenoduodenostomy (in the case of atresia/stenosis), or resection of duodenal membrane.
- Laparotomy also allows exclusion of an external cause of duodenal obstruction such as an annular pancreas (which is bypassed at operation rather than divided) or a malrotation with Ladd's bands or volvulus (see below).

Differential diagnosis

- Malrotation volvulus.
- Annular pancreas.
- Sepsis.

Malrotation volvulus

During fetal life, the developing midgut leaves the abdominal cavity to grow. It returns at week 10, rotating anticlockwise 270° to bring the transverse colon up to its adult position, and the caecum and terminal ileum down into the right iliac fossa. If this process fails (see picture) the midgut mesentery is narrow and susceptible to volvulus. In addition, peritoneal bands that run from the caecum to the posterior abdominal wall (Ladd's bands) cross the duodenum and may cause intermittent obstruction.

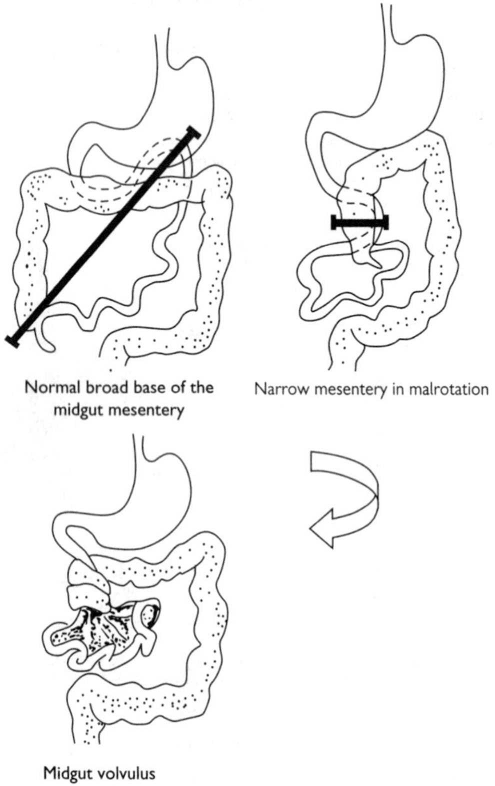

Fig. 14.5 Malrotation volvulus. Adapted from Filston and Kirks: Malrotation—the ubiquitous anomaly. *J Pediatr Surg* 1981; **16**:614.

Ask about

- Vomiting—a history of intermittent episodes of bile-stained vomiting or the sudden onset of bilious vomiting in a previously well baby should raise the possibility of volvulus.
- Recent general health, fever, etc.—an important differential is sepsis.
- Abdominal distension—initially there is little distension because this is a high obstruction, but if the gut is necrotic distension may occur.
- Pain—a sign of progression to intestinal ischaemia.
- Rectal bleeding—a sign of bowel necrosis or venous engorgement.

Look for

- An unwell child—basic assessment (📖 p526). Gangrenous bowel can cause shock.
- Specific features—typically non-distended abdomen and afebrile baby. Abdominal distension, marked tenderness and shock are late signs.

Investigations

- Send FBC, U&Es, LFTs, clotting, blood culture and cross-match 1 unit. Check BM glucose.
- Arrange plain abdominal X-ray. The film is often relatively gasless, with dilated first part of the duodenum (may show 'double bubble') and a little gas more distally.
- If the patient is stable and the diagnosis not clear, arrange an upper GI contrast. This may show complete duodenal obstruction or partial obstruction with the pathognomonic 'corkscrew' appearance of the twisted proximal small intestine.
- USS by experienced radiologists may confirm malrotation, if time permits.

Management

- Urgent senior review and management.
- The patient should be treated in a specialist paediatric surgical centre.
- Neonatal intensive care may be required.
- Volvulus requires urgent laparotomy.

- Admit patient.
- If shocked, attend to ABC. Call for help. Liaise with NICU if necessary.
- Keep nil by mouth.
- Insert NG tube.
- Obtain IV access.
- Commence maintenance fluids/resuscitate as necessary (see IV fluids, 📖 p524).
- Give broad-spectrum antibiotics.
- Liaise with theatres and anaesthetists. Urgent laparotomy is indicated with correction of the volvulus, widening of the small bowel mesentery and division of Ladd's bands. The appendix is also removed, to prevent future diagnostic confusion due to its abnormal position.
- If the small bowel is gangrenous, resection is necessary.

Differential diagnosis

- Duodenal atresia/stenosis.
- Annular pancreas.
- Sepsis.

Meconium ileus

Distal small bowel obstruction may be caused by thick, bulky, abnormal meconium. In the majority of cases (90%) cystic fibrosis, with its resulting abnormally high protein secretions, will be the root cause. The condition starts in utero. Meconium ileus may be simple (obstruction only) or complicated (associated with volvulus, atresia, perforation and meconium peritonitis).

Ask about

- Antenatal USS—prenatal scans may detect dilated loops of small bowel and abnormal meconium.
- Family history of cystic fibrosis.
- Abdominal distension—may be progressive or present at birth. Severe abdominal distension at birth, accompanied by abdominal wall oedema and erythema, is suggestive of complicated meconium ileus. Severe abdominal distension may cause respiratory distress.
- Passage of meconium—absent.
- Vomiting—typically bilious vomiting on first day of life.
- Symptoms and signs of sepsis—indicate complicated meconium ileus.
- Abdominal masses—doughy masses of meconium may be palpable in the abdomen.

Look for

- An unwell child—basic examination and assessment (📖 p526). The neonate with complicated meconium ileus may be in extremis.
- Specific features–abdominal distension; may have palpable lumps of meconium (indents on palpation). Empty rectum. Peritonism, abdominal wall oedema and erythema, and evidence of sepsis are suggestive of complicated meconium ileus.

Investigation

- Send FBC, U&Es, LFTs, clotting and cross-match 1 unit blood.
- Check BM glucose.
- Arrange plain abdominal X-ray. Dilated loops of bowel, with a lack of air–fluid levels (due to the thick meconium) will be seen in simple meconium ileus. Bubbles of air mixing with the thick meconium may give a 'soap bubble' appearance, which is highly suggestive of meconium ileus, although not always seen. Areas flecked with calcium, often on the liver capsule, are indicative of prenatal perforation and meconium peritonitis. Dense calcium-rimmed masses may represent pseudocysts, another consequence of in utero perforation.

Management

- Urgent senior review and management.
- The patient should be treated in a specialist paediatric surgical centre.
- Neonatal intensive care may be required.

- Admit patient.
- If shocked, attend to ABC. Call for help. Liaise with NICU if necessary.
- Keep nil by mouth.
- Insert NG tube.
- Obtain IV access.
- Commence maintenance fluids/resuscitate as necessary (see IV fluids, 📖 p526). Albumin may be needed.
- Give analgesia if required.
- Give broad-spectrum antibiotics.
- Complicated meconium ileus requires urgent laparotomy. Liaise with theatres and anaesthetists.
- Simple meconium ileus may respond to therapeutic Gastrografin® enema under fluoroscopic control. Liaise with radiologists. As patients may subsequently need a laparotomy (if a perforation is found or the enema fails to loosen the meconium), ensure the child has been fully resuscitated, has had antibiotics, and that you have liaised with theatres before sending the patient down to the radiology department.

At laparotomy, the dilated ileum may be washed out with saline or Gastrografin®, the dilated segment resected and re-anastomosed. Alternatively, a temporary ileostomy may be formed through which Gastrografin® or acetylcystine washout can occur postoperatively. Complicated meconium ileus always requires resection and stoma formation.

Postoperatively, *n*-acetylcystine may be given to thin the intestinal secretions. A sweat test and genetic tests for cystic fibrosis should also be performed; liaise with the paediatric CF team.

Differential diagnosis

- Intestinal atresia or stenosis.
- Hirschsprung's disease.

☠ Hirschsprung's disease

Hirschsprung's disease is a gut motility disorder in which the distal bowel is aganglionic. This usually affects the rectosigmoid, but may occasionally affect the descending, transverse or even the whole colon.

Ask about

- The baby's sex—♂ are more commonly affected than ♀.
- Family history—genetic links have been described.
- Down syndrome—present in 5–15% of those with Hirschsprung's disease.
- Passage of meconium—may be delayed beyond the first 24hr of life.
- Abdominal distension following feeds (precedes vomiting).
- Feeding—may be reluctant.
- Vomiting—bilious vomiting may be present after feeding.
- Symptoms of sepsis—Hirschsprung's enterocolitis is a serious complication of the disease and can lead to overwhelming sepsis and death. It also occurs in postoperative Hirschsprung's patients after aganglionic bowel has been resected.
- Diarrhoea, fever, gross abdominal distension and circulatory collapse are all features of Hirschsprung's enterocolitis. *Clostridium difficile* and its toxin may be found in the stools.
- Constipation in the older baby—some patients may present late with chronic constipation.

Look for

- Basic assessment (📖 p526).
- Specific features—rectal examination or saline washout may cause explosive passage of flatus and loose stool, relieving the obstruction temporarily.

Investigation

- Send U&Es if vomiting/dehydration.
- Check BM glucose.
- Arrange plain abdominal X-ray—this shows distended bowel loops with fluid levels.
- Arrange a suction rectal biopsy, the definitive diagnosis. This is usually done on the ward. Rectal mucosa and submusosa are sent for histological examination and histochemical staining for acetylcholinesterase.
- Arrange a contrast enema—this must be 36hr after rectal examination or washout for results to be interpretable. This gives an idea of the length of aganglionic segment. The film shows a 'cone' of transition, where the normal proximal (ganglionic) colon is dilated and the abnormal distal (aganglionic segment) is collapsed.

Management

- Urgent senior review and management.
- The patient should be treated in a specialist paediatric surgical centre.
- Neonatal intensive care may be required.

- Admit patient.
- If septic, attend to ABC. Call for help. Liaise with NICU if necessary.
- Treatment for Hirschsprung's enterocolitis includes rectal irrigation, broad-spectrum IV antibiotic cover including vancomycin (*C. difficile*).
- Otherwise, consider IV access, fluid resuscitation and NG tube in cases of vomiting.

When diagnosis has been confirmed, washouts are continued until surgery. Preoperatively, the baby will require FBC, U&Es and 1 unit crossmatched. Postoperatively, antibiotic cover is given. Surgery may be a 1° pull-through procedure or a defunctioning colostomy/ileostomy with intraoperative frozen section (to ensure the stoma/pull through is in ganglionic bowel). At a later date a definitive procedure, during which normal bowel is pulled through to the anorectal junction, can be performed. Once this is satisfactory, the colostomy is closed.

Differential diagnosis

- Intestinal atresia/stenosis.
- Meconium ileus.
- Imperforate anus.

Small bowel atresia

These absent segments may occur anywhere along the small bowel and are likely to be the consequence of in utero disruption of local blood supply. There are four degrees of atresia (see picture).

- Type I—a mucosal membrane interrupting the continuous bowel lumen.
- Type II—an atretic segment, with proximal and distal bowel held together by a fibrous cord.
- Type III—proximal and distal bowel are blind loops, separated by a mesenteric defect.
- Type IV—multiple atresias.

Ask about

- Antenatal USS—occasionally polyhydramnios and dilated loops of small bowel may have been seen.
- Vomiting—depending on the level of obstruction, bilious vomiting may occur in the first 24hr of life (e.g. high jejunal atresia) or after the first few days of life following abdominal distension (e.g. distal ileal atresia).
- Passage of meconium—may be passed on the first day of life, but is not followed by the passage of normal stools.
- Abdominal distension—gives some indication of level of obstruction.

Look for

- An unwell child—basic examination and assessment (📖 p526).
- Specific features—depending upon the level of obstruction, there may be abdominal distension or a scaphoid abdomen. Empty rectum.

Investigation

- Send FBC, U&Es, LFTs, clotting and cross-match 1 unit.
- Capillary blood gas if unwell.
- Check BM glucose.
- Arrange plain abdominal X-ray. Dilated loops of bowel with fluid levels are seen.
- Arrange contrast enema—shows a microcolon (unused colon) and excludes the presence of a distal colonic atresia (rare).

Management

- Urgent senior review and management.
- The patient should be treated in a specialist paediatric surgical centre.
- Neonatal intensive care may be needed.

- Admit patient.
- If shocked, assess ABC. Call for help. Liaise with NICU if necessary.
- Keep nil by mouth.
- Insert NG tube.
- Obtain IV access.
- Commence maintenance fluids/resuscitate as necessary (see IV fluids, 📖 p540).

- Give broad-spectrum antibiotics.
- Liaise with theatre and anaesthetists. Proceed to laparotomy and resection of atretic segment(s). The bowel proximal to the atresia may be grossly dilated, and may require resection or tapering to the approximate diameter of the distal bowel before re-anastomosis may be achieved. At the end of the procedure, the length of remaining small bowel is measured—if less than 70cm, long-term TPN may be required.

Differential diagnosis

- Meconium ileus.
- Imperforate anus.
- Hirschsprung's disease.

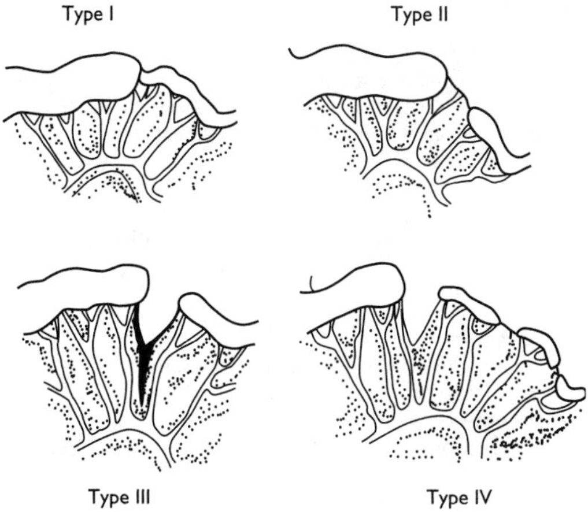

Fig.14.6 Classification of intestinal atresia. After Grosfeld, Ballantine and Shoemaker: Operative management of intestinal atresia and stenosis based on pathologic findings. *J Pediatr Surg*. 1979 Jun; **14**(3): 368–75.

Necrotizing enterocolitis (NEC)

The patient should be treated in a specialist paediatric surgical centre.

NEC is a serious condition of premature babies characterized by intestinal gangrene. Vigorous medical management by neonatologists in a NICU setting is called for, which is beyond the scope of this handbook. If the patient does not respond to medical treatment, the paediatric surgical team may be called to consider surgical management. Important points in surgical management are considered below.

The indications for surgery in NEC are full-thickness bowel necrosis, with perforation or lack of clinical improvement despite appropriate resuscitation and medical treatment (indicating that bowel necrosis is likely to be extensive).

The clinical picture

- Bloody diarrhoea, abdominal distension and bilious vomiting are classic features. Other features include lethargy, poor feeding, apnoeic episodes, unstable temperature, hypotension, hypoglycaemia, abdominal tenderness, and oedema and redness of the abdominal wall (which suggests full-thickness necrosis of bowel wall.)
- The baby shows signs of sepsis and frequently requires ventilatory and/or cardiovascular support. There are known associations between NEC and patent ductus arteriosus and also formula-feeding.

Action

Confirming the diagnosis

- An abdominal X-ray showing intramural gas (pneumatosis intestinalis) or intrahepatic portal venous gas indicates bowel wall necrosis and confirms a diagnosis of NEC.
- Free air (pneumoperitoneum) suggests perforation.
- Other radiological features include thickened bowel wall, dilated loops of gut and a lack of variation in the position of the bowel loops over time from film to film ('fixed loops').

Preoperative management

- Management on NICU will include cessation of oral feeds, insertion of a NG tube, fluid resuscitation, broad-spectrum antibiotics, invasive monitoring and early cardiorespiratory support.
- Patients with NEC are at risk of acidosis, hyperkalaemia, thrombocytopenia and disseminated intravascular coagulation (DIC), so frequent blood monitoring is undertaken.
- Transfusion of blood or blood products may be necessary.
- Investigations include a partial septic screen, clotting, U&Es, LFTs, CRP, cross-match, and serial CXRs and AXRs.

Surgery

The baby is likely to require a laparotomy or peritoneal drain insertion.

Postoperative management

- Supportive treatment on NICU continues with broad-spectrum antibiotics for 7 days postoperatively.
- Bowel rest is usually required for 10 days after surgery—check the operation note.
- Meanwhile TPN is instituted.

☠ Pyloric stenosis

Think about

Congenital hypertrophic pyloric stenosis is one of the most commonly encountered surgical causes of vomiting in infants. It affects 3 children per 1000 live births in the UK, and poses an acute risk to life if left untreated. However, pyloric stenosis can also be cured with relatively simple surgery. For these reasons, it is important for the senior house officer (SHO) covering paediatric surgery to be familiar with the presentation and management of this condition.

Ask about

- Onset and duration of symptoms—vomiting begins between 2 to 8 weeks of life, most commonly at 3–4 weeks. The longer the period of vomiting, the greater the potential severity of water depletion and electrolyte imbalance in the patient.
- Vomiting—typically projectile. May initially be intermittent, but progresses to after every feed.
- Vomitus—non-bile-stained. Coffee-ground material, 2° to oesophagitis, may be present if the infant presents late.
- Appetite and weight—the child seems hungry and is eager to feed. Weight may have reduced or stayed static. Child may look malnourished.
- General well-being—early on, the child is otherwise well and afebrile. Late presentations may be lethargic/listless as dehydration and electrolyte imbalance progress.
- Hydration—number of wet nappies.
- Risk factors—boys more commonly affected than girls (4:1); some familial predisposition; first-born ♂ infants more commonly affected; Caucasians more commonly affected than infants of African, Chinese or Indian ethnic origin.

Look for

- An unwell child—examination and assessment (📖 p526), looking especially for signs and extent of dehydration.
- Specific features—look for two physical signs:
  - Visible peristaltic waves of gastric contraction against the pylorus.
  - A thickened and palpable pyloric muscle (described as an 'olive'), resulting in the pyloric tumour.

The pyloric tumor may be difficult to feel. The following may help:

- Ensure the child is relaxed. Parents may be able to calm a crying child by distraction with a dummy or toy. Passing a NG tube to empty the stomach may also help you to feel the tumour.
- Sit to the child's left and palpate with two fingers of the left hand. The two areas where the tumour is most easily felt are on the lateral border of the rectus abdominis muscle as it rises to meet the liver, and centrally in the gap between the two recti, roughly halfway between the xiphisternum and umbilicus.
- You may need to palpate for a few minutes before the tumour is evident.
- If it is not palpable, feeding may help relax the infant and the peristaltic waves become more prominent too. Feel at the beginning of the feed, before the stomach fills.

Table 14.18 Causes of vomiting in infants

	Comment
Mechanical	
Pyloric stenosis	Non-bile-stained, projectile vomiting in a hungry baby
Gastro-oesophageal reflux	Non-bile-stained, non-projectile vomiting
Incarcerated inguinal hernia	Tense, tender, irreducible groin mass
Malrotation	Intermittent bile-stained vomiting
Malrotation with volvulus	Bile-stained vomiting, shock, passage of blood per rectum
Infective	Common, may present with general or local signs and symptoms. Children often febrile
Meningitis	
UTI	
Gastroenteritis	
Other focal infections	
Other	
Overfeeding	Ask about how much, how often, and how quickly the child is fed
Metabolic	Rare causes, e.g. congenital adrenal hyperplasia
Food intolerance	e.g. cow's milk allergy
Head injury	Don't forget NAI in this age group

Investigation

- Send U&Es, FBC, CRP and G&S.
- Perform capillary blood gas and glucose.
- Arrange an abdominal USS to confirm the diagnosis.

Management

Consider transferring the patient to a paediatric surgical centre if the skills and facilities for surgery and anaesthesia in infants do not exist locally.

- Admit patient.
- Keep nil by mouth.
- Obtain IV access.
- Insert NG tube.
- Commence resuscitation—loss of acid from the stomach results in metabolic alkalosis, with hypokalaemia and hypochloraemia. In the sodium-depleted state, the kidney conserves sodium at the expense of H^+, which is excreted, worsening the alkalosis. Resuscitation in

pyloric stenosis ∴ uses fluids with a higher sodium concentration than is normally given in infants. Many centres have their own fluid regimens for pyloric stenosis—if this exists locally, use it. Otherwise:

- If shocked, give normal saline (0.9%) bolus 20mL/kg as needed.
- Assess percentage dehydration (see IV fluids, 📖 p542).
- Note capillary blood gas results and electrolytes.
- In patients <5% dehydrated with normal electrolyte and normal blood gas, give IV maintenance fluid as dextrosaline: 10% dextrose and 0.18% saline, with 10mmol KCl per 500mL bag at a rate of 100mL/kg/day.
- In patients 5–10% dehydrated with metabolic alkalosis and hypochloraemia give IV maintenance and replacement as dextrosaline (0.45% saline and 5% dextrose) with 10mmol KCl per 500mL bag at a rate of 150mL/kg/day. Re-evaluate gases and electrolytes after 12hr and, if improved, change to dextrosaline: 10% dextrose and 0.18% saline, with 10mmol KCl per 500mL bag at a rate of 100mL/kg/day.
- In patients severely volume depleted (>10%) give replacement as dextrosaline: 0.45% saline and 5% dextrose with 10mmol KCl per 500mL at 150mL/kg/day. You will also need to give additional fluid boluses 20mL/kg of normal saline titrated to response.
- In all cases, replace NG losses mL for mL with normal saline 0.9% with 10mmol KCl per 500mL bag.
- Monitor plasma K^+ during resuscitation and adjust replacement if necessary. (See worked example below.).

- Once the patient is fully resuscitated (which may take days), proceed to pyloromyotomy. This may be performed open or laparoscopically.
- Postoperatively, a small feed (15mL formula or a short breast-feed) is given. If the child tolerates this, a full feed is offered 1hr later. If this is tolerated too, IV fluids may be discontinued and feeds given every 3hr (but it is wise to leave the cannula in until the child has taken two full feeds successfully). The child may be discharged once two consecutive feeds have been tolerated without vomiting.
- If the child has a significant vomit, wait 3hr and then give that volume of feed again. If successful, proceed as above; if unsuccessful, repeat the feed in a further 3hr.

Differential diagnosis

- Gastro-oesophageal reflux.
- Overfeeding.
- Infective causes.

Example

Six-week-old Aaron (who was 4kg when weighed at the health centre 2 weeks ago) presents after 10 days of worsening non-bilious, projectile vomiting. He is alert and eager to feed but has dry mucous membranes, sunken eyes and reduced skin turgor. He is not exhibiting clinical signs of shock. His weight today is 3.8kg.

Clinically Aaron is 5–10% dehydrated. This is corroborated by a known weight loss of 5% of his weight. He ∴ needs 0.45% saline/ 5% dextrose (with K^+) at 150mL/kg/day, as well as replacement of NG losses mL for mL.

His fluid prescription will read:

- 500mL dextrosaline (0.45% saline, 5% dextrose) + 10mmol KCl to be given IV at a rate of 25mL/hr (150mL/kg/day using his pre-morbid weight of 4kg).
- 500mL normal saline (0.9% saline) + 10mmol KCl to replace NG losses mL for mL.

This may need adjusting depending on the results of Aaron's U&E and capillary blood gas results.

Post-Pyloromyotomy feeding regimen

Some hospitals have their own re-feeding protocols, but, in the absence of local protocol, the following may be used as a guide.

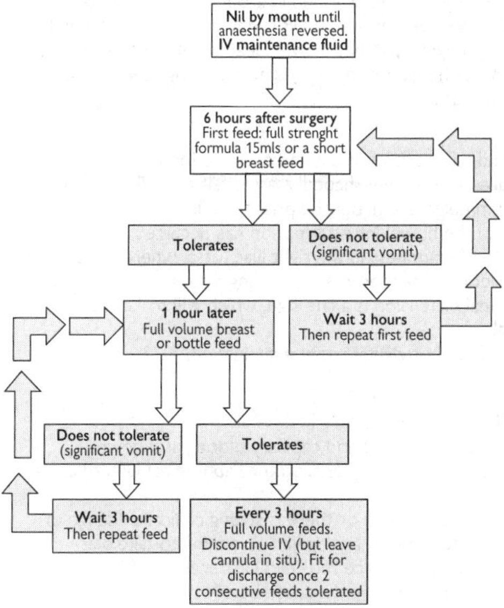

Fig. 14.7 Refeeding pyloric stenosis flowchart.

☠ Intussusception

Think about

Intussusception refers to the invagination of a section of bowel (the intussusceptum) into adjacent distal bowel (the intussuscipiens). Partial and, later, complete intestinal obstruction results and bowel necrosis may occur. Infants in whom intussusception has been present for several days may be very unwell.

Ask about

- The child's age—intussception is rare in children >2yr. Peak incidence is reported between 5 and 9 months. In older children, it is important to exclude a pathological lead point to the intussusception.
- Vomiting—often occurs in the first few hours with onset of pain, abates, then returns once complete obstruction has been established, at which time it is typically bile stained.
- Pain—sudden-onset colicky pain, lasting for a few minutes. The infant screams and draws up the knees. Mothers state that the child's cry is different from their usual one. The spasms occur ~ every 20min and are associated with facial pallor.
- Diarrhoea—patients may have an episode of loose stools shortly after the onset of symptoms.
- Rectal bleeding—less than half present with grossly bloody stool. The classic 'redcurrant jelly' stool is found in around 5% of patients.
- Recent health—gastroenteritis and URTI have been associated with intussusception (Peyer's patches provide lead points). Post-laparotomy intussusception, although much rarer, is also a recognized entity.
- Altered mental status.

Look for

- An unwell child—basic assessment and examination (📖 p536).
- Specific features—a 'sausage-shaped' mass is felt typically in the right hypochondrium/epigastrium, but the position will vary depending on which region of the bowel intussusception has occurred in. Dance's sign is a feeling of emptiness in the right iliac fossa, where the caecum should be. Abdominal tenderness ± guarding may be present over the mass. Abdominal distension is a late sign, which will make the mass difficult to palpate.
- Blood may be found on digital rectal examination.

Investigation

- Send FBC, CRP and U&Es.
- Consider G&S, blood culture and capillary blood gas if unwell.
- If there is doubt over the diagnosis, arrange abdominal USS to confirm intussusception.
- When diagnosis is confirmed or there is strong clinical evidence of intussusception and if stable, arrange an air enema to take place in the radiology department once the child has received IV fluids and antibiotics. (For details of air enema, see below.)

Management

If you do not have appropriate paediatric radiology, surgical and anaesthetic skills locally, transfer the patient to a paediatric surgical centre.

- Admit patient.
- If shocked, attend to ABC. Call for help.
- Keep nil by mouth.
- Insert NG tube.
- Obtain IV access.
- Give analgesia (📖 p546) as needed.
- Commence maintenance fluids/resuscitate as necessary (see IV fluids, 📖 p540).
- Give intravenous antibiotics—metronidazole 7.5mg/kg and Augmentin 30mg/kg IV. If penicillin allergic, use amikacin 10mg/kg.
- If there is clinical evidence of peritonitis or septicaemia (which signify necrotic bowel) liaise with theatres and anaesthetists to arrange emergency laparotomy. Make sure blood has been cross-matched. Routine preoperative preparation. If the patient is very unwell, you may need to liaise with PICU.

Air enema is both diagnostic and therapeutic. The radiologist would usually allow three attempts at reduction under fluoroscopic guidance. If this fails to reduce the intussusception and the child remains in good clinical condition, the radiologist may have a further attempt after 2–3hr. Laparotomy is indicated if:

- Reduction is still unsuccessful.
- There is perforation—free intraperitoneal gas is seen.
- There is a pathological lead point—e.g. Meckel's diverticulum or a polyp.

Differential diagnosis

- Simple colic ('wind')—this rarely lasts more than a couple of hours and is not usually associated with vomiting.
- Gastroenteritis—severe gastroenteritis may cause abdominal pain, diarrhoea, vomiting and passage of blood and mucus, mimicking intussusception. Diarrhoea seen in intussusception is usually small amounts, whereas in gastroenteritis it is a prominent feature. If in doubt, arrange a USS.
- Henoch–Schönlein purpura—although intussusception can occur in this condition, patients may have abdominal pain, abdominal distension and even rectal bleeding, 2° to submucosal haematomas.
- Look for a purpuric rash ± joint swelling, check BP and dipstick urine looking for nephritis. Further assessment by an experienced clinician and radiologist is required to manage these patients.

☠ Appendicitis

This is the most common condition requiring emergency abdominal surgery in childhood. Although the signs and symptoms of appendicitis are similar in children and adults, diagnosis can be difficult, especially in preschool children in whom they can be subtle. Do not send home small children with abdominal pain and tenderness unless an alternative diagnosis is absolutely certain. In cases of uncertainty, the best course of action is admission for observation and re-examination at intervals.

Think about

Is it appendicitis? If so, has the appendix perforated? The paediatric appendix has often perforated by the time of presentation.

Ask about

- Pain—this is usually the first symptom, and may begin either in the right iliac fossa (RIF) or centrally (midgut pain), later localizing to the RIF once local peritoneal inflammation has occurred.
- Vomiting—can be seen in appendicitis in children, occurring early after the onset of pain. NB: Unlike bowel obstruction, it does not progress.
- Fever—may be high- or low-grade as in adults. A high temperature is common in younger children with uncomplicated appendicitis, but in older children may indicate perforation.
- Appetite—unlike adults with appendicitis, children may be hungry.
- 'Dysuria'—although true dysuria is a symptom of UTI, if the appendix lies close to the bladder there may be pain on emptying the bladder. Try to distinguish between pain in the urethra (UTI) and lower abdominal pain on micturition.
- Duration of symptoms—it is generally accepted that perforation is likely to occur within 48hr on onset of symptoms. Young children often present late as they are unable to communicate their symptoms.
- Diarrhoea—an important Δ of appendicitis is gastroenteritis. However, diarrhoea lasting >24hr should suggest the possibility of a pelvic, retrocaecal or retroileal appendicitis.
- Masses—as young children and children with learning difficulties present late, an inflammatory mass may be palpable in the RIF.
- Gynaecological PID and ectopic pregnancy are important to exclude in girls. A gynae history including cycle length, regularity, LMP and a sensitive enquiry about sexual activity should be made. If you have any child protection concerns, contact the paediatric SpR and follow local protocol.

The presentation of appendicitis varies with the age of the child:

- <2yr—non-specific presentation with vomiting, diarrhoea, lethargy, fever, diffuse abdominal pain.
- 2–5yrs—more specific but late presentation, with vomiting and fever. Abdominal pain may be diffuse or periumbilical/RIF tenderness. Appendiceal masses.
- >5yrs—more specific presentation, similar to that in adults. High fever and diffuse tenderness are more indicative of perforation in this group.

Look for

- An unwell child—basic assessment and examination (📖 p526).
- Specific features—in older children the signs of appendicitis may be similar to those in adults, but in infants and young children localized and general peritonitis may be difficult to identify. Tenderness may be poorly localized and poorly communicated; rigidity and guarding may not be present despite peritonitis; and, as peritonitis progresses, RIF signs can be harder to elicit in the distended, diffusely tender abdomen. Rebound tenderness is unreliable in children, although percussion tenderness can be useful. An appendiceal mass may be felt. Rectal examination is not performed routinely in children: if the diagnosis is obvious from abdominal examination, it adds little. However, if the signs are equivocal, if ovarian pathology is suspected, if there is low diffuse tenderness (suggestive of a pelvic appendix) or if a pelvic collection is suspected, rectal exam may give vital information about the diagnosis. Discuss your preliminary examination findings with your registrar before performing a PR. Parental consent and the presence of a chaperone (in addition to the parent) are mandatory.

Investigations

- Useful investigations include CRP, FBC, BM to exclude diabetic ketoacidosis (DKA) and urine microscopy to exclude UTI.
- Note that, although a raised CRP and neutrophilia give weight to a diagnosis of appendicitis, the diagnosis remains primarily clinical.
- Note also that the inflamed appendix lying next door to the bladder may give rise to mild pyuria (20–50wbc/mm^3).
- The presence of ketonuria on urine dipstick (2° to loss of appetite and fasting) can be a useful finding. In cases of ketonuria with glucosuria, consider DKA.
- USS may be used to exclude other suspected diagnoses (e.g. gynaecological causes).
- AXR is useful if a mass is felt.
- Don't forget to do a pregnancy test in ♀—ectopic pregnancy is a potentially fatal Δ in a sexually active girl.

Management

- Check with your seniors if you have the surgical and anaesthetic skills and facilities locally to perform an appendicectomy in a child.
- If the child has advanced disease or is very young, the patient should be referred to a paediatric surgical centre.

- If appendicitis is suspected, even if no firm diagnosis has been made, admit the patient.
- If shocked, attend to ABC. Call for help.
- Nil by mouth.
- Consider NG tube if vomiting.

- Obtain IV access. Commence maintenance fluids/resuscitate as necessary (see IV fluids, p542).
- Give analgesia as needed (see Analgesia, p546).
- Give IV antibiotics—Augmentin 30mg/kg IV except if penicillin allergic. If allergic, give amikacin 10mg/kg and metronidazole 7.5mg/kg.
- Book theatres for appendicectomy. This may be open or laparoscopic depending on the skills available and the consultant's preference.
- If a mass is palpated, arrange a USS to confirm the diagnosis. Discuss the patient's individual case with your senior to determine subsequent management. A course of antibiotics (initially IV) followed by interval appendicectomy some 6 weeks later may be appropriate if the patient is stable. However, if the patient is unstable, laparotomy may be required.

Differential diagnosis

Appendicitis may present in a variety of ways. In each scenario, the following Δ should be considered:

- RIF tenderness:
  - Gastroenteritis.
  - Acute constipation.
  - Mesenteric adenitis.
  - Renal stone.
  - Deep iliac lymphadenitis.
  - PID.
- Local peritonitis (guarding in RIF):
  - Meckel's diverticulitis.
  - Ruptured luteal cyst (apoplectic ovary).
  - Torsion of ovarian cyst/ovary.
  - Suppurating deep iliac lymph nodes.
- Generalized peritonitis:
  - 1° peritonitis.
  - Perforated Meckel's diverticulum.
- Mass (appendiceal mass):
  - Intussusception.
  - Duplication cyst.
  - Ectopic kidney.
  - Retroperitoneal mass.
  - Ectopic pregnancy.
- Intestinal obstruction:
  - Adhesions.
  - Meckel's diverticulum (band causing obstruction).
- Diarrhoea (retroileal/pelvic appendicitis):
  - Gastroenteritis.
- Dysuria/pyuria (appendix/inflammation close to ureters):
  - Urinary tract infection.
  - Acute pyelonephritis.
- Acute scrotum (see The groin).

A mass in the groin

Think about

- Is it in the scrotum or inguinal region?
- Is it painful or painless?

Remember that scrotal and inguinal problems may be the source of abdominal pain. It is also worth bearing in mind that boys sometimes complain of tummy pain rather than groin pain due to embarrassment or limited levels of communication.

Table 14.19 Causes of a lump in the groin

	Scrotal	Inguinal
Painful	Torsion of testicular appendage Torsion of the testis Hydrocele of the cord *Rarer:* Epididymo-orchitis Mumps orchitis Malignancy (older patients) Fournier's gangrene Trauma	Incarcerated inguinal hernia
Non-tender	Idiopathic scrotal oedema Hydrocele Varicocele Malignancy (older patients)	Reducible inguinal hernia Undescended testis Inguinal lymphadenopathy

Inguinal hernia

Think about

With an incidence of 1–5% in boys, this is the commonest condition requiring surgery in children. An incarcerated inguinal hernia is a surgical emergency which you must identify during patient assessment.

Ask about

- Duration of symptoms—when did the parent first notice the swelling?
- Incarceration—is the swelling always present, or does it come and go? (typically appearing when crying/straining, seen on nappy changes).
- If the swelling is always present, can it be reduced manually? If it currently can't be reduced, how long has it been this way?
- Have there been previous episodes of incarceration—when, for how long, and how did they resolve?
- Pain or discomfort—reducible hernias are usually painless, but may cause discomfort. Incarcerated hernias are generally painful.
- Features of intestinal obstruction or strangulation colicky abdominal pain, vomiting, abdominal distension, constipation, PR bleeding (concerning).
- Predisposing conditions—♂ sex (5–10:1 ♂:♀), prematurity, connective tissue defects, congenital urological abnormalities, ↑ abdominal pressure (ventriculoperitoneal [VP] shunt, peritoneal dialysis).
- Contralateral side—distribution is right 60%, left 30%, bilateral 10%.

Look for

An unwell child (📖 p526).

Reducible inguinal hernia

- The child is not usually distressed.
- Groin examination:
  - You may not be able to see or feel a swelling if the hernia is reduced at the time of examination. Place your index finger over the spermatic cord as it lies against the pubic crest, and roll from side to side. You may feel a thickened cord compared with the non-affected side, and detect a 'rustle' as the walls of the hernial sac rub together (the 'silk purse' sign).
  - If the hernia is not currently reduced, you will be able to demonstrate a swelling overlying the superficial inguinal ring. It may be painless (usually) or tender, with an impulse felt on crying. It is not possible to get above the swelling. It may extend down into the scrotum (inguinoscrotal hernia), but can be felt separate from the testis. Use gentle pressure along the line of the inguinal canal to reduce the hernia (often with a gurgle if the sac contains bowel). If the hernia cannot be reduced, it is a surgical emergency (see below).

Incarcerated inguinal hernia

- The child is usually distressed and inconsolable.
- Groin examination—the swelling over the superficial inguinal ring is tense, tender and irreducible by gentle manipulation.
- Abdominal examination—generalized tenderness/abdominal distension may be present with obstruction.
- Peritonism, induration of the skin overlying the hernia, a history of PR bleeding and a long period of delay in diagnosis are associated with necrotic bowel within the hernial sac.
- Emergency surgery is indicated—do not attempt to reduce manually if these features are present.

Management

All inguinal hernias in children require surgery.

Reducible inguinal hernia

Although immediate admission may not be required, your SpR will want to confirm your diagnosis and make arrangements for rapid elective admission.

Premature babies on NICU/special care baby unit (SCBU)

- Continue care as given by neonatologists.
- Take patient's details.
- Liaise with SpR to arrange for the baby to undergo an inpatient hernia repair at a paediatric surgery centre just before discharge home.

<1yr

- Take patient's details.
- Liaise with SpR to arrange emergency clinic review and admission within the next few days for hernia repair at a paediatric surgery centre.

>1yr

- Take patient's details.
- Liaise with SpR to arrange for an urgent outpatient appointment and admission within next few months for hernia repair. This may be at a paediatric surgery centre or locally, depending on available skills.

Spontaneously reduced inguinal hernia, with history of incarceration

- Transfer to paediatric surgical centre—an incarcerated hernial sac is friable and must be treated by an experienced paediatric surgeon.
- Your SpR will want to review this patient as soon as it is convenient.

- Admit patient.
- If shocked, attend to ABC and call for help.
- Assess pain—give analgesia if needed (see Analgesia, p546).

- Assess hydration state. Site cannula and commence fluid resuscitation if needed (see IV fluids, 📖 p542).
- Investigations—consider U&Es if history of vomiting or clinically dehydrated.
- Surgery may be delayed for 24hr to allow oedema of the sac and tissues to subside, but repair is usually performed during this admission.

Irreducible inguinal hernia

- Transfer to a paediatric surgical centre—an incarcerated hernial sac is friable and must be treated by an experienced paediatric surgeon.
- Very rarely, gangrenous bowel will necessitate segmental excision and anastomosis.

- Admit patient.
- Keep nil by mouth as surgery may be required.
- If shocked, attend to ABC and call for help.
- Give analgesia (📖 p546).
- Establish IV access.
- Send U&Es, CRP and FBC. Consider capillary blood gas if unwell.
- Asses hydration state—give fluid bolus if needed. Commence maintenance fluids. (see IV fluids, 📖 p542).
- Give antibiotics.
- Investigations—consider AXR (obstruction/ perforation).
- With the SpR, attempt to reduce the hernia manually (unless clinical evidence of necrotic bowel):
  - Consider analgesia with 0.1mg/kg IV morphine, or sedation with chloral hydrate 15 mg/kg. Ensure appropriate monitoring.
  - Place finger and thumb of the left hand over the external ring, and finger and thumb of the right hand on the fundus of the hernia.
  - Moving your right hand downwards, disimpact the hernial sac from the external ring.
  - Manipulate the sac up with the right hand in the line of the inguinal canal.
  - Wait a moment. You may then feel a gurgle as the hernia contents are reduced.
  - Several attempts may be necessary.
- If reduction is successful, proceed to semi-elective herniotomy during this admission.
- If the hernia cannot be reduced, book theatre for an emergency herniotomy/exploration.

? Undescended testes

Think about

During normal development, the testes descend through the inguinal canal into the scrotum. An undescended testis may be present as a painless lump in the groin.

Ask about

- The contents of the scrotum—the scrotum may be empty on one or both sides. Although the scrotum may have been empty since birth, in some cases the testes re-ascend as the child grows.
- A groin mass—the undescended testis may or may not be palpable in the inguinal region. If it is impalpable, the testis may be absent, atrophied to a remnant, intra-abdominal or in an ectopic position.
- Age—after the age of 4 months, the testes are unlikely to descend on their own.
- Predisposing conditions—undescended testes are common in premature newborns.

Look for

- An unwell child (📖 p526). Children with undescended testes are well and comfortable. If unwell, strongly reconsider your diagnosis.
- Examine the scrotum and groin with the child lying down in a warm, comfortable environment. On inspection, the affected side(s) of the scrotum lies empty, place your left hand at the top of the inguinal canal, and run it down the line of testicular descent towards the scrotum, milking down any mass encountered into the scrotum and between the waiting finger and thumb of the right hand. If the testis cannot be brought to the bottom of the scrotum, or if it will not remain in the sac once released, surgery is required. If the testis is palpable, check carefully for ectopic position (away from the normal line of descent). This will need exploration. Examine also the descended testis. If this is larger than expected, it may be a sign that the contralateral testis is missing or too small to function.

Management

- Can be managed on an outpatient basis.
- Inform the SpR, who may want to confirm your diagnosis.

Orchidopexy is usually undertaken around the age of 1yr. It is performed to avoid impairment of fertility, to normalize the appearance of the scrotum, because of the risk of malignancy in undescended testis (although it is not clear whether early orchidopexy actually reduces the risk of malignancy, it does make surveillance easier) and to prevent testicular torsion.

If patient is ≥1yr

- Take the patient's details and liaise with the SpR to organize elective admission for orchidopexy (if testis is palpable) or exploratory laparoscopy and Fowler–Stephens procedure/orchidectomy (if testis is impalpable).
- During laparoscopy, the surgeon checks the abdominal cavity for an undescended testis. The abdominal testis is then prepared for mobilization by disconnection of the testicular vessels. The testis is left for 6 months to establish an alternative blood supply via the vas, then mobilized into the scrotum during a second procedure. If the testis cannot be seen intra-abdominally, the surgeon follows the vas and vessels, to find it or its remnant, and inguinal exploration may be necessary. Any testicular remnants found are removed.

If the patient is <1yr

- Take the patients details and liaise with the SpR to organize outpatient follow-up so that timely surgery can be arranged if the testes do not descend naturally.

ⓘ Inguinal lymphadenopathy

Think about

This is an important differential for a lump in the groin.

Ask about

- Recent minor skin infections in the region drained by the superficial inguinal lymph nodes—the lower limbs and the 'napkin area' (buttocks/perineum).
- Systemic symptoms—fever, poor appetite, 'not himself'.

Look for

- An unwell child—basic assessment and examination (📖 p526).
- Specific features—abscesses may form in infected lymph nodes. Look for signs of generalized lymphadenopathy (axilla, cervical nodes, spleen).

Management

- Incision and drainage of abscesses.
- Treat any local causes of lymphadenopathy.
- Refer patients with generalized lymphadenopathy for further investigation.

Other conditions in the groin

Testicular torsion/torsion of testicular appendage

See Testicular torsion in Chapter 12 (📖 p466).

Malignancy

Operations

Sutures

Having sutures removed and dressings changed can be traumatic for a child, and in recognition of this absorbable sutures, tissue glue and minimal dressings are used wherever possible in paediatric surgery.

Bowel preparation

Suitable measures you might take to prepare the bowel for surgery are suggested below. However, hospitals often have their own protocols for bowel preparation regimens, so check your local policy before prescribing.

Cross-matching

The amount of blood you might need for each operation is suggested below. However, do follow your local blood-ordering schedule, which should be available from your hospital blood bank.

The following paediatric surgical operations may be helpful to know about. However, the list is necessarily limited. If you have any questions about the operations your patients are having, do ask your senior to explain matters as it is important that you understand procedures in order to prepare patients for theatre, care for them after surgery and assist effectively in the operating theatre.

ACE procedure (Malone procedure for antegrade continence enemas)

- Indications:
  - Faecal incontinence, failed conventional management.
  - Chronic constipation.
- Anaesthetic—general.
- Incision/scars—right lower quadrant transverse incision, small right iliac fossa stoma (although position may vary). If laparoscopic, laparoscopy post scars.
- Complications—stoma stenosis, leakage, infection, persistent incontinence/constipation. Parents of patients undergoing laparoscopic procedure should be aware that it might be necessary to convert to an open procedure.
- Preop—FBC, U&Es, 1 unit cross-match, full bowel prep (e.g. laxatives 1 day preop, rectal washouts, clear fluids 24hr preop—see local guidelines), stoma nurse specialist review and stoma site marking.
- Postop—5 days of antibiotics, IV fluids and nil by mouth until postoperative ileus has resolved, Foley catheter remains in situ until healed. The first enema is given at around 24hr. After about 2 weeks, the patient returns, the Foley is removed and the patient learns to catheterize the stoma. Enema regimens vary from patient to patient, but are often performed every other day.

Appendicectomy

As in adults. See Chapter 2 (📖 p52).

Congenital diaphragmatic hernia repair

- Indication—congenital diaphragmatic hernia in a patient whose ventilatory status has been optimized.
- Anaesthetic—general.
- Incision/scar—subcostal scar on side of defect.
- Complications—malrotation volvulus, perforation/gut ischaemia, recurrence, wound infection, wound dehiscence, respiratory complications (hypoplastic lungs).
- Preop—specialist management on NICU; cross-match 1 unit.
- Postop—specialist management on NICU.

Closure of exomphalos (1°)

- Indication—small to moderate exomphalos.
- Anaesthetic—general.
- Incision/scar—existing defect.
- Complications—gut necrosis, short bowel syndrome, wound dehiscence and infection, fistula, absence of umbilicus, ventral hernia.
- Preop—group and save.
- Postop—IV antibiotics (5 days), nil by mouth, NG and TPN until bowel function has returned.

Exomphalos staged repair/silo

- Indication—large exomphalos.
- Anaesthetic—general.
- Incision/scar—existing defect.
- Preop—cross-match 1 unit.
- Postop—IV antibiotics (5 days or until the sac has been removed), nil by mouth, NG and TPN until bowel function has returned.

Gastroschisis repair

- Indication—gastroschisis.
- Anaesthesia—general.
- Incision/scar—existing defect is extended superiorly.
- Complications—gut necrosis, short bowel syndrome, wound dehiscence and infection, fistula, absence of umbilicus, ventral hernia.
- Preop—cross-match 1 unit.
- Postop—IV antibiotics (5 days or until the sac has been removed), nil by mouth, NG and TPN until bowel function has returned.

Nissen fundoplication

- Indication—gastro-oesophageal reflux with failed medical management, an established stricture, congenital anatomical anomaly predisposing to reflux, recurrent aspiration or life-threatening apnoea.
- Anaesthetic–general.
- Incision/scars—upper midline abdominal incision, xiphisternum to umbilicus.
- Complications—respiratory complications (pneumonia/atelectasis) especially in those already compromised, dysphagia, recurrence of reflux (wrap disruption/migration up into posterior mediastinum), paraoesophageal hernia, wound infection/dehiscence, and retching, dumping symptoms, gas bloat and hiccups (usually transient). Parents must be aware that as the fundoplication renders the child unable to vomit, bowel obstruction may present atypically.
- Preop—contrast swallow, pH study, group and save.
- Postop—nil by mouth, NG, IV fluids for 2–4 days (until postop ileus has resolved).

Gastrostomy—open (Stamm)

- Indication—a child with a functioning upper GI tract, who has a long-term (at least 3 months) need for enteral feeding. Gastrostomy feeds may be required either because the child cannot swallow, or because they are unable to consume adequate nutrients by the oral route alone.
- Anaesthetic—general.
- Approach/scar—small transverse upper abdominal incision.
- Complications—bleeding, wound infection/dehiscence, leaking of gastrostomy site, tube displacement, natural wear of the tube means it will need replacing in time.
- Preop—investigations as indicated by child's underlying condition, group and save.
- Postop—nil by mouth and IV fluids until postop ileus has resolved.

Gastrostomy—percutaneous endoscopic gastrostomy (PEG)

- Indications—as above, but PEG is contraindicated in patients in whom endoscopy cannot be performed, and in cases of anatomical abnormality which make it difficult to identify structures transabdominally (malrotation, scoliosis, etc.).
- Approach/scars—upper GI endoscopy, gastrostomy exit site upper abdomen.
- Anaesthetic—usually general, although older children without airway compromise may have the procedure under sedation and local anaesthetic.
- Complications—as above.
- Preop—investigations as indicated by child's underlying condition.
- Postop—feeds usually commence next day.

Hickman line insertion

- Indication—a long-term need for central venous access.
- Incision/scar—short transverse incision in the left or right neck.
- Anaesthetic—general. A soft roll is placed under the patient's shoulders and the neck is extended and head turned to the contralateral side.
- Complications—line infection, wound infection, bleeding, pneumothorax, cardiac arrhythmia, thrombosis, dislodgement/migration, line fracture.
- Preop—FBC, coagulation, screen, if >3kg group and save, if <3kg cross-match 1 unit. Check that a radiographer will be available to perform an on-table check X-ray once the line is inserted.
- Postop–careful line care.

Inguinal herniotomy

- Indication—inguinal hernia.
- Anaesthetic—general.
- Incision/scar—small transverse incision on left/right in groin crease.
- Complications—injury to spermatic cord or vessels, wound infection, scrotal haematoma, recurrent hernia. nerve damage, testicular atrophy.
- Preop—investigations as indicated by individual circumstance.
- Postop—analgesia, may feed immediately, keep wound dry for 48hr; older children should refrain from vigorous activity for a month.

Pyloromyotomy

- Indication—pyloric stenosis, in a patient with corrected electrolytes.
- Approach/scars—small transverse right upper quadrant or small umbilical or laparoscopy ports.
- Anaesthetic—general.
- Complications—wound infection, wound dehiscence, recurrence.
- Preop—U&Es, FBC, capillary blood gases, group and save, abdominal USS.

Index

G

H

I

P

Common haematology values *If outside this range, consult:*

Haemoglobin	men:	13–18g/dL
	women:	11.5–16g/dL
Mean cell volume, MCV	76–96fL	
Platelets	150–400 × 10^9/L	
White cells (total)	4–11 × 10^9/L	
neutrophils	40–75%	
lymphocytes	20–45%	
eosinophils	1–6%	

Blood gases	*kPa*	*mmHg*
pH 7.35–7.45		
P_aO_2	>10.6	75–100
P_aCO_2	4.7–6	35–45
Base excess ± 2mmol/L		

U&E etc (urea and electrolytes) *If outside this range, consult:*

Sodium	135–145mmol/
potassium	3.5–5mmol/L
creatinine	70–150μmol/L
urea	2.5–6.7mmol/L
calcium	2.12–2.65mmol/L
albumin	35–50g/L
proteins	60–80g/L

LFTs (liver function tests)

bilirubin	3–17μmol/L
alanine aminotransferase, ALT	3–35iu/L
aspartate transaminase, AST	3–35iu/L
alkaline phosphatase	30–35iu/L *(adults)*

'Cardiac enzymes'

creatine kinase	25–195iu/L
lactate dehydrogenase, LDH	70–250iu/L

Lipids and other biochemical values

cholesterol	<6mmol/L *desired*
triglycerides	0.5–1.9mmol/L " "
amylase	0–180*somorgyi* u/dL
C-reactive protein, CRP	<10mg/L
glucose, fasting	3.5–5.5mmol/L
prostate specific antigen, PSA	0–4ng/mL
T4 (total thyroxine)	70–140mmol/L
TSH	0.5– ~5mu/L